Behavioral Economics and Public Health

Behavioral Economics and Public Health

Edited by **CHRISTINA A. ROBERTO
AND ICHIRO KAWACHI**

OXFORD
UNIVERSITY PRESS

OXFORD
UNIVERSITY PRESS

Oxford University Press is a department of the University of
Oxford. It furthers the University's objective of excellence in research,
scholarship, and education by publishing worldwide.

Oxford   New York
Auckland   Cape Town   Dar es Salaam   Hong Kong   Karachi
Kuala Lumpur   Madrid   Melbourne   Mexico City   Nairobi
New Delhi   Shanghai   Taipei   Toronto

With offices in
Argentina   Austria   Brazil   Chile   Czech Republic   France   Greece
Guatemala   Hungary   Italy   Japan   Poland   Portugal   Singapore
South Korea   Switzerland   Thailand   Turkey   Ukraine   Vietnam

Published in the United States of America by
Oxford University Press
198 Madison Avenue, New York, NY 10016

Library of Congress Cataloging-in-Publication Data
Behavioral economics and public health / edited by Christina A. Roberto and Ichiro Kawachi.
p. ; cm.
Includes bibliographical references.
ISBN 978–0–19–939833–1
I. Roberto, Christina A., editor.   II. Kawachi, Ichiro, editor.
[DNLM: 1. Health Behavior.   2. Behavior Control—methods.   3. Choice Behavior.
4. Economics, Behavioral.   5. Health Promotion—methods. W 85]
RA427.8
362.1—dc23
2015006806

9 8 7 6 5 4 3
Printed in the United States of America
on acid-free paper

For Alida and Louis Roberto

CONTENTS

ACKNOWLEDGMENTS

There are many people to thank in the development of this book. We offer special thanks to our colleagues who attended the Harvard exploratory workshop on applying social science insights to public health held in the spring of 2014. The workshop brought together a diverse group of experts in the fields of behavioral economics, psychology, marketing, epidemiology, medicine, and public health and many of those experts are authors who have contributed to this book. We would also like to thank our colleagues from the Harvard Behavioral Insights Group, many of whom participated in the workshop.

We would like to thank Lisa Berkman, the Director of the Harvard Center for Population and Development Studies for providing support for and hosting the workshop as well as Laura Price and Kayla Small for helping to plan and facilitate such a successful event.

We thank our family and friends for supporting our scholarship. Most important we thank the book chapter authors for contributing their work. Each is doing innovative work to help solve some of the world's greatest public health problems. We are grateful they found time in their busy schedules to share their insights for this book.

CONTRIBUTORS

Jason Block
Obesity Prevention Program,
  Department of Population
  Medicine
Harvard Medical School, Harvard
  University
Boston, MA

Zoë Chance
Yale School of Management,
  Yale University
New Haven, CT

Ravi Dhar
Yale School of Management,
  Yale University
New Haven, CT

William H. Dow
Division of Health Policy and
  Management
University of California at
  Berkeley
Berkeley, CA

Rebecca Ferrer
Basic Biobehavioral and
  Psychological Sciences Branch
Behavioral Research Program
Division of Cancer Control and
  Population Sciences
National Cancer Institute
Rockville, MD

Michael Hallsworth
Behavioural Insights Team
Imperial College London
London, England

Michelle Hatzis
Global Food, Heath and Wellness
  Program
Google, Inc.
Mountain View, CA

Kim Huskey
Food Services Director
Google, Inc.
New York, NY

Ichiro Kawachi
Department of Social and
   Behavioral Sciences
Harvard T.H. Chan School
   of Public Health, Harvard
   University
Boston, MA

Dacher Keltner
Department of Psychology and the
   Greater Good Science Center
University of California
   at Berkeley
Berkeley, CA

William Klein
Behavioral Research Program
Division of Cancer Control and
   Population Sciences
National Cancer Institute
Rocksville, MD

Jennifer Lerner
Harvard Kennedy School of
   Government
Harvard University
Cambridge, MA

Kristina Lewis
Division of Public Health Sciences
Wake Forest Baptist Medical Center
Winston-Salem, NC

Brent McFerran
Marketing Area
Beedie School of Business
Simon Fraser University
Burnaby, CA

Rebecca K. Ratner
Department of Marketing
Robert H. Smith School
   of Business
University of Maryland
College Park, MD

Valerie Reyna
Department of Human
   Development
Cornell University
Ithaca, NY

Jason Riis
Department of Marketing
The Wharton School
University of Pennsylvania
Philadelphia, PA

Christina A. Roberto
Assistant Professor
Medical Ethics and Health
   Policy Perelman School of
   Medicine
University of Pennsylvania
Philadelphia, PA

Dennis Rünger
Department of Psychology
University of Southern
   California
Los Angeles, CA

Michael Sanders
Behavioural Insights Team
Harvard Kennedy School of
   Government, Harvard University
Cambridge, MA

Brian Wansink
Department of Applied Economics
   and Management
Cornell University
Ithaca, NY

Justin S. White
Philip R. Lee Institute for
   Health Policy Studies
UCSF School of Medicine
San Francisco, CA

Wendy Wood
Department of Psychology
University of Southern California
Los Angeles, CA

Frederick J. Zimmerman
Department of Health Policy
   and Management
UCLA Fielding School
   of Public Health
Los Angeles, CA

[Handwritten annotations at top of page:]

Standart model
— invariant choices
not altered by the
context
— constant through the
time

behavioral
— influenced by
the context
— focused on
here and now

1 | An Introduction to Behavioral Economics and Public Health

CHRISTINA A. ROBERTO AND ICHIRO KAWACHI

HEALTH BEHAVIORS AND PRACTICES CONSTITUTE the foundation of good physical and mental health. The leading contributors to the global burden of disease include tobacco smoking, low-quality diets, alcohol abuse, physical inactivity, and obesity (Murray & Lopez, 2013). Accordingly, encouraging people to adopt—and maintain—healthy behaviors is a major objective of public health. According to the Nurses' Health Study, 90% of type 2 diabetes could be prevented if people would adopt just five daily practices: avoid smoking, exercise regularly, eat a healthy diet, abstain from alcohol, and maintain a healthy weight (Hu et al., 2001). But the fact of the matter is that less than 10% of the population engages in all five recommended behaviors (King, Mainous, Carnemolla, & Everett, 2009). Worse, the proportion of the population adhering to a healthy regimen of behaviors appears to be declining over time. Despite gains in smoking cessation since 1964 (when the first Surgeon General's report on smoking and health was issued), the trends for healthy eating, physical activity, and overweight/obesity have been moving in the wrong direction (King et al., 2009).

Advances in medical technology have helped to offset some of these adverse population trends. For example, advances in the treatment of heart disease have led to a dramatic decline in cardiovascular *mortality* rates over time, even while obesity and diabetes rates have continued to soar. Improvements in surgical techniques have also allowed bariatric surgery, once a treatment of last resort, to be offered to an increasing number of overweight individuals (Encinosa, Bernard, Du, & Steiner, 2009). To wit, we have become increasingly sophisticated in medical rescue. Mass medical treatment, in the form of a "Polypill" (a low-dose combination of lipid-lowering and antihypertensive drugs), is even being developed to short-circuit the need to make painful behavioral changes (Wald & Wald, 2010). Instead of relying on individuals to start exercising regularly or to follow a healthy diet, the Polypill strategy is to medicate the population to bring down their cholesterol and blood pressure levels.

Yet there is a limit to medical rescue. Even the Polypill—should it become widely prescribed—involves an unavoidable behavioral component: the challenge of getting patients to adhere to their medication. The problem is not a dearth of medical technology to address public health problems; the challenge is how to ensure that patients adopt—and stick to—the treatments that already exist. For example, evidence-based guidelines recommend that post–myocardial infarction patients receive treatment with a beta-blocker, a lipid-lowering agent, an angiotensin-converting enzyme (ACE) inhibitor, and aspirin. Randomized trials have demonstrated that these drugs in combination can reduce the risk of reinfarction by 80% (Choudhry & Winkelmayer, 2008). Yet, out of all patients prescribed these medications after hospital discharge, typically only half of them are still sticking to their regimens 2 years later. In one study that tracked medical and pharmacy claims from a large health plan, 7% of post–myocardial infection patients had stopped their ACE inhibitors within 1 month, 22% at 6 months, 32% at 1 year, and 50% at 2 years (Akincigil et al., 2008). It is easier to grasp why New Year's resolutions get quietly dropped after 2 weeks (we have all been there), but harder to comprehend why patients fail to adhere to life-saving medication after a brush with a near-death experience. How can we explain the gap between knowledge and action, and how might we use that knowledge to improve health behaviors?

What Behavioral Economics Adds

This book is about behavioral science insights into human behavior—why we behave the way we do, and why our actions frequently fail to align with our intentions. In the past four decades we have witnessed a remarkable convergence of theories and evidence about human judgment and decision making across psychology, economics, and neuroscience. The field of behavioral economics began as an attempt to infuse psychological realism into theories of economic behavior, thereby explaining aspects of human decision making that violated predictions made by the standard economic model, which assumes that people are fully rational, that imperfect self-control does not interfere with people's ability to carry out their *the challenge is how to ensure that patients adopt and stick to treatments that already exits*

intentions, and that they act in their self-interest. For example, ~~the stan-dard economic model assumes that people's preferences are invariant, that their judgments and choices are not altered by irrelevant features of the decision context.~~ But behavioral economists suggest that people are heavily ~~influenced by the way choices are presented~~. For example, a medical procedure that seems risky when thought about in isolation may seem safe when presented alongside an even riskier procedure. The standard economic model ~~also assumes that people have dynamically consistent time preferences:~~ that if they place a 5% premium on delaying a reward (say, eating a yummy piece of chocolate fudge) for one day, they will apply the same discount rate for all future delays. However, behavioral economics suggests that people are disproportionately focused on the here and now, and that their valuations fall very rapidly for small delay periods, but then fall slowly for longer delay periods. That is, my preference to eat the chocolate now instead of 1 day from now is far greater than my preference to eat the chocolate 27 days from now instead of 28 days from now. These anomalies—or "errors" as neoclassical economics would prefer to think of them—turn out to be quite widespread, and incorporating them into behavioral models could improve forecasts about what people are likely to decide and do, and about which interventions are most likely to help them.

The goal of this introductory chapter is to provide a broad overview and to introduce the nuts and bolts of behavioral economics and the terms that are used throughout the chapters. In the next section, we outline the aspects of human decision making that contribute to our tendencies to pursue unhealthy lifestyles and choices. We then briefly describe a series of insights from behavioral economics that can be leveraged to address these vulnerabilities. Each of these insights is discussed in depth in the chapters that follow. Finally, we conclude with a discussion of the strengths and limitations of behavioral economics in improving population health.

How can we explain the gap between knowledge and action?

Vulnerabilities to Unhealthy Habits

Psychologists have converged on the idea that there are two systems of thought operating simultaneously in the human brain, commonly referred to as *System 1* and *System 2* (Kahneman, 2003; Sloman, 1996; Stanovich & West, 2000). System 1 thinking is faster (i.e., impulsive, reflexive, emotional, and impatient), whereas System 2 thinking is slower (i.e., more deliberative, controlled, analytical, and patient). System 1 produces an automatic response, whereas System 2 produces a reasoned response.

For example, consider the decision to drink soda. System 1 may draw on associations from advertisements to make me want to drink soda, whereas System 2 may draw on the knowledge that soda is unhealthy to make me not want to drink soda.

The function of System 2 is to monitor the activities of System 1, which requires attention and effort. However, as most of us know, when our cognitive resources are stretched (e.g., we are thirsty, hungry, stressed, or in a distracted state), System 1 wins out (Kahneman, 2003). This fact has long been appreciated by the advertising industry, especially firms whose clients include the tobacco, alcohol, and food industries. The direct appeal to "feel-good" emotions in tobacco, alcohol, and junk food advertisements (think of the McDonald's "Happy Meal") is, in fact, an appeal to System 1. For example, a full-page color advertisement for cigarettes might try to develop positive, easily accessed associations with smoking (e.g., an ad depicting a group of friends "alive with pleasure" as they canoodle near a campfire, often without even depicting them in the act of smoking) (California State University, Northridge, http://www.csun.edu/~vceed002/health/tobacco/Pages/3.html). In contrast to commercial marketing tactics, System 1 appeals have tended to be underutilized by official government warning labels, which seek to primarily educate the consumer about long-term costs, such as developing cancer years down the line. These reason-based appeals to System 2 stand little chance against emotional appeals to System 1.

Part of the reason we rely so heavily on System 1 is because humans are *boundedly rational*, in the sense that we have a limited ability to attend to, process, and remember the information in our environment (Kahneman, 2003; Simon, 1955). We are simply unable to carefully process most of the information we come across. Indeed, it is even adaptive from an evolutionary perspective that humans evolved to take mental shortcuts in making hundreds of snap decisions throughout the course of a day. If we let System 2 do all the thinking, we would be literally paralyzed (e.g., "Should I have butter with my toast? What are the consequences of spreading two pats of butter on my toast rather than just one?"). One implication of bounded rationality is that we typically fail to remember, and act upon, information that is overly complex. Unfortunately, public health information is all too often communicated in a complex manner. Consider the case of communicating nutrition information. Although we know that people have difficulty quickly processing numeric information (Dehaene, 1997; Paulos, 1988), most health-related nutrition information is presented in numbers that require onerous calculations. Nutrition labels

humans are boundedly rational (BD)
limited habality to attend, process and remember

contain information in grams and milligrams with percentages that may not be easy to interpret. Ounces, cups, or grams are used to convey serving sizes. Doctors communicate with patients about their body mass index (BMI), which is calculated by dividing weight by height squared. And the cornerstone of many weight-loss programs is for patients to count calories (Roberto & Kawachi, 2014). Even when information is conveyed in an apparently simple manner, it is often susceptible to framing effects that mislead consumers. For instance, many consumers think "2% milk" means "98% fat-free" (which it decidedly is not, considering that "full-fat" milk is 3.25% fat).

In short, it is time for public health experts to recognize the importance of System 1 thinking as a driver of health behavior and to understand how System 1 works to increase human vulnerability to engage in unhealthy behaviors. In the section that follows, we review the heuristics and biases that characterize System 1 thinking, exposing how a reliance on System 1 leads people to (1) develop faulty perceptions and beliefs about health-related actions, (2) have preferences for behaviors that make them less healthy in the long term, and (3) choose unhealthy behaviors even when they know and prefer not to. We then review the ways in which policy makers and public health practitioners can leverage these insights to design policies and interventions that more effectively "nudge" people's behaviors in directions that are in their long-term interests.

BD—D We fail to remember and act upon information that is overly complex.

Heuristics and Biases

Although people can, and often do, engage in thoughtful, calculated behavior, much of our everyday behavior is less thoughtful and more automatic. We rely on *heuristics,* or mental shortcuts, to make quick decisions throughout the day, rather than pausing to conduct cost-benefit analyses each time we make a decision. This frees up cognitive resources to focus on tasks requiring more attention and thought. Although these heuristics are generally useful, they can bias our thinking in ways that lead to predictable errors in our beliefs, predictable preferences for options that may not benefit us in the long term, and a predictable susceptibility to the manner in which options are presented or described.

It is difficult to make wise choices when you do not know the consequences of those choices. First, and most obviously, sometimes people do not know which options are healthier than others, simply because they lack information. Take the case of the food environment, where even consumers

Although people can, and often do engage in thoughtful, calculated behavior, much of everyday behavior is automatic.

who pay careful attention to information can be misled. For example, the packages of largely unhealthy foods may prominently display claims that mislead consumers into believing that their products are healthy—claims such as "zero trans fat," "gluten-free," or "organic." Consumers are also frequently faced with information asymmetry, with suppliers having knowledge that consumers lack. For example, at many restaurants, people do not know the nutrition composition of the food they are eating, because nutrition facts such as calorie content and serving sizes are not easily or at all available. Addressing information asymmetry requires consumer education and, at times, direct regulation (e.g., mandating the disclosure of trans fatty acid content on package labels, requiring chain restaurants to post the caloric content of menu items).

People's health is also heavily influenced by their *lay theories* of health (Dweck, 1996), especially their beliefs about the causes and consequences of health problems (McFerran, 2015). For example, as McFerran discusses in Chapter 5, he studied the relationship between lay theories of obesity and BMI (McFerran & Mukhopadhyay, 2013). They found that people tend to fall into one of two categories: people who believe that a poor diet is the primary cause of obesity (diet theorists) and those who believe lack of physical activity is the primary cause of obesity (exercise theorists). McFerran and Mukhopadhyay found that diet theorists had lower BMIs than exercise theorists, even when controlling for variables known to be associated with BMI. This makes sense given the considerable evidence that excessive caloric intake, rather than limited exercise, is more to blame for the obesity epidemic (Swinburn, Sacks, & Ravussin, 2009). This is important because it suggests that it may actually be harmful to teach people that obesity is primarily caused by a lack of exercise rather than poor diet.

More generally, the pervasiveness of false beliefs about health suggests that public health experts ought to be working to correct those beliefs, preferably through simple, concrete, memorable messaging. Toward this aim, in Chapter 6, Riis and Ratner offer guidance on how best to design guidelines and other communication tools for the public that are both memorable and actionable. But the problem of faulty beliefs is not due simply to ignorance or informational asymmetry; instead, it is reinforced by the vagaries of System 1. For example, consider human susceptibility to *the planning fallacy*, which captures our tendency to overestimate our ability to perform future tasks (Buehler, Griffin, & Ross, 1994). When we are given the choice as to whether or not to eat a delicious but fattening brownie, we may think it is OK because we have planned to start an exercise program the next day. However, when the next day arrives, we find that we cannot summon the willpower to start exercising. Such *optimistic biases* also extend beyond planning and to our perceptions of risks. Although people may be educated about the health risks associated with various behaviors, they may nevertheless believe they have a below-average chance of being harmed by the behavior (Weinstein, 1982, 1987). For example, Weinstein and colleagues found that smokers believed they had a lower risk of developing lung cancer than the average smoker; moreover, they dramatically underestimated their actual cancer risk, and this was especially true of heavy smokers (Weinstein, Marcus, & Moser, 2005).

The *affect heuristic*, our tendency to judge risks based on how we feel toward a behavior or object, also contributes to our inability to accurately assess risks (Finucane, Alhakami, Slovic, & Johnson, 2000). If we have positive feelings toward a behavior, we tend to assume that its risks are low. If we have negative feelings toward a behavior, we tend to assume that its risks are high. For example, Finucane and colleagues (2000) found that telling people that a technology (e.g., nuclear power) had low risks made them believe it has more benefits, even though no actual information was conveyed to them about the benefits. Conversely, telling them that a technology had many benefits made people think that the technology was less risky. This tendency to see an *inverse* association between risks and benefits runs counter to most real-world scenarios. For example, people are prey to engaging in risky behavior—such as smoking, drug abuse, unprotected sex—precisely because they are pleasurable in the moment (and therefore high in "benefit"). Conversely, many behaviors that are low risk also tend to have low benefits (e.g., playing solitaire on the PC in between editing a book chapter). It follows that the risks and benefits of various activities in life are *positively* correlated, contrary to System 1 thinking. Indeed, if activities existed having the profile of low benefit *and* high risk, societies would tend to ban them.

Favorable attitudes that arise from a consideration of one attribute can lead people to develop favorable attitudes about other attributes of the same object, even if those favorable assessments are unfounded. The affect heuristic results in a "halo" effect, imbuing all aspects of a behavior with the same evaluation. In this case, viewing a policy as low risk created a halo around it that also led people to view it as having greater benefits. The consequences of this heuristic pose a challenge for public health, as it suggests that marketers' attempts to create a positive feeling toward an

H it difficult to take a wise desicion when you dont know the consequences.

unhealthy product can lower the perceived risks associated with that product. This is one reason why advertisements for unhealthy products often resort to positive affective appeals ("alive with pleasure," "life is good," "Happy meals," and so forth).

The distorting effects of feelings are not limited to evaluations of specific policies and behaviors but can also arise from the discrete emotions the decision maker is experiencing at the time. Moreover, the impact of different emotions on judgment and decisions are much more subtle and complex than suggested by the traditional categorization of emotions according to their valence (positive vs. negative). As Ferrer and colleagues describe in Chapter 4, Lerner and Keltner's (2000), *appraisal tendency framework* suggests that different emotions generate different cognitive and motivational processes that influence judgment and decision making. The theory makes specific predictions about the effects of specific emotions on risk appraisals and decision making. For example, although fear and anger are both negative emotions, they can lead to different appraisals of a situation's controllability. When people experience fear in response to a situation, such as getting cancer, they will be more likely to view that situation as beyond their control and to be more pessimistic and risk averse. In contrast, if they experience anger in response to a cancer diagnosis, they are more likely to view the situation as in their control (Lerner & Keltner, 2000) and to be more optimistic and risk seeking. Thus, a person who is angry about her cancer may be more likely to pursue a risky but promising treatment option than a person who is fearful.

The field is still in its infancy when it comes to leveraging specific emotions to influence health-related judgment and decision making. In the past, public health experts—just like clinicians—have tended to resort to the fear appeal to persuade the public to quit smoking, avoid driving after drinking, use condoms during casual sexual encounters, or apply sunscreen when going outdoors. Fear appeals certainly seem to raise people's risk perceptions about a target behavior, but whether they are effective in changing behavior is far less certain (Witte & Allen, 2000). More recently, graphic warning labels on cigarette packages have begun to appeal to a broader palette of emotions—including sadness, anger, and disgust, as well as some positive ones such as pride or hope. However, the science of understanding the impacts of specific emotions on health-related decision making remains underdeveloped and is an important topic of future research.

Present-Biased Preferences and Problems of Intertemporal Choice

Even if our beliefs about health-related behaviors were perfect, we would still be vulnerable to preferences that drive us to choose unhealthy options. In particular, much research shows that we have *present-biased preferences*: We place disproportionately more weight on present concerns than on future concerns (O'Donoghue & Rabin, 1999). Thus, we tend to prioritize immediate goals over long-term goals, and immediately available rewards over delayed rewards. For example, for a smoker the decision to reach for the next cigarette pits the immediate benefit of smoking (i.e., it is pleasurable) against the future benefit of not smoking (i.e., you will live longer). Because the immediate benefits are more vivid relative to the intangible promise of future health gains, the smoker is likely to reach for the next cigarette. The problem is compounded by what behavioral economists call the *peanuts effect,* which is the tendency to discount very small individual losses without considering the cumulative effect of these small, but multiple, losses (Prelec & Loewenstein, 1991). For example, smoking just one more cigarette is unlikely to cause cancer ("it's mere peanuts"), and hence smokers are apt to cave into temptation repeatedly during the course of a day (Downs & Loewenstein, 2011).

Present-biased preferences give special weight to the here and now, and are different from preferences that merely prioritize sooner time periods over later ones. For example, present-biased preferences mean that we will choose immediate over future rewards and thus decide to smoke the next cigarette now. However, when smokers are asked about their long-term preferences, most of them would prefer to quit (it is just that they would rather quit tomorrow than today). It is as if two individuals coexist within the same person (i.e., tomorrow's self is rather patient and would prefer the "self" to stop smoking for one's long-term benefit). However, today's "self" demands a huge premium on putting off the pleasure of smoking. Often the smoker may be self-aware of his *dynamic inconsistency* (i.e., the contradictory preferences between today and tomorrow) and choose to *precommit* himself to the long-term goal of smoking cessation. For example, a man might commit his future self to stop smoking by setting a quit date and instructing his spouse to get rid of all smoking paraphernalia in the house (e.g., matches, ashtrays) ahead of the set date.

As this example illustrates, present-biased preferences are time inconsistent, meaning that the decisions we would make for our present selves are different from the decisions we would make for our future selves. Most health behaviors are plagued by time-inconsistent preferences—those that our present selves want to do but our future selves would like to avoid (such as smoking, alcohol consumption, drug use, unhealthy food choices, risky sexual behavior) or vice versa (behaviors that our present selves ought to be doing, but we would rather put off, such as dental flossing, going to the gym, getting the seasonal flu shot).

Chapter 2 of this book is about making *intertemporal choices*, decisions made when preferences are time inconsistent. As White and Dow discuss, overcoming present-biased preferences is challenging, but especially when people are under the influence of visceral factors. Such factors include drive states (e.g., hunger, thirst, sexual desire), moods and emotions, and physical pain (Loewenstein, 1996). Visceral factors put people into an emotionally charged "hot state" that motivates decisions that serve that state. For example, shopping while you are hungry (a hot state) will make you want to buy more food than will shopping while you are full (a cold state).

Importantly, people in hot states are susceptible to *projection bias*, which is our tendency to project our current state—whether it be hot or cold—onto our future selves (Loewenstein, O'Donoghue, & Rabin, 2003). This creates an *empathy gap* between our present and future selves, leading us to underestimate the extent to which our preferences will change when we move from one state to another (Loewenstein, 2005). Thus, when we are in a cold state, we often fail to appreciate how much a future hot state will influence our decision making. For example, a person who is not addicted to cigarettes may underestimate the power of addiction on his future behavior, leading him to start by having an occasional cigarette when out at a bar with friends, and to falsely assume that he will be able to stop whenever he wants to (Loewenstein, O'Donoghue, & Rabin, 2003). It is easy to be optimistic about one's ability to ward off a temptation when one is not being tempted.

Status Quo Bias and Default Options

Even when beliefs and preferences encourage choices that improve the public's health, people may continue to choose unhealthy options if the choice context promotes it. This is seen most dramatically in the case of the *status quo bias*, the strong tendency to stick with whatever options happen to be the current default (Samuelson & Zeckhauser, 1998). A famous example of the power of defaults occurs in organ donation.

Those countries that automatically enroll people as organ donors have dramatically higher donor rates versus countries where people must opt-in to be a donor (Johnson & Goldstein, 2003). Unfortunately, when it comes to health behaviors, unhealthy options tend to be the default. For example, french fries is the default side dish at many restaurants; if you would prefer a salad, you have to ask. Similarly, the default portion in many American restaurants is large, requiring consumers to ask for smaller portions, which almost no one does unprompted (Schwartz, Riis, Elbel, & Ariely, 2012).

Defaults work for a lot of reasons. First, it is usually more effortful to switch from a default than to stay with it. Second, even if it does not take more effort to switch from a default, there is an asymmetry in the need for a justification: Although one does not need a reason to choose a default, one needs a reason to switch away from it. Thus, in the absence of a good reason for choosing either option, people are likely to choose the default. For example, if you are indifferent between french fries and a salad, you are likely to stick with the one that is the default. Third, defaults can be interpreted as a signal that it is the "normal" or recommended option. In the case of portion sizes, consumers may assume that the portion that they are given is the portion they should eat. In one study, participants used 30% more pasta when they were given a 2-lb box than a 1-lb box, and they used 23% more oil when they were given a 32-oz bottle of oil than a 16-oz bottle of oil (Wansink, 1996). This effect may stem from participants' beliefs that the amount they were given is normal, or near-normal, and that they should use approximately that amount.

The important insight from behavioral economics is that we are surrounded by default options in daily life without being aware of their influence on our choices and behaviors. For example, the dining defaults in Japanese culture tend to promote lower caloric intake. Portions sizes at meals are small (at least by American standards) because Japanese cuisine tends to divide the elements of a meal into separate itty-bitty serving containers. For example, rice is served in a bowl that fits snugly in the hollow of one's palm. The default is one serving per meal (you have to trouble the host for a refill—called *okawari*—if you want more). Candy in Japan tends to be sold in individual wrappers so that it is difficult to grab a fistful (as one does with a bag of loose M&Ms). No doubt Japanese candy manufacturers are not attempting to restrain the appetites of consumers in the public health interest (the individual wrappers are there to preserve freshness), yet the resulting default option is in the direction of sensible snacking portions. As Richard Thaler has argued, we can be much more systematic in our use of default options to shift people's behaviors in directions that serve their long-term interests. In short, we can become active "choice architects" to nudge people in a healthy direction.

Social Norms

Finally, our behaviors are influenced by *social norms* (Cialdini & Trost, 1998). Most health behaviors are performed within a social context. For instance, most of us do not eat alone; as McFerran argues in Chapter 5, we tend to eat our meals in the presence of others. To the extent that we do, we are likely to be unconsciously influenced by the eating behaviors of our companions. We are more likely to eat more when we observe that a companion (especially a thin person) is overeating at a meal. Conversely, when others at the table order just the soup and salad for lunch, we are unlikely to order the 24-oz. steak and fries on the menu. A *subjective norm* is defined as an individual's perception of whether other people think the behavior should be performed. According to the theory of planned behavior (Montano & Kasprzyk, 2008), our intentions to perform (or not perform) a behavior are shaped in part by perceived peer norms. For instance, a teenager is more likely to experiment with puffing on her first cigarette if she thinks her friends will view her negatively for not joining them while they smoke. Thus, the social norms people are exposed to can shape health behavior in either the positive or negative direction depending on the social norms associated with the context.

A change in the social norm is often at the root of some of the most successful behavioral interventions in the history of public health. A case in point is legislation to restrict indoor smoking adopted by many countries beginning in the 1990s. Although originally intended to protect the health of nonsmokers from inhaling secondhand smoke, by far the greater impact of the legislation has been to persuade smokers to quit their habit in droves. Whereas a generation ago, it was quite acceptable to light up in enclosed spaces without asking for permission, the norm these days has shifted to the extent that it would be regarded as rude to do so even in the privacy of a friend's home (Nyborg & Rege, 2003). The example in this instance illustrates how the passage of laws can trigger a change in social norms as an unintended and collateral benefit of legislation. The limitation of this approach is that changing social norms through legislation can seem heavy-handed and paternalistic. The question is whether we can also leverage the power of social norms without going to the extent of changing behavior via legislative action.

Leveraging Behavioral Insights to Improve Health

In the first half of this chapter, we discussed insights from psychology and behavioral economics that help explain why maintaining healthy behaviors can be challenging. We now turn to the ways in which behavioral insights can inform solutions to behavior change. We discuss how the lessons of behavioral economics can be leveraged to design psychologically informed interventions and policies to promote public health. We first outline interventions designed to change people's faulty beliefs and perceptions and then outline interventions that directly change their behavior.

Changing Perceptions and Beliefs

As we have discussed, human beings have important cognitive limits. We do not perfectly process information or even usually remember the information that we do process. Thus, message design to impart the beliefs required to make healthy choices must be both easy to process and easy to remember. That is, messages must be simple, concrete, and emotional (Heath & Heath, 2007), as well as repeated and relatable.

In Chapter 6, Riis and Ratner discuss the importance of designing public health messages that are simple and easy to visualize. For example, the "Friends Don't Let Friends Drive Drunk" campaign repeatedly conveyed one simple message. It is no surprise then that the message was highly memorable, as more than 90% of Americans were aware of it more than 20 years after its introduction (Ad Council, 2014). Messages that are simple will stick and potentially influence behavior, whereas messages that are too complex will either be ignored or forgotten (Heath & Heath, 2007). Health messages that ignore this principle will themselves be ignored.

The example of food labeling illustrates how behavioral economics can inform the design of public health interventions. As we have noted, much of the nutrition information we encounter is communicated through numbers that are hard to find, hard to process, and hard to understand. Consequently, in the United States there has been a push to move key nutrition information from the back or side of packaged food to the front so that it is more likely to be seen by consumers at the time they are deciding whether to buy it. Persuading legislators to mandate nutrition information on the front of packaged foods poses one challenge, but another challenge is how to most effectively communicate that information at the point of purchase.

Consider two different approaches to the communication of nutrition information. In the United States, cereal food manufacturers have recently endorsed and implemented a labeling system called Facts Up Front (http://www.factsupfront.org), which displays grams of saturated fat, grams of sugar, and milligrams of sodium, along with percent daily value metrics, on the front of the box. Some labels list up to two additional (positive) nutrients, such as fiber or vitamins. Moreover, the labels appear in different locations for different products, and sometimes on the *top* of a cereal box rather than the *front*, and they often appear in the same color as the box. Clearly, this system, with its difficult-to-find, difficult-to-understand labels, does not represent the most effective way to communicate these products' nutrition information.

In contrast, the United Kingdom Food Standards Agency developed a traffic light labeling system used by some food manufacturers there (Malam et al., 2009). The label uses red, yellow, and green circles to indicate low, medium, or high levels of different key nutrients. This approach leverages existing, automatic associations between "red" and "stop" and "green" and "go" and is thus very easy to understand (Liu et al., 2014). The traffic light is also likely more eye catching than monochromatic labeling systems and might also serve as a reminder of health goals. A study that tested the effectiveness of traffic light labels in a US hospital cafeteria observed a significant increase in purchases of "green" items as well as a significant decrease in purchases of "red" items (Thorndike, Sonnenberg, Riis, Barraclough, & Levy, 2012).

Unfortunately, the most effective labeling systems are those the food industry is most likely to lobby against. This is true not only of traffic light labels but of other labeling systems as well. The US Food and Drug Administration had proposed graphic warning labels to cover the top 50% of the front and back of cigarette packs (*R.J. Reynolds v. FDA*, No. 11–1482). The warnings targeted a range of emotions, including fear, sadness, and disgust, as well as positive emotions such as pride from having quit smoking. However, a lawsuit by US tobacco companies has prevented the graphic warning labels from being implemented. A quote from the US District Judge's ruling explains why: "it is abundantly clear from viewing these images that the emotional response they were crafted to induce is calculated to provoke the viewer to quit or never to start smoking—an objective wholly apart from disseminating purely factual and uncontroversial information" (*R.J. Reynolds v. FDA*, No. 11–1482). The requirement that government warnings must only be factual messages devoid of emotional appeal means that their messages will be less likely to be noticed and remembered, and thus greatly diminishes their ability to influence consumers.

Solutions to the problems of limited attention and memory go beyond the design of simple and memorable advertisements and labels. As White and Dow describe in Chapter 2, studies have found that text-message reminders are effective for promoting smoking abstinence (Free et al., 2011; Rodgers et al., 2005). More and more hospitals are now using *checklists* as tools for doctors to ensure that they carry out all steps required for complicated medical procedures (Haynes et al., 2009). And asking people to specify where, when, and how they plan to engage in healthy behaviors—a practice known as *implementation intentions*—has also been shown to be effective (e.g., Gollwitzer & Sheeran, 2006; Milkman, Beshears, Choi, Laibson, & Madrian, 2011). Such plans reduce forgetfulness and prevent procrastination, making people more likely to carry out their best intentions.

Changing social norms is another way to change behavior. For example, college administrators might seek to reduce binge drinking on campus by telling them, truthfully, that most students do not endorse the practice (Schroeder & Prentice, 1998). Social norms can also be created through laws and policies. A case in point is legislation to restrict indoor smoking, as referred to earlier. Although some studies show that social norm information can backfire—especially when it suggests that it is acceptable to engage in fewer health-related activities (John & Norton, 2013)—its potential as a positive avenue for intervention seems promising.

Changing Behaviors

In Chapter 3, Rünger and Wood explain that we form habits by performing a behavior over and over again in the same circumstances. Eventually, automatic associations are made between cues in the environment where the behavior is performed and the actual behavior. If Sam begins eating ice cream while watching television at night, then eventually watching television might prompt him to get up and grab some ice cream, even in the absence of a conscious goal or intention to eat ice cream (Gardner, 2014; Wood & Neal, 2007). Habits can be difficult to change because our intentions fail to predict habitual behavior. This was illustrated when Wood and colleagues studied fast-food consumption among college undergraduates. They found that intentions to eat fast food predicted actual consumption *only* among those who had not developed a habit of eating it. For those who had developed the habit of eating fast food, their intentions to either eat fast food or to not eat fast food did not predict their actual behavior (Ji & Wood, 2007). Based on a daily diary study, Wood and colleagues estimate that 40% of our daily behaviors are habits (Wood, Quinn, & Kashy, 2002). This means 40% of behaviors will be hard to alter by changing people's intentions. Although habits are difficult to change because of their automatic nature, one promising time to intervene is when people are changing a context in which they perform a habit. In a study of 115 students transferring from one university to another, Wood and colleagues (2005) found that when the context in which someone exercises was changed, exercise habits were disrupted. The students with strong exercise habits maintained them after they transferred schools only if they kept exercising in the same location, such as at home or at the gym, or they perceived little change in their exercise context. But this was not the case if students with strong habits changed the location of where they exercised; then exercise became under intentional control, rather than habitual control. In contrast, for those who had weak exercise habits from the start, the location change had little impact on their behaviors (Wood, Tam, & Witt, 2005). These results suggest that interventions targeting habitual behaviors might have a greater chance of success if they are timed when people are changing contexts. Key intervention points might be when a child switches schools or an adolescent goes off to college, a person starts a new job or moves to a new city, or a family has a baby. These changes all bring with them disruptions in the contextual cues that help to maintain habits.

In addition to changing the context in which people *behave*, we can also change the *choice architecture* or context in which people make *decisions*. Richard Thaler and Cass Sunstein (2008) have popularized the idea of altering the choice environment through "nudging." Their philosophy of "libertarian paternalism" espouses the idea that we can alter choice environments in ways that preserve freedom, while encouraging people to make choices that are aligned with their long-term self-interest. For example, we discussed earlier that people are prone to stick with default options. In the case of the food environment, this is problematic because many default options are for less healthy foods or beverages. In one study, Schwartz and colleagues (2012) tested a small, behavioral nudge to see if they could counter the unhealthy default of large portion sizes. Patrons of a large, Chinese, fast-food restaurant were randomly assigned to one of two conditions. In one condition, the customers who ordered a high-calorie side dish were asked if they wanted a half portion of the dish instead, which would cut their calories by approximately 200. In two experiments,

33% and 21% of patrons, respectively, agreed to downsize their saving an average of 100 and 76 calories in each instance. In add.. offering a $0.25 discount for the smaller portion did not influence whether customers wanted it. The authors also examined a subset of patrons in a third study and found that those who downsized their orders did not compensate by ordering or eating more (Schwartz et al., 2012). In one of the studies, calorie information was also presented in conjunction with the downsize option. They found that fewer people opted to downsize their meal in the presence of calorie information (14% versus 21%) when it was not provided. This suggested that the two interventions in combination did not have positive additive effects, as one might predict. In Chapter 7, Chance and colleagues present a framework that explains how different aspects of choice architecture can influence decision making. They call the framework the four P's and it refers to possibilities (what choices are offered), process (how choices are made), persuasion (how choices are communicated), and person (how intentions are reinforced). The authors provide numerous examples of how these levers of change can be used to nudge people toward healthier decisions. This book has two in-depth examinations of promoting healthier food choices. First, Chance and colleagues describe a case study of interventions in a worksite cafeteria to promote healthy eating. In Chapter 9, Brian Wansink puts forth the CAN framework, which advocates for making "choices more convenient (physically and cognitively), more attractive (comparatively and absolutely), and more normative (actual and perceived)." He describes the Smarter Lunchroom movement to illustrate how these concepts can be applied to promote healthier foods in school cafeterias.

In short, social epidemiology research can be informative about *what* we should be doing to improve health behaviors—such as encouraging public–private partnerships to open grocery stores in low-income communities (RWJ Commission to Build a Healthier America, 2008)—but they do not provide guidance on *how* to increase the purchase of more fruits and vegetables in stores; for example, by the use of choice architecture to display fresh produce in prominent and easy-to-reach locations. The principles of Chance et al.'s four P's model could be equally applied to environmental interventions in neighborhood grocery stores.

In addition to a growing interest in altering worksite environments, many companies have become interested in paying people to engage in healthier behaviors. The hope is that this will help companies save on longer term healthcare expenses. Lewis and Block review the literature on financial incentives in Chapter 8. A randomized, controlled trial by

Volpp et al. (2009) found that paying individuals to stop smoking, for example, has been more successful at encouraging cessation than simply imparting information. At 15–18 months follow-up, the incentive group had significantly higher cessation rates compared to an information-only group (9.4% vs. 3.6%). In this chapter, we provide one example of how principles of behavioral economics have been used to design incentives offered through workplace wellness interventions. In one workplace study, Volpp and colleagues (2008) randomized 57 obese individuals between the ages of 30 and 70 years old to one of three weight-loss interventions: (1) monthly weigh-ins, (2) a lottery incentive program, or (3) a deposit contract with a weight-loss goal of 1 lb (0.45 kg) per week over 16 weeks. These three study arms were informed by behavioral economics in a few ways. First, the lottery arm was designed to leverage people's tendency to place greater weight on small probabilities occurring, like winning a lottery. Lottery participants were eligible for a daily lottery if their weight was at or below their goal. Frequent, small payoffs were offered such as a 1 in 5 chance of winning $10 as well as infrequent, larger payoffs such as a 1 in 100 chance of winning $100. Lottery results were texted to participants to cater to present-biased preferences and provide immediate feedback. This is in contrast to other programs that reward individuals with money in their monthly paychecks and is arguably much less salient.

Second, a deposit contract was used as a *commitment device* to encourage people to change their behaviors (see Bryan, Karlan, & Nelson, 2010). The classic illustration of a commitment device is when Odysseus decides to tie himself to the mast so that he can hear the song of the sirens without jumping to his death. The rationale behind commitment devices is that people are more willing to commit their future selves to an action that they would prefer not to do in the present moment. In the deposit contract arm of the study, participants could deposit between $0.01 and $3.00 for each day of the month. As an added incentive, the employer matched all employee contributions and added a fixed payment of $3 per day. If the target weight was met at the monthly weigh-in, the participant received the accumulated money (up to a maximum of $252 per month). If the target weight was not met, the participant lost the deposited money, which went into an office pool of money that was divided equally among deposit contract participants who lost 20 lb or more over the 16 weeks. These types of precommitment devices aim to leverage people's dislike of losing something they already possess to motivate behavior change.

At the end of the 4-month trial, those receiving incentives lost significantly more weight than the control group, but the two incentive groups did not differ from one another. About half of participants in the incentive groups had met the 16-lb weight-loss target, whereas 10.5% of the control group met the target. However, when the researchers looked to see what had happened 3 months after the intervention ended, between a third to a half of the lost weight had been regained. The total weight lost at 7 months was larger in the incentive groups (9.2 lb in the lottery group and 6.2 lb in the deposit contract group), but it did not significantly differ from the control group (4.4 lb).

In this section we reviewed a number of ways in which insights from the behavioral sciences can be applied to health-related policies and interventions to change perceptions, beliefs, and behaviors. In the next section, we talk about some of the exciting developments in the field of behavioral economics as well as some of the limitations of what these insights can offer.

The Strengths and Limitations of Behavioral Economics

One of the most exciting developments in the field of behavioral economics is the interest from world governments to create behavioral insight teams. In Chapter 10, Sanders and Hallsworth describe the creation of the most famous of these units, the Behavioural Insights Team in the United Kingdom. The mission of this group, often referred to as the "Nudge Unit," is to take insights from the behavioral sciences and apply them to public policy problems. Their efforts are advancing evidence-based policy making in two very important ways. Not only are they linking behavioral science with public policy, but they are also testing these insights using large-scale, randomized, controlled trials. Sanders and Hallsworth briefly describe their framework and methods for running these trials, along with the results from two randomized controlled trials they have run to test behavioral interventions to increase organ donation and promote smoking cessation. There is growing interest around the world in developing such teams from countries such as the Netherlands, Israel, and the United States.

Although the "nudge" approach has received a lot of interest and enthusiasm, it has also been met with skepticism and criticism. Some worry that behavioral nudges will be implemented in lieu of potentially more effective government regulations that are less politically palatable (Rayner &

Lang, 2011). In their critique of the UK nudge unit, Rayner and Lang (2011) argued that the behavioral economics approach:

> dispenses with the complexity of real life contexts and acknowledges only the immediate proximal horizons of consumer choice. At a stroke, policy is reduced to a combination of cognitive and "light" environmental signals, such as location of foods within retail geography. Nudge ... is presented as the alternative to regulation, or in the media jargon, the "nanny state." Our worry is that nudge becomes collusion between the state and corporations to hoodwink consumers. At least nannies are overt. (BMJ 2011;342:d2177)

In other words, although changing choice architecture is appealing, it is important to understand that there are also long-term and structural barriers to achieving optimal health in people's lives. For example, research on residential neighborhoods suggests that built environment characteristics influence health behaviors over and above the characteristics of individual residents. The walkability of neighborhoods (the presence of sidewalks, adequacy of street lighting) can influence levels of walking for both leisure and transport. Furthermore, the correlation between built environment and physical activity has been shown to be independent of people's personal preferences for living in a walkable environment (i.e., the association cannot be explained away by the selective movement of physically active people into more walkable neighborhoods) (Frank, Saelens, Powell, & Chapman, 2007). Similarly, features of the local retail environment, such as the proximity of off-premise alcohol outlets, have been shown to affect the risk of binge drinking and heavy alcohol use among residents (Halonen et al., 2013). A decrease in distance to the nearest alcohol retail outlet (e.g., because a liquor shop opened next door) was found to correlate with an increase in heavy alcohol use over time, net of observed and unobserved individual characteristics in a fixed effects analysis (Halonen et al., 2013). These findings have prompted suggestions to improve the quality of residential environments such as by building bike paths or applying zoning restrictions as an avenue for health promotion. Such interventions would require more durable and extensive investments in our communities than those suggested by nudging alone.

We do not believe behavioral economics should be viewed as a replacement to more paternalistic strategies used to protect the public's health. Instead, it can be a powerful complement to these approaches. The value added by behavioral economics is in "supercharging" the traditional approaches used in public health. For example, if traditional economics suggests that we should have a larger price difference between sugar-free and sugared drinks, behavioral economics can guide us on whether consumers would respond better to a subsidy on unsweetened drinks or a tax on sugary drinks (Loewenstein & Ubel, 2010). In Chapter 11, Zimmerman has proposed a multilevel theoretical model that incorporates the knowledge of how our behavioral choices are shaped by heuristics and habits but also recognizes how power imbalances across social, political, and economic structures shape our choices. There is a need for research to integrate the insights generated from the behavioral sciences to form multilevel policies and interventions that will promote public health.

Another hope is that the use of behavioral economics might help to improve health across the socioeconomic gradient. People, especially from low-income households, face constraints on their monetary and time budgets to adhere to healthy behaviors. Even if they have a latent preference for exercising daily and eating healthy, they may not be able to practice these behaviors on a consistent basis due to lack of time or money. The differential ability to afford to engage in healthy behavior forms an important part of the explanation for the existence of health disparities. Accordingly, the public health approach to tackle socioeconomic inequalities in health has focused on subsidizing the price of desirable behaviors, such as making seasonal flu vaccinations free, or lowering the price of healthy food options in low-income neighborhoods. In addition to these manipulations based on standard economic principles, the behavioral economics approach suggests the use of low-cost approaches to enhance behavioral uptake, which may be especially effective among low-income populations. For example, the uptake of seasonal flu vaccinations remains discouragingly low with coverage rates in the United States falling well below the Healthy People 2020 goals for all demographic groups. Coverage rates are particularly low among low-income households (Linn, Guralnik, & Patel 2010). Given the constraints on their time and money budgets, it makes good sense to bring the flu clinic into workplaces (instead of expecting employees to take time off work to travel to the clinic) and to make the vaccinations free of charge under their health plans. On top of these sensible steps, we saw that the behavioral economics approach suggests adding a "Post-it" sticker to an advertisement for a free on-site flu clinic that prompted people to make a plan to get the shot (Milkman et al., 2011). Although still a long way to go from fixing the issue of low coverage rates, the intervention demonstrated that meaningful gains (from a population health perspective) can still be achieved for very little additional cost. In addition, to the extent that high-income earners are already likely to be looking after themselves, the behavioral economic approach holds promise for helping to narrow the socioeconomic gap in vaccination coverage.

In summary, in this introductory chapter, we have reviewed insights from the behavioral sciences that shed light on why it can be difficult to maintain healthy behaviors. We also introduced a number of ideas from psychology and behavioral economics that can be applied to bolster public health policies and interventions. These ideas are referred to throughout the chapters in this book. Finally, we have argued that there is no tension or opposition between the existing tactics to engender behavior change in public health and the approaches suggested by behavioral economics. The behavioral insights described in this book are unlikely to supplant the strategies traditionally deployed in public health, including health education, taxation, and direct regulation. Instead, the future likely holds the development of behavioral insight teams within government that can merge insights from academic scholarship with policy making and test those insights in large-scale, real-world studies to create psychologically informed, evidence-based policies.

References

The Ad Council. *Buzzed driving prevention.* Retrieved March 2014, from http://www. adcouncil.org/Impact/Case-Studies-Best-Practices/Drunk-Driving-Prevention

Akincigil, A., Bowblis, J. R., Levin, C., Jan, S., Patel, M., & Crystal, S. (2008). Long-term adherence to evidence based secondary prevention therapies after acute myocardial infarction. *Journal of General Internal Medicine, 23,* 115–121.

Buehler, R., Griffin, D., & Ross, M. (1994). Exploring the "planning fallacy:" Why people underestimate their task completion times. *Journal of Personality and Social Psychology, 67,* 366–381.

Bryan G., Karlan, D., & Nelson, S. (2010). Commitment devices. *Annual Review of Economics, 2,* 671–698.

California State University, Northridge. (n.d.). *Cigarette ads.* Retrieved January 2015, from http://www.csun.edu/~vceed002/health/tobacco/index.html

Choudhry, N. K., & Winkelmayer, W. C. (2008). Medication adherence after myocardial infarction: A long way left to go. *Journal of General Internal Medicine, 23,* 216–218.

Cialdini, R. B., & Trost, M. R. (1998). Social influence: Social norm, conformity, and compliance. In D. T. Gilbert, S. T. Fiske, & G. Lindzey (Eds.), *Handbook of social psychology* (Vol. 2, pp. 151–192). New York, NY: McGraw-Hill.

Dehaene, S. (1997). *The number sense: How the mind creates mathematics.* New York, NY: Oxford University Press.

Downs, J. S., & Loewenstein, G. (2011). Behavioral economics and obesity. In J. Cawley (Ed.), *The Oxford handbook of the social science of obesity*. New York, NY: Oxford University Press.

Dweck, C. S. (1996). Implicit theories as organizers of goals and behavior. In P. M. Gollwitzer & J. A. Bargh (Eds.), *The psychology of action: Linking cognition and motivation to behavior* (pp. 69–90). New York, NY: The Guilford Press.

Encinosa, W. E., Bernard, D. M., Du, D., & Steiner, . (2009). Recent improvements in bariatric surgery outcomes. *Medical Care, 47*, 531–535.

Finucane, M. L., Alhakami, A., Slovic, P., & Johnson, S. M. (2000). The affect heuristic in judgments of risks and benefits. *Journal of Behavioral Decision Making, 13*, 1–17.

Frank, L. D., Saelens, B. E., Powell, K. E., & Chapman, J. E. (2007). Stepping towards causation: Do built environments or neighborhood and travel preferences explain physical activity, driving, and obesity? *Social Science and Medicine, 65*, 1898–1914.

Free, C., Knight, R., Robertson, S., Whittaker, R., Edwards, P., Zhou, W., . . . Roberts, I. (2011). Smoking cessation support delivered via mobile phone text messaging (txt-2stop): A single-blind, randomised trial. *Lancet, 378*, 49–55.

Halonen, J. I., Kivimäki, M., Virtanen, M., Pentti, J., Subramanian, S. V., Kawachi, I., & Vahtera, J. (2013). Proximity of off-premise alcohol outlets and heavy alcohol consumption: A cohort study. *Drug Alcohol Dependence, 132*, 295–300.

Gardner, B. (2014). A review and analysis of the use of 'habit' in understanding, predicting and influencing health-related behaviour. *Health Psychology Review*, 1–19. Epub ahead of print.

Gollwitzer, P. M., & Sheeran, P. (2006). Implementation intentions and goal achievement: A meta-analysis of effects and processes. *Advances in Experimental Social Psychology, 38*, 69–119.

Haynes, A. B., Weiser, T. G., Berry, W. R., Lipsitz, S. R., Breizat, A. H., Dellinger, E. P., . . . Gawande, A. A. (2009). A surgical safety checklist to reduce morbidity and mortality in a global population. *New England Journal of Medicine, 360*, 491–499.

Heath, C., & Heath, D. (2007). *Made to stick: Why some ideas survive and others die*. New York, NY: Random House.

Hu, F. B., Manson, J. E., Stampfer, M. J., Colditz, G., Liu, S., Solomon, C. G., & Willett, W. C. (2001). Diet, lifestyle, and the risk of type 2 diabetes mellitus in women. *New England Journal of Medicine, 345*, 790–797.

John, L. K., & Norton, M. I. (2013). Converging to the lowest common denominator in physical health. *Health Psychology, 32*, 1023–1028.

Johnson, E. J., & Goldstein, D. (2003). Do defaults save lives? *Science, 302*, 1338–1339.

Ji, M. S., & Wood, W. (2007). Purchase and consumption habits: Not necessarily what you intend. *Journal of Consumer Psychology, 17*, 261.

Kahneman, D. (2003). Maps of bounded rationality: Psychology for behavioral economics. *American Economic Review, 93*, 1449–1475.

King, D. E., Mainous, A. G., 3rd, Carnemolla, M., & Everett, C. J. (2009). Adherence to healthy lifestyle habits in US adults, 1988–2006. *American Journal of Medicine, 122*, 528–534.

Lerner, J. S., & Keltner, D. (2000). Beyond valence: Toward a model of emotion-specific influences on judgment and choice. *Cognition and Emotion, 14,* 473–493.

Linn, S. T., Guralnik, J. M., & Patel, K. V. (2010). Disparities in influenza vaccine coverage in the United States, 2008. *Journal of the American Geriatrics Society, 58,* 1333–1340.

Liu, P. J., Wisdom, J., Roberto, C. A., Liu, L. J., & Ubel, P. A. (2014). Using behavioral economics to design more effective food policies to address obesity. *Applied Economic Perspectives and Policy, 36,* 6–24.

Loewenstein, G. (1996). Out of control: Visceral influences on behavior. *Organizational behavior and human decision processes, 65,* 272–292.

Loewenstein, G. (2005). Hot-cold empathy gaps and medical decision making. *Health Psychology, 24,* S49–S56.

Loewenstein, G., O'Donoghue, T., & Rabin, M. (2003). Projection bias in predicting future utility. *Quarterly Journal of Economics, 118,* 1209–1248.

Loewenstein, G., & Ubel, P. (2010, July 14). Economics behaving badly. *New York Times.* Retrieved September 2014, from http://www.nytimes.com/2010/07/15/opinion/15loewenstein.html?_r=0

Malam, S., Clegg, S., Kirwan, S., & McGinigal, S. (2009). *Comprehension and use of UK nutrition signpost labelling schemes.* Retrieved August 2011, from http://www.food.gov.uk/multimedia/pdfs/pmpreport.pdf

Milkman, K. L., Beshears, J., Choi, J. J., Laibson, D., & Madrian, B. C. (2011). Using implementation intentions prompts to enhance influenza vaccination rates. *Proceedings of the National Academy of Sciences USA, 108,* 10415–10420.

McFerran, B., & Mukhopadhyay, A. (2013). Lay theories of obesity predict actual body mass. *Psychological Science, 24,* 1428–1436.

Montano, D. E., & Kasprzyk, D. (2008). Theory of reasoned action, theory of planned behavior, and the integrated behavioral model. In K. Glanz, B. K. Rimer, & K. Viswanath (Eds.), *Health behavior and health education. Theory, research, and practice* (pp. 67–96). San Francisco, CA: Wiley.

Murray, C. J. L., & Lopez, A. D. (2013). Measuring the global burden of disease. *New England Journal of Medicine, 369,* 448–457.

Nyborg, K., & Rege, M. (2003). On social norms: The evolution of considerate smoking behavior. *Journal of Economic Behavior and Organization, 52,* 323–340.

O'Donoghue, T., & Rabin, M. (1999). Doing it now or later. *American Economic Review, 89,* 103–124.

Paulos, J A. (1998). *Innumeracy: Mathematical illiteracy and its consequences.* New York, NY: Hill and Wang.

Prelec, D., & Loewenstein, G. (1991). Decision making over time and under uncertainty: A common approach, *Management Science, 37,* 770–786.

Rayner, G., & Lang, T. (2011). Is nudge an effective public health strategy to tackle obesity? No. *British Medical Journal, 342,* d2177.

R. J. Reynolds v. FDA, No. 11–1482, 2012 WL 653828. United States District Court for the District of Columbia.

Roberto, C. A., & Kawachi, I. (2014). Using psychology and behavioral economics to promote healthy eating. *American Journal of Preventive Medicine, 47,* 832–837.

Rodgers, A., Corbett, T., Bramley, D., Riddell, T., Wills, M., Lin R., & Jones, M. (2005). Do u smoke after txt? Results of a randomised trial of smoking cessation using mobile phone text messaging. *Tobacco Control, 14,* 255–261.

RWJ Commission to Build a Healthier America. (2014). Time to Act: Investing in the health of our children and communities. Retrieved September 2014, http://www.rwjf.org/en/research-publications/find-rwjf-research/2014/01/recommendations-from-the-rwjf-commission-to-build-a-healthier-am.html

Samuelson, W., & Zeckhauser, R. (1998). Status quo bias in decision making. *Journal of Risk and Uncertainty, 1,* 7–59.

Schroeder, C. M., & Prentice, D. A. (1998). Exposing pluralistic ignorance to reduce alcohol use among college students. *Journal of Applied Social Psychology, 28,* 2150–2180.

Schwartz, J., Riis, J., Elbel, B., & Ariely, D. (2012). Inviting consumers to downsize fast-food portions significantly reduces calorie consumption. *Health Affairs (Millwood), 31,* 399–407.

Simon, H. (1955). A behavioral model of rational choice. *The Quarterly Journal of Economics, 69,* 99–118.

Sloman, S. A. (1996). The empirical case for two systems of reasoning. *Psychological Bulletin, 119,* 3–22.

Stanovich, K. E., & West, R. F. (2000). Individual differences in reasoning: Implications for the rationality debate. *Behavioral and Brain Sciences, 23,* 645–665.

Swinburn, B., Sacks, G., & Ravussin, E. (2009). Increased food energy supply is more than sufficient to explain the US epidemic of obesity. *American Journal of Clinical Nutrition, 90,* 1453–1456.

Thaler, R. H., & Sunstein, C. R. (2008). *Nudge. Improving decisions about health, wealth, and happiness.* New York, NY: Penguin Books.

Thorndike, A. N., Sonnenberg, L., Riis, J., Barraclough, S., & Levy, D. E. (2012). A 2-phase labeling and choice architecture intervention to improve healthy food and beverage choices. *American Journal of Public Health, 102,* 527–533.

Volpp, K. G., John, L. K., Troxel, A. B., Norton, L., Fassbender, J., & Loewenstein, G. (2008). Financial incentive-based approaches for weight loss: A randomized trial. *Journal of the American Medical Association, 300,* 2631–2637

Volpp, K. G., Troxel, A. B., Pauly, M. V., Glick, H. A., Puig, A., Asch, D. A., ... Audrain-McGovern, J. (2009). A randomized, controlled trial of financial incentives for smoking cessation. *New England Journal of Medicine, 360,* 699–709.

Wald, D. S., & Wald, N. J. (2010). The polypill in the primary prevention of cardiovascular disease. *Fundamental and Clinical Pharmacology, 24,* 29–35.

Wansink, B. (1996). Can package size accelerate usage volume? *Journal of Marketing, 60,* 1–14.

Weinstein, N. D. (1982). Unrealistic optimism about susceptibility to health problems. *Journal of Behavioral Medicine, 5,* 441–460.

Weinstein, N. D. (1987). Unrealistic optimism about susceptibility to health problems: Conclusions from a community-wide sample. *Journal of Behavioral Medicine, 10,* 481–500.

Weinstein, N. D., Marcus, S. E., & Moser, R. P. (2005). Smokers' unrealistic optimism about their risk. *Tobacco Control, 14,* 55–59.

Witte, K., & Allen, M. (2000). A meta-analysis of fear appeals: Implications for effective public health campaigns. *Health Education and Behavior, 27*, 591–615.

Wood, W., & Neal, D. T. (2007). A new look at habits and the habit-goal interface. *Psychological Review, 114*, 843–863.

Wood, W., Quinn, J. M., & Kashy, D. A. (2002). Habits in everyday life: Thought, emotion, and action. *Journal of Personality and Social Psychology, 83*, 1281.

Wood, W., Tam, L., & Witt, M. G. (2005). Changing circumstances, disrupting habits. *Journal of Personality and Social Psychology, 88*, 918–933.

Many health behaviors such as Smoking involve the accretion of a series of incremental desicions

2 | Intertemporal Choices for Health

JUSTIN S. WHITE AND WILLIAM H. DOW

T IS NEW YEAR'S EVE. In keeping with tradition, many revelers resolve to lose weight, to find time for exercise, or to kick some unpleasant habit. When we encounter these individuals many months later, we find their lives and their health behaviors unchanged. Why is it so difficult for individuals to follow through on their plans and goals? What might we as social scientists and public health researchers conclude about the preferences and choices of these individuals? This chapter addresses the wedge between the health-related plans and goals of individuals and their subsequent actions. In so doing, we also consider the wedge between how economists have traditionally understood issues of intertemporal choice and how newer cohorts of economists have applied the principles of behavioral economics to understand the topic. In comparing standard economic theory and behavioral economic theory, we highlight the unique contributions of behavioral economic insights to a fuller conception of intertemporal choices for health.

By intertemporal choice, we refer to any decision that impacts a person's future welfare. The consumption of many health-related goods does not take place in a single instance, but over time. Take smoking as an example. A typical life-course trajectory might be the following. At a young age, Maria decides to take a first puff. Soon, she sneaks a cigarette after school every day. In 5 years, she has developed a habit of smoking half a pack each day. Many health behaviors such as smoking involve the accretion of a series of incremental decisions. Each day, Maria wakes up and chooses whether or not to smoke, in essence whether to sustain the habit or to try to kick it. Economists theorize that in making these daily decisions Maria is solving a series of intertemporal choice problems in which she trades off the current pleasures and harms of smoking against the future pleasures and harms of having smoked. The difference between how traditional economics and behavioral economics view Maria's smoking behavior boils down to certain assumptions about how Maria arrived at a decision to smoke. We consider those assumptions in detail next.

The field of behavioral economics arose to help understand anomalies that are difficult to explain using the framework of standard (i.e., "neoclassical") economic theory. Among the most prominent anomalies are those pertaining to intertemporal choices, and many of the most glaring examples relate to health. The Nobel Prize–winning economist Thomas Schelling (1980) wrote, "People behave sometimes as if they had two selves, one who wants clean lungs and long life and another who adores tobacco, or one who wants a lean body and another who wants dessert" (pp. 95–96). In the intervening decades, we have learned a great deal about how this time-inconsistent behavior pervades an assortment of health-related activities. Behavioral economic concepts have been applied in health most frequently to the consumption of habit-forming goods such as alcohol and unhealthy foods, although the power of these concepts extends far beyond this subset. For example, nonadherence to medications can often be attributed to the intertemporal choices of patients: an inability or unwillingness to weather the short-term side effects of medications, a miscalculation about the harms caused by nonadherence, or a limited ability to remember when or how much medication to consume. The implications for public health practitioners of not addressing problems of intertemporal choice are significant. For example, nonadherence may have serious consequences for personal health and the health system as a whole, accounting for one third to two thirds of all medication-related hospital admissions in the United States (Osterberg & Blaschke, 2005).

To take another example, more than one in three patients is not screened for colorectal cancer as recommended by federal guidelines (Klabunde et al., 2012). This situation shares some of the same characteristics as medication nonadherence. Individuals may not wish to undergo an invasive and unpleasant colonoscopy; they may not fully realize the value of the screening; or they may not remember when it is time for a screening exam or how often to get one. Elucidating the existence and importance of each of these pathways for health-related activities is an important challenge for researchers.

Our focus in this chapter is on the systematic—that is, potentially foreseeable—ways in which individuals' intertemporal health choices depart from the predictions of standard economic theory. By "standard" theory we refer to a model (elaborated in the next section) of the rational agent from neoclassical economics who is perfectly informed, forward-looking, and consistent in his or her preferences. The first section, "Rational Choice Theory," begins with a description of the standard economic model of rational choice. We then describe three classes of deviations from the standard model, relying on a framework developed by DellaVigna (2009): (1) nonstandard preferences, (2) nonstandard beliefs, and (3) nonstandard decision making. We often adopt the first-person voice in our illustrations in recognition that we are as susceptible to cognitive mistakes as anyone.

The first and most studied class is the apparent display of preferences that are inconsistent with the standard model. We focus on time preferences that generate self-control problems. Situations that result in immediate pleasure or pain often lead to self-control problems, as discussed in the section "Self-Control Problems." A desire to avoid immediate pain may lead us to delay quitting smoking or to avoid our annual flu shot. Likewise, a desire to indulge in immediate pleasures may lead us to overeat or to engage in drug use or unprotected sex.

The second class of deviations involves nonstandard beliefs that individuals hold about the future. In the section "Mistaken Beliefs," we consider two types of mispredictions that impact health decisions. First, when in a state of heightened emotion, arousal, or hunger, we fail to predict how we will feel in the future after we have emerged from the state. While hungry, we fail to consider how many entrées we would have ordered in a more sated state. In the heat of the moment, we fail to consider fully our underlying preferences for using contraception. Second, we tend to be overly confident about our abilities. For example, we tend to view ourselves as impervious to illness and perfectly capable of resisting temptations in the future.

The third class of deviations from the standard model involves nonstandard decision making. In "Limited Attention and Memory," we tackle the cognitive limitations of human attention and memory and the ways that limited attention and memory can undermine our health behavior.

After introducing and illustrating the ways that our preferences, beliefs, and decision making may systematically diverge from the standard model, in the section "Implications for Policy and Behavior," we turn to the implications for policy and the design of decision aids. What tools can be leveraged to help individuals deal with complex and challenging choice environments? First, we discuss one of the most celebrated approaches to promoting time-consistent choices: a strategy of precommitment. Next, we consider more broadly how public health programs, and in particular the incentives within programs, can be designed to combat cognitive biases, or decision errors that fail to promote the person's well-being. Then, we discuss the special role played by taxation as a counterweight to the urges to partake in undesirable health behaviors. Finally, we concentrate on vulnerable populations to discuss how cognitive biases can perpetuate disparities across socioeconomic strata and lead to lifelong consequences when initiated in adolescence and young adulthood.

This chapter considers several theoretical constructs from behavioral economics that affect intertemporal choices for health. Yet there are many more that we do not have space to explore, such as heuristic thinking, social preferences, and reference dependence. These topics are considered in other chapters in this volume. Daniel Kahneman and Amos Tversky's (2000) *Choices, Values, and Frames* is a good starting point for a general discussion of these topics. We have also tried to be somewhat selective in our presentation of the literature, as it has grown in recent years. We direct most of our attention to evidence drawn from field settings, rather than laboratory settings. By doing so, we hope to make clear the applicability of this line of inquiry for real-world public health research and practice and the expansive implications of behavioral economics for intertemporal choices across the entire spectrum of health behavior.

Rational Choice Theory

Rational choice underpins much of microeconomic theory. In this section, we provide a brief overview of the standard economic theory of rational choice and its application to public health. Then, we describe certain critiques of the theory that have led in part to the emergence of alternative models of behavior.

Description of the Standard Model

Individuals are considered to be rational if they make choices so as to obtain the most utility (satisfaction) from a given set of resources. Satisfaction or utility depends on tastes or preferences for different goods.

Individuals are assumed to have well-defined preferences. This means that for any pair of goods, say fish and steak, a person can always say that fish is preferred to steak, steak is preferred to fish, or the two are equally attractive. These preferences are often assumed to be stable over time, because this assumption simplifies the researcher's job.

Individuals trade off present utility for future utility using a weighting function called the discount factor. The same resource is more valuable in the present than in the future, and the discount factor represents the degree to which a person down-weights future consumption relative to present consumption. A peculiar feature of the standard model is that the discount function is typically assumed to be constant, such that short-run tradeoffs are treated the same as long-term tradeoffs. This implies that individuals have time-consistent preferences. If a rational consumer prefers to visit the gym tomorrow but not today, then all else equal he will always go to the gym when tomorrow comes. Time inconsistency, or preference reversals, in which a person sleeps in tomorrow, are not usually possible in the standard model.[1]

The standard model also makes assumptions about the beliefs of individuals. They are forward-looking individuals who plan ahead, with full information about available options. Moreover, individuals hold rational expectations about their own future behavior. This means that individuals' predictions of the likelihood of future outcomes and the payoffs that future outcomes yield are correct on average.

Decision making in the standard model involves the maximization of lifetime expected utility. A person uses all available information, factoring in the uncertainty surrounding all possible events, to choose the consumption plan that will produce the maximum level of utility over the person's lifetime. A person is assumed to behave as if he follows this principle, even if he does not explicitly perform such calculations in his head. If a new alternative presents itself, the person integrates it into his current consumption plan before making a choice.

A Simple Utility Model

To show how economists apply the assumptions of the standard model in practice, we present a simple model of utility. Suppose that a person lives for T periods, $t = 0, 1, 2, \ldots, T$. For simplicity, you may think of each period as 1 day. In each period t, a person receives instantaneous utility as a function of the goods consumed during that period. Imagine a person only derives utility from a single good, x. The person's instantaneous utility at time t is denoted $u(x_t)$, which we shorten to u_t for simplicity. Thus, in periods 1, 2, and T, a person's instantaneous utility would be u_1, u_2, and u_T.

Building on this framework, we can determine a person's lifetime utility U as a function of consumption in each time period $U = U(x_0, x_1, ..., x_T)$. The person's lifetime utility function is the sum of utility in period 1 and discounted future utility in periods 2 through T.

$$U = u_0 + \delta u_1 + \delta^2 u_2 + \delta^3 u_3 + \cdots + \delta^T u_T$$

$$= \sum_{t=0}^{T} \delta^t u_t \tag{1}$$

The most commonly used discount function is the exponential function δ^t, as used here. The discount factor δ represents the degree to which a person discounts future consumption relative to current consumption. For example, owning a bicycle today is more valuable than owning one tomorrow by a factor δ; owning the bicycle tomorrow is more valuable than the day after tomorrow by a factor δ; and owning one today versus the day after tomorrow by a factor $\delta^2 = \delta \times \delta$.

A key property of *exponential discounting* is that the discount factor from any period t to the subsequent period $t + 1$ is constant.[2] A person will discount the same between today and tomorrow as between tomorrow and the day after tomorrow. An implication of this constant discount factor is that the choices of an "exponential discounter" are always time consistent.

A Standard Model Incorporating Uncertainty
(Casual Readers may Skip this Section!)

We now add one more layer of complexity to our utility function in order to capture the notion that choices have uncertain outcomes. Individuals make choices based not only on the outcomes of a choice but also on the probability of that outcome being realized. For example, Anya is a 40-year-old woman trying to decide whether to get a mammogram for breast cancer screening. She must consider the benefit from a mammogram in the presence and absence of cancer. She also needs to consider her probability of having breast cancer.

Suppose that Anya has a 25% probability of being diagnosed with breast cancer. Further assume that if she gets a mammogram her instantaneous utility is 2 if diagnosed with cancer and 10 if not diagnosed with cancer. Anya's expected utility from the mammogram would be: $(0.25 \times 2) + (0.75 \times 10) = 8$. Assume that her expected utility if she does not get a mammogram is 10. In this case, Anya would choose not to get a mammogram, as it yields greater utility.

Formally, let $p(s)$ be the probability of outcome s, and let $u(x|s)$ be the person's instantaneous utility from consuming x given outcomes $s = 1, 2, ..., S$. In this simple case, where we have omitted any time component, expected utility $E(U)$ is the product of the payoff from each outcome and the probability of each outcome, just as for Anya earlier:

$$E(U) = p(1)u(x|1) + p(2)u(x|2) + \cdots + p(S)u(x|S)$$

$$= \sum_{s=1}^{S} p(s)u(x|s) \tag{2}$$

Under rational expectations, a person's beliefs about the probability of each outcome $p(s)$ are accurate. In other words, Anya is fully informed about her cancer risk. If we extend the model to capture future mammography choices as well (as in Equation [3]), Anya is also assumed to accurately predict her future cancer risk.

We combine the concepts from Equations (1) and (2) to show a simple model of how a person makes intertemporal choices according to the standard model. A person who is about to enter period 0 faces uncertain choices in each time period $t = 0, 1, ..., T$ that are subject to probabilities $p(s_t)$ for outcomes s_t. This person maximizes lifetime expected utility by maximizing expected utility in each period.

$$\max_{x_t} \underbrace{\sum_{s_0} p(s_0)u(x_0|s_0)}_{\substack{\text{Expected utility} \\ \text{in period 0}}} + \delta \underbrace{\sum_{s_1} p(s_1)u(x_1|s_1)}_{\substack{\text{Discounted expected} \\ \text{utility in period 1}}} + \cdots + \delta^T \underbrace{\sum_{s_T} p(s_T)u(x_T|s_T)}_{\substack{\text{Discounted expected} \\ \text{utility in period } T}}$$

$$= \max_{x_t} \sum_{t=0}^{T} \delta^t \sum_{s_t} p(s_t)u(x_t|s_t) \tag{3}$$

Equation 3 states that a person maximizes the expected utility from her current and future consumption of good x, where future utility is discounted by discount factor δ.

Criticisms of the Standard Model

Standard utility theory has been criticized along several lines. Some researchers have pointed to the long list of apparently self-defeating behaviors that are at odds with the predictions of the theory. The sheer prevalence of drug addiction, gambling, unsafe sexual behavior, obesity, and many others belies the existence of utility-maximizing behavior. Individuals who struggle with these conditions often feel regret and shame, and often invest large sums of money and time trying to change their behavior, as evidenced by the profitability of the weight-loss and self-help industries and the popularity of programs such as Alcoholics Anonymous. Throughout this chapter, we highlight evidence that does not conform to the predictions of the standard model.

Proponents of the standard model have tried to marshal evidence in support of the standard model. A notable case is the application of rational choice theory to addictive behavior. In the "rational addiction model," individuals choose to become addicted and to maintain an addiction after determining that it enhances their utility (Becker & Murphy, 1988). As in the standard model, rational addicts are forward looking. Thus, one test of the rational addiction model is to see if individuals reduce current levels of consumption of addictive goods in response to anticipated price changes (Becker, Grossman, & Murphy, 1994). Critics have pointed out that this prediction of forward-looking behavior is not unique to the standard model. In fact, it accords with "all plausible psychological theories of people's errors," with the exception of a model of complete myopia (Rabin, 2013). Evidence in favor of the standard model may be weaker than its proponents have claimed.

Another line of criticism has been leveled specifically against the rational addiction model. Critics have pointed out that supportive evidence for this model has been drawn largely from analyses that look for positive consumption levels such that a person would choose to remain addicted, rather than scrutinizing the decision to become addicted in the first place (Rabin, 2013). If addictions are as powerful as suggested, then the decision to become addicted is of far greater relevance to understanding the addictive process. As earlier, the evidence base is not fully persuasive.

Self-Control Problems

A Bias for the Present

Self-control problems may be thought of as intrapersonal conflicts that pit a present self against a stream of future selves. For example, Stu feels an urge to binge on the chocolate ice cream in his freezer, but he knows that his future self will regret it. Moreover, had we asked Stu yesterday about whether he wanted his present self to eat the ice cream, he would have said no. Stu's various incarnations are in conflict, a clear indication that his preferences are time inconsistent. Another way to put it is that eating the ice cream would represent a preference reversal. Yesterday he would have preferred for his today's self to avoid the ice cream, but today the chocolate Sirens are calling.

Economists refer to self-control problems as *present-biased preferences*, or simply present bias, because they are the outcome of placing too much weight on present costs and benefits and too little on future costs and benefits. All self-control problems involve this feature of revising our consumption plans. We make plans for tomorrow that we revise once tomorrow comes. There are two ways that we tend to revise our plans. First, consider the case of "investment goods" that have an immediate cost and a future benefit. These are healthy goods that we wish to consume but lack the motivation or willpower to do so, such as physical exercise and preventive services such as cancer screening. A present-biased person will tend to delay the consumption of investment goods, going to the gym and getting cancer screening too infrequently. The gym members plan to work out but revise those plans when it comes time to peel themselves off the couch. For most people, working out is a chore. We would much rather loaf on the couch than deal with the immediate unpleasantness that the workout brings, and the potential benefits involving weight loss and improved health are far in the future. Our present self places far more importance on those immediate costs than the long-run benefits, and so we skip the gym workout today in hopes that we will make a different choice tomorrow. Often, we make the same choice tomorrow and delay the activity yet again.

The second scenario of revising our plans involves "leisure goods" that have an immediate benefit and a future cost. These are unhealthy goods that we wish to consume in moderation or not at all but then overindulge in, such as junk food, recreational drugs, and risky sexual behavior. Present-biased individuals will overconsume leisure goods because of the urge to realize the immediate gratification. We want to smoke cigarettes today and cut back or quit tomorrow. When tomorrow comes, we revise our plan and consume as we did the day before. In this way, we may maintain a bad habit indefinitely, even though we would prefer to kick it.

There are a number of telltale signs that self-control problems are commonplace in the general population. Rational choice theory may be able to account for some of these aspects of behavior, for example, Orphanides and Zervos's (1995) attempt to incorporate regret. Taken as a whole, however, these patterns are highly suggestive that models that allow for self-control problems constitute a more parsimonious explanation.

First, individuals often express a desire not to partake in the unhealthy behaviors in which they then engage, and they often make unsuccessful attempts to quit or reduce consumption of unhealthy goods. For example, 69% of current US smokers reported in 2010 that they would like to stop smoking completely (Malarcher, Dube, Shaw, Babb, & Kaufmann, 2011). More than half of smokers made a quit attempt in the prior year, but only 6% of smokers quit successfully (Malarcher et al., 2011). Failed quit attempts can exact hefty costs in terms of cravings, withdrawal symptoms, and a bruised ego. Most individuals would not voluntarily subject themselves to this pain unless they really wanted to succeed. Moreover, individuals frequently make repeated failed attempts to change behavior. In one typical study, a sample of smokers had a mean of four past failures (Zhou et al., 2009). This pattern of behavior would be a highly inefficient path to maximizing utility.

Second, individuals who succeed in changing their behavior often succumb to high rates of recidivism. Studies find that as many as 40% to 60% of patients treated for drug dependence return to active use within a year of discharge from treatment (McLellan, Lewis, O'Brien, & Kleber, 2000). Addictions in general are characterized by a chronic risk of relapse.

A third piece of evidence that self-control problems are common is the prevalence of regret that individuals express about past behavior. For example, 90% of smokers in Australia, Canada, the United Kingdom, and the United States agree or strongly agree that they would not have started smoking if they could do it over again (Fong et al., 2004). It is no wonder that individuals often turn to professionals for help, as seen by the proliferation of behavioral and cognitive therapies to modify lifestyles.

Beyond the existence of anomalous behavioral patterns, a large body of research has directly elicited the time preferences of individuals and found them to be dynamically inconsistent. This research consistently shows the tendency of individuals to discount delayed rewards according to a hyperbolic function, in contrast to the exponential function assumed by standard economic theory (Ainslie, 1992; Frederick, Loewenstein, & O'Donoghue, 2002). Relative to the exponential function, the hyperbolic function has a steeper decline over small delays but levels out into a smaller decline over long delays. For example, in trading off a tempting snack now versus tomorrow (small delay) and tomorrow versus next week (long delay), a person would be expected to heavily discount the value of the snack between now and tomorrow but to modestly discount the value of the

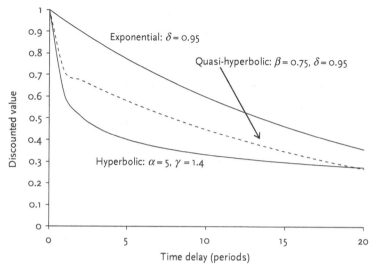

FIGURE 2.1 Discount functions.

NOTE: The hyperbolic discount function is $(1+\alpha t)^{-\gamma/\alpha}$, as used in Loewenstein and Prelec (1992).

snack between tomorrow and next week. Figure 2.1 depicts the shape of these discounting functions, as well as the quasi-hyperbolic function discussed in the next section.

Dozens of empirical studies have linked hyperbolic discounting to health behaviors, such as tobacco use, alcohol use, and illicit drug use (Chabris, Laibson, & Shuldt, 2008). These studies typically calculate discount rates by asking individuals about their willingness to accept varying amounts of money in exchange for varying delays of gratification. To take one example, Kirby, Petry, and Bickel (1999) observe the responses of heroin users and matched controls to offers of smaller immediate rewards ($11 to $80) and larger delayed rewards ($25 to $85). They show that a hyperbolic discounting function provides a good fit for the data, and heroin users hold discount rates about twice as large as the control group. Similar patterns have been found for users of nicotine, alcohol, cocaine, and other substances.

A Model of Self-Control Problems

In the section "A Simple Utility Model," we presented a utility function that assumes individuals are exponential discounters. Economists have suggested other discount functions that do not embed an assumption of time consistency. R. H. Strotz (1956) pointed out that any discount function other than an exponential function could produce time-inconsistent preferences, although he did not advocate any specific functional form. David Laibson (1997), drawing on work by Phelps and Pollak (1968), proposed an easy-to-use model of time-inconsistent preferences that has a quasi-hyperbolic discount function. Much like the hyperbolic discount function advocated by Ainslie (1992) and others, the Laibson model allowed for steeper discounting in the short term than in the long term:

$$U = u_0 + \beta\delta u_1 + \beta\delta^2 u_2 + \beta\delta^3 u_3 + \cdots + \beta\delta^T u_T$$

$$= u_0 + \beta\sum_{t=1}^{T} \delta^t u_t \tag{4}$$

The only difference between Laibson's β-δ model in Equation (4) and the standard model in Equation (1) is that the β-δ model embeds an additional discount factor $\beta \leq 1$ on all future utility. In fact, the standard model is a special case of the β-δ model, where $\beta = 1$. If $\beta = 1$, then Equation (4) simplifies to Equation (1), and the person becomes an exponential discounter with time-consistent preferences. If $\beta < 1$, then the person gives less weight to all future time periods relative to the present and is a hyperbolic discounter with time-inconsistent preferences.

To see this, consider that a person in the β-δ model discounts utility tomorrow (period 1) relative to today (period 0) by a factor of $\beta\delta$. Now, consider that a person discounts any two consecutive future periods, such as tomorrow (period 1) versus the day after tomorrow (period 2), by a factor of $\beta\delta^2 / \beta\delta = \delta$. This is the same discount factor as in the standard model. In other words, the model predicts that a person is not subject to self-control problems when comparing the future to the more distant future. Only in the present does the person feel the pull of temptation. Thus, we want to eat candy today but avoid it tomorrow. However, when tomorrow comes, we again indulge ourselves and decide to avoid candy the day after tomorrow. Once the day after tomorrow comes, we again revise our plans. This is the essence of time-inconsistent preferences for a hyperbolic discounter.

As an aside, it is as yet unclear the extent to which self-control problems are domain specific. Does a person's propensity to succumb to glazed donuts imply that the person will have poor self-control at work or at the pub? We do not know whether we should speak of individuals having a self-control parameter β or many βs, one for each type of action. We hope that future research will clarify this point.

Sophistication Versus Naiveté

An important distinction is to be made between individuals who are aware of their self-control problems and individuals who are not. Behavioral economists refer to those who are self-aware as "sophisticated individuals" and those who are not as "naïve individuals" (O'Donoghue & Rabin, 1999a, 2001). In practice, many individuals do not fit neatly into either category. Self-awareness might be better conceived of as a continuum with full sophistication and full naïveté as the poles. Most of us fall somewhere in the middle, partially aware of our self-control problems; we recognize that we lacked self-control today but nevertheless remain overly optimistic about our ability to show self-control in the future. A present-biased person's place on this continuum of self-awareness has major implications for how he deals with a self-control problem.

Sophisticated individuals may give in to temptation, but only for a limited period of time. Eventually, a sophisticate will search for strategies that precommit herself to following through on a goal. Consider a sophisticate who is trying to avoid overconsuming alcohol, a leisure good that has a present benefit and a future cost. She may pursue a few different strategies that precommit her to lower consumption of alcohol. The person may try to remove environmental cues that trigger drinking. For example, she may avoid hanging out with drinking buddies or avoid spending time in pubs. Or she may try to diminish the pleasure she gets from alcohol. An extreme example would be the use of disulfiram, a drug that makes a person vomit when taken with alcohol. Needless to say, the unpleasant effects of the drug may be a powerful motivator for decreasing alcohol use.

In contrast to sophisticates, individuals who are naïve about their self-control problems will not recognize the need to precommit themselves to a path. In the extreme case, an aspiring gym-goer may delay working out day after day, year after year, always planning to go tomorrow. Likewise, the naïve dieter will perpetually plan to start a diet tomorrow, that is, until tomorrow comes and the grocery store has a sale on chocolate bars. If these individuals truly believe that they have the willpower needed to exercise or diet, they will fail to adopt self-control strategies or to seek out external support, and they will inevitably fail to reform their ways.

We can represent sophistication and naïveté in the β-δ model presented in the last section. Recall that $\beta < 1$ is an indicator of present bias. Let $\hat{\beta}$ be a person's prediction of his or her future self-control, that is, a prediction of β. A fully sophisticated person, who perfectly predicts the degree to which she will lack self-control, will have $\beta=\hat{\beta}<1$. A fully naïve person, who predicts that he will show total self-control, will have $\beta<\hat{\beta}=1$. A partially naïve person underestimates her future self-control, such that $\beta<\hat{\beta}<1$.

One conundrum of the sophistication-naïveté distinction is why individuals would not learn about their degree of present bias over time. After breaking a diet 100 times, wouldn't a dieter have learned by the 101st attempt? Moreover, can we educate naïfs about their self-control problems, for example, by offering them feedback about past behavior, in order to increase their level of sophistication? More research is needed to understand the degree to which learning about self-control occurs over time. If we examine our own experiences, we find many instances in which our self-control problems have persisted over long stretches of time. Thus, we must theorize some reason that learning is incomplete, namely a reason that individuals do not adjust their beliefs to take self-control problems into account. One hint may lie in what psychologists refer to as a self-serving bias. We tend to blame our failures on external factors outside of our control, on the situation in which we were placed rather than on our failings. We binged on snacks at the holiday party, but it was the party planner's fault, not due to our own self-control. If we perceive each situation to be sufficiently different from the last situation—the holiday party is only once a year—then we may be able to convince ourselves that such instances are not learning opportunities.

Field Evidence of Self-Control Problems

The empirical literature on present bias has multiplied in recent years. In this section, we present several lines of economic research that highlight individuals' self-control problems related to health.

Exercise

Exercise is a prime example of a health application in which many individuals fail to meet their own goals. DellaVigna and Malmendier (2006) show that individuals make suboptimal decisions about gym attendance. Gym members often purchase monthly passes yet attend the gym so infrequently that per-visit passes would be a cheaper alternative. Such inefficient behavior is incongruous with a standard model, although it can be reconciled with a model of present bias. The authors conclude that sophisticates who recognize their self-control issues may purchase monthly passes as a precommitment to exercise more often.

Acland and Levy (2015) show that infrequent gym visits may also involve a high degree of naïveté about present bias. As part of a field experiment, participants were eligible to win cash in exchange for meeting attendance targets in a randomly assigned week. Comparing participants' predictions about attendance and actual attendance, the authors find that participants are highly overoptimistic (i.e., naïve) about future gym attendance. Participants expect their future selves to be two-thirds less present-biased than they actually are now.

Tobacco Use

Several economists have noted the link between present bias and the consumption of addictive goods. Satisfying one's immediate gratification today for an addictive good, such as tobacco, makes a person more likely to become addicted tomorrow than that person would have preferred in advance.

Gruber and Köszegi (2001) reassess the evidence in favor of the rational addiction model, such as the work of Becker, Grossman, and Murphy (1994) based on the forward-looking behavior of smokers. They show that observed smoking patterns fit a model in which smokers have present-biased preferences. In particular, present-biased smokers, like "rational" smokers, would respond now to expected future increases in excise taxes, although they may respond less than the rational addiction theory would predict.

Another piece of evidence comes from subjective ratings of happiness before and after the passage of tobacco control legislation. Gruber and Mullainathan (2005) find that smokers report having greater life satisfaction after the regulations take effect, as would be the case if smokers view smoking as a bad habit that they regret. In this context, the tobacco control laws function as a precommitment that aids smokers in following through with their own plans to quit smoking.

Levy (2010) finds more direct evidence on the present bias of smokers. He is able to separate the short-run and long-run discount factors, β and δ, by using short-run and long-run changes to cigarette prices. Price variation due to taxes represents a long-run price change, and fluctuation in tobacco leaf prices represents a short-run change. Assuming that smokers are sophisticated about their present bias, Levy finds that on average smokers exhibit a moderate level of present bias that leads many to start a welfare-reducing, lifelong smoking habit.

Default Effects

Another line of evidence comes from the potency of default options in influencing individuals' decision making. One of the most notable examples of default effects is organ donation. Some countries require citizens to register to become organ donors (opt-in system), whereas others require citizens to register if they do not want to donate their organs (opt-out system). Johnson and Goldstein (2003) find that more than 85% of citizens donate in countries that have an opt-out system, and over 99% in most of opt-out countries, as compared to 4% to 28% under an opt-in system. At least one aspect of these sizable default effects is likely the role of present bias.[3] Opting into the system involves time and mental effort to complete and submit the requisite forms. This process may be unpleasant, as individuals are asked to contemplate their wishes if they die. As we have discussed, situations that carry upfront costs and long-term benefits are apt to be put off, sometimes indefinitely.

Default effects have also been found for vaccination (Chapman et al., 2010), advance directives (Halpern et al., 2013), and HIV testing (Montoy, Dow, & Kaplan, 2014). Moreover, they likely apply to many other aspects of health, such as choice of a health insurance plan, contributions to health savings accounts, health worker flu shots, and treatment decisions like the removal of a catheter after 72 hours in order to avoid urinary tract infections. Halpern, Ubel, and Asch (2007) discuss many other examples of default policies that may improve health.

Payday Effects

Many health-related programs dispense regular cash or in-kind benefits. Examples include food assistance programs and conditional cash transfer programs that make payments conditional on criteria such as regular check-ups or vaccinations. In many programs, the purchasing behavior of recipients shows signs of a regular cycle, in which recipients make larger or more frequent purchases around the time of receipt of income but then run out of money by the end of the cycle. The consumption cycle is highly suggestive that individuals have a short-run impatience, or present bias.

A good example is the monthly food stamp cycle in which some families that receive monthly benefits through the Supplemental Nutrition Assistance Program (SNAP) consume relatively more food and calories at the start of the month and run out of food by the end of the month (Hastings & Washington, 2010; Shapiro, 2005; Wilde & Ranney, 2000). Food insecurity from this cycling may put diabetic SNAP recipients at higher risk of end-of-month hypoglycemia and hospital admissions (Seligman, Bolger, Guzman, López, & Bibbins-Domingo, 2014). This monthly cycling cannot be explained under the standard model, although it is quite consistent with behavior under a model of quasi-hyperbolic discounting.

Another consequence of payday effects is that individuals may be more likely to purchase "temptation goods," such as alcohol and sweets immediately after the receipt of income. Dasso and Fernandez (unpublished data) find that recipients of a conditional cash transfer in Peru are more likely to spend the income on sweets, soft drinks, and meals in restaurants, relative to nonrecipients and relative to themselves during other times of the month. This behavior violates the assumption from the standard model—known as the permanent income hypothesis—that receiving previously anticipated sources of income should not affect a household's consumption.

Deadline Effects

Another line of evidence, largely unexplored for health-related decisions, is the way in which individuals respond to deadlines or time-limited offers. Individuals will often prefer to defer a costly action until the future, although individuals who are overoptimistic (i.e., somewhat naïve) about their future self-control may procrastinate. Setting a deadline or making a time-limited offer, if sufficiently large to overcome the immediate cost, may be able to prevent present-biased individuals from procrastinating on the action. Duflo, Kremer, and Robinson (2011) offer a time-limited discount on fertilizer to Kenyan farmers right after the harvest when they are flush with cash and find that the deadline significantly helps to ward off procrastination. Ariely and Wertenbroch (2002) show that deadlines help workers not only to complete a task but also to do a more thorough job. Moreover, they find that evenly spaced, externally imposed deadlines are more effective than self-imposed deadlines. While many health settings feature deadlines, such as the open enrollment period for selecting a health insurance plan, these aspects have not been studied in depth.

Precommitment

Perhaps the most notable area of research on self-control problems is individuals' demand for precommitment. These are strategies that make it more costly for a person to deviate tomorrow from a person's preferred choices today. Individuals need to be at least somewhat self-aware (at least partially sophisticated) about their future self-control in order to seek out precommitment strategies. For example, a person who recognizes her weakness for ice cream may avoid buying any at the grocery store, thereby making it more difficult to binge when she craves ice cream tomorrow. In a world of rational choice, that is, in a world of perfect self-control, individuals would have no need for precommitment. We take up further discussion of precommitment in the section "Commitment Devices."

Microfoundations of Self-Control Problems

As yet, we have not discussed in depth the biological and psychological underpinnings of self-control problems, except to say that they involve intertemporal tradeoffs. Behavioral economists lean on two overlapping frameworks for understanding the deeper underpinnings, or microfoundations, of self-control problems, as captured by hyperbolic and quasi-hyperbolic discounting. The first framework looks at the neurological foundations of self-control problems. This burgeoning field, known as neuroeconomics, points to an interplay between multiple systems in the brain that process information on rewards. The second framework focuses on the psychological foundations of self-control problems, notably the dual cognitive processes that lead to preference reversals.

Neuroeconomics

Multiple neurological systems process information on rewards, each of which handles time delays differently. The mesolimbic dopamine system is "impatient"; the fronto-parietal system is "patient." Although the neurobiological evidence is still subject to multiple interpretations (Sellito, Ciaramelli, & di Pellegrino, 2011), one view is that the balance between levels of activation of these two systems determines the degree of resulting patience or impulsivity. For example, McClure et al. (2004) use functional magnetic resonance images (fMRIs) to measure brain activity during experiments in which subjects were offered monetary choices between smaller amounts of varying immediacy and larger delayed amounts. Regardless of the immediacy, there was activation of regions of the prefrontal cortex commonly associated with higher cognitive function, such as computation. However, when choices involved more immediate rewards, there was disproportionate activation of midbrain limbic structures associated with the dopamine system, that is, areas that have been implicated in impulsive behavior. Research by Albrecht et al. (2011) building on this study further found immediate awards disproportionately associated with increased activity in the anterior cingulate cortex, which they interestingly note has also been found to be activated in risky decision problems that involve large gains. Relatedly, studies from patients with brain lesions that reduce emotional responsiveness find that those patients display lower levels of myopic loss aversion (Shiv, Loewenstein, Bechara, Damasio, & Damasio, 2005). This is consistent with the hypothesis that individuals may make decisions that better correspond to standard rational choice models when the parts of the brain engaging in executive function have less competition from emotional centers.

Dual-Process Models

Psychologists have advanced a number of frameworks describing cognitive processes in conflict. While the shorthand used to describe the processes has varied by author, the concepts are relatively stable. Humans have one cognitive process that is impulsive, reflexive, impatient, and irrational and another that is deliberative, analytical, patient, and rational. For example, Shiffrin and Schneider (1977) referred to automatic and controlled processing; Epstein (1994), to the experiential system and the rational system; Sloman (1996), to associative thought and rule-based reasoning; Metcalfe and Mischel (1999), to hot and cool cognitive systems; and Kahneman (2011), simply to System 1 and System 2. The conflict between these processes waylays a person from any premeditated plans and induces self-control problems.

In recent decades, behavioral economists have incorporated dual-process thinking into their own models under the broad category of "dual-self models." These assume that preferences can be represented by multiple selves within the person, whose interests are only partially aligned. This tradition dates back to Adam Smith (1759), who recognized in *The Theory of Moral Sentiments* the internal struggle between the "passions" and the "impartial spectator." Only since the emergence of behavioral economics have economists revived this work. Here, we introduce a handful of dual-self models to provide a flavor for their distinguishing and overlapping features and implications. This discussion draws heavily on a review of precommitment by Bryan, Karlan, and Nelson (2010).

Thaler and Shefrin (1981) propose a dual-self model comprised of a planner and a doer. The planner is a farsighted agent who wishes to maximize the person's lifetime utility but does not actually make any consumption decisions; rather, she derives utility from the choices of the doer. The doer lives for one period and is completely selfish and myopic. At times, the planner may try to modify the preferences or incentives of the doer. For example, a planner on a diet may increase monitoring of the doer by counting calories. Keeping track of the calories acts as a tax on the doer's decision to break the diet. At other times, the planner may wish to constrain the choices of the doer by imposing certain rules. These may be flexible rules, such as a dieter who aims to cut refined sugar from her diet, or stringent rules, such as checking herself into a weight-loss clinic that will enforce a strict diet. We come back to these rules in our discussion of precommitment in the section "Commitment Devices."

There are several variants of the planner-doer model. One difference arises due to different assumptions about the short-run self. Fudenberg and Levine (2005) assume that the short-run self is myopic. Bernheim and Rangel (2004) describe a short-run self, an addict, who is helpless to cue-triggered impulses. Each dual-self model implies that individuals have different abilities to control impulses. The long-run self may be able to incur a cost in exchange for exerting control over the short-run self (Fudenberg & Levine, 2006; Thaler & Shefrin, 1981) or may face a random shock that determines whether the long-run self or short-run self has complete cognitive control (Bernheim & Rangel, 2004). In each case, the models predict that precommitment strategies would be helpful to the long-run self.

A debate in the literature involves whether dual-self models are consistent with an alternative model of self-control problems developed by Gul and Pesendorfer (2001). In their temptation model, individuals have preferences regarding menus, or choice sets, of items. The canonical example is a customer at a restaurant who is choosing between, say, a hamburger and a salad. The person receives a certain level of utility from choosing from a menu where salad is the only entrée listed. However, once the hamburger is also on the menu, the salad provides less satisfaction, as the self-control needed to choose the salad and overcome the tempting hamburger is costly. More generally, a person's welfare may diminish if a tempting option is added to the choice set. Unlike the β-δ model, the temptation model implies that choices are always consistent with preferences. A person who gives in to temptation does so because the cost of temptation outweighs the cost of exerting self-control. In the β-δ model, utility depends only on actions; costly self-control does not factor into a person's utility function. Yet, as in the β-δ model, Gul and Pesendorfer's model predicts that a person will seek out precommitments to remove tempting options from the person's future choice set.

Mistaken Beliefs

In this section, we discuss situations in which a person's beliefs deviate from rational expectations. We consider two forms of mistaken beliefs: (1) mispredictions about future preferences and (2) overconfidence.

Mispredicting Preferences

An old adage is never to shop on an empty stomach. In a classic experiment, Read and van Leeuwen (1998) studied the food choices of office workers in different hunger states, either when hungry late in the afternoon or when sated immediately after lunch. Subjects in each hunger state were asked to order a snack from a menu of healthy snacks (e.g., apples and bananas) and unhealthy snacks (e.g., candy bars and potato chips) 1 week in advance. Hungry subjects would be expected to have less self-control and to choose the unhealthy option. Some subjects were told that the food would be delivered late in the afternoon when they were hungry, while others were told that the food would be delivered right after lunch when they were sated. Thus, in making the choice, subjects had to grapple with their current hunger state and their predicted hunger state in 1 week's time. The study revealed that subjects correctly anticipated being less likely to want an unhealthy snack in a future state of satiety (last row of Table 2.1), although subjects allowed their current state of hunger to heavily influence this decision. In particular, subjects projected their current state of hunger onto their predicted future hunger. Whereas 78% of hungry subjects ordered an unhealthy snack to be delivered when hungry in a week, only 42% of sated subjects did so. The same holds for those predicting snack preference for a future state of satiety: Hungry subjects were twice as likely as sated subjects to prefer the unhealthy snack to be delivered when sated in a week.

TABLE 2.1 Percentage of Subjects Who Chose an Unhealthy Snack, by Current and Future Hunger

	HUNGRY IN A WEEK (%)	SATED IN A WEEK (%)
Hungry now	78	56
Sated now	42	26
Total	60	46

SOURCE: Read and van Leeuwen (1998).

The tendency to project one's current state onto one's predictions for the future is a general phenomenon called *projection bias* (Loewenstein, O'Donoghue, & Rabin, 2003). In the earlier example in which subjects are asked to predict their future hunger state, they are making a mistake by projecting their current state onto points in the future when their current state is no longer relevant. An important case of projection bias occurs when a person's state of being is affected by visceral factors, such as emotions (e.g., fear, anger), drive states (e.g., hunger, sexual desire), and feeling states (e.g., pain). Loewenstein (2005) refers to these visceral factors as affectively "hot" states, as opposed to affectively "cold" states when a person is not affectively aroused.

Loewenstein describes two general forms of projection bias involving visceral factors. When visceral factors grip our minds, we fail to appreciate the extent to which the affective state influences our preferences and behavior. This leads to a *hot-to-cold empathy gap*, in which we underestimate how our preferences will change once we exit the temporary hot state. Put differently, we overestimate how stable our preferences are when in a hot state. We saw this in the Read and van Leeuwen article; hungry workers had trouble divorcing their current hunger from their snack choice for a future state of satiety. We may also suffer from a *cold-to-hot empathy gap*. In our more sober moments, we do not predict the extent to which our decision making will be distorted in an affectively hot state. For example, on a full stomach, we may recognize that hunger would push us toward choosing an unhealthy snack, but we underestimate the degree to which this force will drive us.

Many important health decisions occur once we have entered a hot state. The undue influence that visceral factors exert on our decision-making process often leads to errors. In the next section we sample from the evidence on projection bias and health.

Addiction

Addiction is one of the most important arenas in which projection bias comes into play. Addicts in a state of craving may underestimate how good they would feel if unaddicted. Addicts may exaggerate how long the pain of quitting will last. Moreover, nonaddicts may not fully appreciate the motivational force of addiction, contributing to initial decisions to experiment with drugs. All of these forces could contribute to the development of harmful addictions.

Several studies provide evidence on the projection bias of addicts. Giordano et al. (2002) and Badger et al. (2007) assessed the time preferences of longtime heroin addicts who were receiving a less potent substitute, buprenorphine, to reduce cravings for heroin and alleviate opioid withdrawal symptoms. The addicts typically received a single maintenance dose per day. The researchers offered the addicts a choice between different amounts of money and a second dose of buprenorphine, which is still pleasurable, to be delivered after the initial dose. Some would receive the dose that day and others in 5 days. The key experimental manipulation was that half of the subjects were asked when "deprived," 2 hours before receiving their initial daily dose, and half were asked when "sated," right after receiving their initial daily dose. The authors found that, for doses to be delivered that day, subjects were willing to pay an average of $75 when currently deprived and $50 when currently sated. For those asked about a second dose to be delivered in 5 days, the authors found a similar pattern; deprived subjects were willing to pay $60 for the second dose and sated subjects were willing to pay $35. Note that all subjects were to receive the second dose when in the same craving state, that is, right after the initial dose. Thus, these findings reveal that even experienced addicts did not fully appreciate how much their preferences for drugs would change after the cravings subside.

Levy (2010) studied projection bias in cigarette smokers. He finds that younger smokers do not fully appreciate their likelihood of becoming addicted in the future, underestimating by 40% the degree to which their preferences for being addicted will change once addicted.

Good Habits

It is also the case that we may not realize the extent to which we would enjoy developing good habits. For example, we may underappreciate how much we would enjoy including more vegetables in our diet. Acland and Levy (2015) test whether a group of college students predict how much they would enjoy developing a habit for attending the gym. The authors paid non–gym attenders assigned to the treatment group to attend the gym at least twice a week for a month, thereby developing a "gym habit." The authors elicited predictions from subjects about their future gym attendance in order to compare the treatment group's valuation of going to the gym before and after developing the habit, relative to that of the control group. The authors found that subjects displayed near-total myopia—that is, projection bias—regarding the enjoyment they received from going to the gym after forming the habit. This suggests that researchers might place more emphasis on interventions that develop good habits, as they can help individuals to realize benefits that they otherwise would ignore.

Overconfidence

Individuals consistently overestimate their ability to perform tasks. A corollary to this statement is that individuals often see themselves as being less at risk of harm compared with other people. Psychologists have termed this phenomenon *optimism bias*.

The origins of overconfidence include a combination of cognitive and motivational processes (Armor & Taylor, 1998). Cognitively, individuals rely on scenarios for how the future will unfold. These scenarios tend to be overly simplistic, to assume that individuals will engage in all actions necessary to obtain the outcome under consideration, and to neglect potential impediments such as situational factors and the actions of others. In comparing one's abilities to others, the person also may draw on reference groups that are not actually representative. Motivationally, individuals may maintain overly optimistic beliefs as part of a self-serving tendency in social comparisons. Affective states may also alter the degree of overconfidence a person holds.

Individuals display an unrealistic optimism about their susceptibility to a wide variety of health problems. Comparing individuals' objective health risk to their average perceived risk, individuals consistently report having a below-average perceived risk. This holds for the risk of lung cancer, tooth decay, ulcers, and a variety of other health risks (Weinstein, 1980, 1987). The result is that individuals may take more risks with their health than they realize and more than they would if better informed about the objective risk of a health behavior.

An important question is whether individuals accurately perceive their likelihood of becoming addicted to an addictive substance. The question bears on whether policy makers ought to educate the public or regulate addictive substances. The largest body of work in this area has focused on whether individuals accurately realize the addictive nature of tobacco use. While smokers seem to understand the health risks of smoking in general and in some cases may even overestimate those risks (Viscusi, 1992), that understanding does not necessarily translate into how smokers view their personal risk. Research shows that smokers underestimate their own personal risk relative to the risk of other smokers and nonsmokers (Slovic, 2001). In addition, smokers may perceive little or no risk from smoking individual cigarettes, even if they recognize the cumulative risks as high. Overconfident individuals, who underestimate their likelihood of becoming addicted, are likely to consume more cigarettes than they ever intended to consume.

In the section "Sophistication Versus Naiveté," we discussed overconfidence about an ability to show self-control. Individuals who are not fully aware of their self-control problems—that is, (partially) naïvely present-biased individuals—will overestimate the amount of self-control they will exert in the future. As discussed, naïveté can perpetuate a self-control problem over a long period of time and substantially harm the present-biased person.

Overconfidence would not be of great concern if it could be easily eliminated through education or some other means. However, the available research indicates that it is surprisingly difficult to "debias" a person who is overconfident (Weinstein & Klein, 1995). More research is needed on the ways that researchers and policy makers might temper overconfident beliefs. One approach may lie in learning from situations in which individuals do not display overconfidence, such as for events that are perceived to be uncontrollable (Harris, 1996).

Limited Attention and Memory

Description

Individuals have a limited ability to attend to and process stimuli in their environment. Moreover, individuals lack the cognitive bandwidth to integrate all available information as part of some utility-maximizing procedure, as assumed by the standard model. Herbert Simon (1957) was one of the first to note these constraints, referring to them as the human capacity for *bounded rationality*. Subsequently, psychologists such as Kahneman, Slovic, and Tversky (1982) have catalogued some of the heuristics, or cognitive shortcuts, that individuals use to arrive at decisions when constrained by bounded rationality. We focus in this section on attention and memory as limited resources, as they are especially germane to intertemporal choices for health. Underweighting or wholly neglecting relevant information compromises our ability to make decisions in our own best interest. However, we acknowledge that other forms of nonstandard decision making, such as a reliance on heuristics and a dependence on how choices are framed (e.g., as gains versus losses), are critical elements of decision theory more generally, not only for intertemporal choice.

When we make plans for the future, such as a weight-loss plan, a critical prerequisite for success is that we remember the plan when the moment of truth arrives. In our busy lives, we might not remember the plan if we are buried under a pile of work or tending to a family crisis. Thus, memory poses one set of challenges. Even if we manage to remember the plan, we might not have an ability to attend to it amid multitasking or dealing with more pressing issues. It is important to recognize that attentional deficits are not always "irrational," especially if the acquisition of information needed to inform a decision is costly. We may want to lose weight, but it would require a heroic effort to make sense of the conflicting information in the popular media and scientific literature about the best way to lose weight. As such, we may be better off attending to other aspects of our diet, such as how often we should eat or in what quantity. The combination of memory and attentional failures is able to compromise even the best-laid plans.

A close cousin of attention is salience, the degree to which certain features of a choice or choice environment rise to the top of a person's mind. Some features appear more visible, or more salient, to a consumer, while other features appear more opaque. Assume that we have settled on a plan to lose weight by limiting the amount of refined sugars in our diet. The nutritional content in our food is not always obvious. Nutritional labels on packaged foods have not traditionally made it easy to discern nutritional content, and prepared foods make it even harder to monitor our dietary intake. The nutritional value of our food is often less salient than other features, such as the colors on the package or the brand name. (See Chapter 6 by Riis and Ratner for further discussion of salient front-of-package nutritional labeling.)

In some cases, attributes of choices are shrouded from consumers. For example, the cost of visiting a clinic or a hospital in the United States is hidden from patients, meaning that patients do not typically take these costs into account when deciding where to seek care. Shrouding is often a deliberate profit-seeking strategy on the part of the companies that supply the good. In our example, the administrators of clinics and hospitals are able to charge higher prices to patients and health insurers if uninformed patients cannot direct their business toward more affordable facilities. In other cases, a person may overlook items when making plans. We have already noted that multitasking and bounded rationality hinder our ability to absorb relevant information. The end result is that limited attention and memory often prevent us from making health decisions that promote our well-being.

Applications

Researchers have studied limited attention and salience across a variety of health situations. In this section, we describe several areas of study.

Prices and Taxes of Health Products

Chetty, Looney, and Kroft (2009) study whether consumers are attentive to the prices of beer. The authors use the fact that state sales taxes are not factored into the posted prices of goods but only assessed at the cash register, whereas excise taxes are included in posted prices. Thus, an excise tax may be considered more salient to the consumer than is a sales tax. The authors analyze cross-state differences in beer taxes and find that consumers are far more responsive to alcohol-specific excise taxes than to sales taxes. The authors rule out that customers are uninformed about the sales taxes. They run a survey of grocery shoppers indicating that they are informed about the sales tax. Rather, salience effects led consumers to underreact to taxes that are not included in posted prices. The broader lesson is that the salience of taxes and of incentives more generally may have a large impact on their effectiveness.

Reminders

Models of inattention make a key prediction about the responsiveness of individuals to reminders. Reminders can be used to draw attention to the future consequences of choices. Due in part to their simplicity, reminders have been an active area of investigation. The advancement of digital technology has made reminder systems increasingly easy to implement. It is now simple and inexpensive to send reminders to groups of people, and many individuals have access to phone and computer applications that can set reminders.

A natural application of reminders is to improve medication adherence. Vervloet et al. (2012) review the evidence on electronic reminders that are automatically sent to patients. Delivery mechanisms have included text message reminders and electronic reminder devices that alert users with lights or sounds. Most studies document short-run improvements in adherence, although the long-term impact of electronic reminders is not well established.

Several studies find that text message reminders are effective for promoting smoking abstinence (Free et al., 2011; Rodgers et al., 2005). This approach is easily transferrable to other attempts at behavior modification, including dieting and physical activity. Moreover, reminders could be effective for regularly scheduled activities, such as primary care visits, Pap smears, and colonoscopies.

Checklists

A growing movement of medical professionals has advocated for the use of checklists as a quality improvement intervention in medical settings

(Haynes et al., 2009). Medical diagnoses and procedures routinely involve complicated and extensive lists of activities. In settings where clinicians are overwhelmed and systems of coordination are often inadequate, it is easy for mistakes to creep in. A simple checklist can be the difference between clinicians adhering to a protocol and committing gross negligence.

Planning Prompts

One way to encourage individuals to follow through on a plan is to prompt them for details about how they intend to implement the plan. By prodding people to think through specific aspects of a task, it can reduce forgetfulness and prevent procrastination. Creating a plan forms an association between the future moment and the plan to be implemented. When the moment arrives, it cues the person to follow through on the plan.

Milkman et al. (2011, 2013) have found that simple planning prompts modestly increase preventive screening rates. Sending a planning prompt to get a flu shot by mail increased the share who received a flu shot by 4 percentage points above the 33% of control group members who got the shot, that is, a 13% increase in relative terms. Similarly, a mailing that reminded people to get a colonoscopy increased the percentage of those who got the test by 1 percentage point above the 6% in the control group who got the test, that is, a 16% relative increase. Like text message reminders, these are low-cost interventions that could easily be expanded population-wide.

Implications for Policy and Behavior

The Role of Policy

Under the standard model, there are two economic rationales for policy intervention into health-related behavior. First, policy makers may wish to correct a market imperfection that impedes the ability of individuals to fulfill their own preferences. Second, policy makers may wish to correct for costs that individuals impose on others, so-called negative externalities. Behavioral economic models suggest that there is also an important role for policy makers to address "internalities" that individuals impose on themselves from making suboptimal choices. Several researchers have promoted policy making that nudges individuals toward better choices without mandating change. This idea has been referred to as asymmetric paternalism or libertarian paternalism (Camerer, Issacharoff, Loewenstein, O'Donoghue, & Rabin, 2003; Thaler & Sunstein, 2003).

Many public health efforts involve the provision of information and education to individuals. Where imperfect information is a major contributor to poor decisions, these interventions may be effective at changing behavior. However, in instances where cognitive biases are responsible for unhealthy behavior, educational campaigns are not likely to achieve large gains. More robust behavioral interventions would be needed.

More generally, policy makers need to recognize the limits of human rationality. To take one example, US lawmakers have taken a hard stance on drug use, including banning needle-exchange programs in many states on the grounds that they send the wrong message to the public about the acceptability of drug use. A heroin addict who is due for a hit but lacks a clean needle is unlikely to think deeply about the consequences of injecting himself with a dirty needle. In the throes of a craving, he will feel an overpowering bias for the present and an inability to think beyond his preferences at that moment, not to mention potentially being overconfident about the likelihood of infection and being inattentive to where to access public health resources. Under these circumstances, the addict will often choose the dirty needle if a convenient alternative is not at hand. For any number of similar policies, there is a strong behavioral case for government action.

In the following subsections, we delve into some specific implications of behavioral economics for policy and behavior.

Commitment Devices

A major contribution of behavioral economics to public health research has been the clearer direction it has provided about how to ameliorate self-control problems. Behavioral economists have highlighted the potential of self-management techniques, known as precommitments or commitment devices, in which individuals make it more costly for themselves to choose tempting options in the future.

Commitment devices have made their way outside of the ivory tower of academia. A number of Web sites, such as http://www.StickK.com and http://www.healthywage.com, have sprung up offering willing customers the opportunity to bet on whether or not they can follow through on a health goal of the person's choice. The customers put their own money at risk, to be forfeited if they fail. To further raise the stakes, StickK.com even offers customers the option of donating forfeited money to an "anti-charity" of the person's choice, such as the National Rifle Association for a customer who believes in gun control. Some governments have also taken notice of these approaches. The UK government established an agency called the Behavioural Insights Team to investigate behavioral economic applications, and one of its efforts has involved testing the scale-up of commitment devices in a drug store chain in the United Kingdom.

One way to classify commitment devices is as "soft commitments" or "hard commitments." The former are nonbinding agreements to follow through on a goal, whereas the latter are binding agreements that typically carry a prespecified penalty. We probe the difference between these two categories next.

Soft Commitments

Soft commitments are promises that a person makes to oneself, or occasionally to others. As such, they tend to be self-enforcing contracts that a present self makes with his or her future self. An example might be a New Year's resolution where a person promises today to take some action tomorrow. Such personal rules may be helpful by boosting motivation and making certain types of behavior particularly salient. The challenge is that soft commitments can be difficult to enforce. In addition, the penalties, such as disappointment with oneself, may not be concrete enough to dissuade someone from breaking a personal rule.

Soft commitments may take different forms. They may involve attempts to avoid environmental cues that trigger temptation. Recovering alcoholics may avoid social events where alcohol is served, or dieters may avoid walking down the candy aisle of the grocery store. Soft commitments may also be personal rules that guide a set of behaviors, such as resolutions to smoke only after meals or to work out twice a week. Bénabou and Tirole (2004) argue that we create personal rules because we fear creating behavioral precedents that our future selves will follow. In the famous "marshmallow experiment," researchers showed that 4-year-olds who could delay immediate gratification in exchange for a larger reward—forgoing one marshmallow now in exchange for two later—experienced improved educational and social outcomes later in life (Mischel, Shoda, & Rodriguez, 1989). It is possible that these children had set a behavioral precedent for self-control that they followed throughout their lives.

To deter ourselves from allowing too many exceptions to a personal rule, we sometimes define "bright lines." Recovering alcoholics are often advised to avoid even a sip of alcohol. Dieters may avoid even a morsel of a forbidden food. Defining the boundaries of a rule may be useful for self-enforcement. A danger is that bright-line rules will cause a person to forgo large benefits, such as a dieter who gives up a turkey feast on Thanksgiving. More generally, personal rules sometimes lead us to overregulate our behavior, occasionally turning a rule into an obsession or compulsion. Some people are able to carve out exceptions where it is acceptable to deviate from the rule, putting a diet on hold for Thanksgiving, without self-signaling that a lack of willpower is acceptable.

Behavioral economists have focused most of their attention on hard commitments, although there has been some work on soft commitments. Khwaja, Silverman, and Sloan (2007) surveyed US smokers and found that 81% had used a soft commitment device to limit tobacco consumption. Strategies included keeping busy by doing yardwork, banning smoking at home or at work, and avoiding other smokers. Some smokers also report "self-rationing," purchasing cigarettes in smaller quantities, such as by the pack rather than by the carton, in order to avoid consuming more than they prefer (Wertenbroch, 1998). Self-rationing may also occur for food choices, as in the case of consumers who only buy junk food in small quantities, knowing that it will limit the amount consumed during binges. Smokers may view tobacco control laws as a form of commitment device to limit tobacco consumption. Gruber and Mullainathan (2005) find that the passage of higher cigarette excise taxes increased the overall happiness of smokers, as would be predicted from a model of self-control problems but not from the standard model.

Hard Commitments

These are binding commitments in which a predefined penalty for failing to reach a goal is enforced. Often called commitment contracts, these agreements typically put a person's own money at stake, which is contingent on meeting a health goal. Some permutations, called deposit contracts, ask people to deposit money on a regular basis as part of the monetary commitment. The money is typically forfeited if the person cannot reach the health goal. Other permutations earmark money for certain expense items, such as health emergencies, and the money cannot be withdrawn for other purposes. Though less tested, some contracts put a person's reputation at stake, as in the case of a public declaration to accomplish a task.

Hard commitments have been tested for a variety of health behaviors, including weight loss, smoking cessation, exercise, health savings, and use of antimalarial bednets. Overall, the contracts have been effective at promoting behavior change across these domains. Weight loss is the one area where the results have not been consistently positive. The literature on commitment contracts is reviewed in greater detail in Chapter 8 of this volume by Lewis and Block. We briefly discuss several important features of these contracts here.

Commitment contracts have been promoted and criticized on a number of grounds. A major argument in their favor is their potential cost-effectiveness. Relative to clinical approaches, commitment contracts do not have the same reliance on skilled personnel and often use less expensive inputs. Commitment contracts may even generate net revenue, thanks to the forfeited deposits from users who fail to achieve their goal.

An outstanding question in the literature is the magnitude of demand for commitment contracts. Take-up rates of commitment products have varied greatly across setting and application, though they have tended to be modest. Some survey data suggest that most individuals have unfavorable views toward the use of commitment contracts for health behavior change (Promberger, Brown, Ashcroft, & Marteau, 2011). More research is needed to understand whether the approach is scalable and acceptable to the general public.

Commitment contracts are designed to be a "libertarian paternalistic" solution, leaving individuals without present bias unharmed, providing needed help to sophisticated present-biased agents, and leaving fully naïvely present-biased individuals unharmed but also unhelped. In practice, partial naïfs may fail to put enough money at stake to motivate themselves—undercommitting—because they underestimate their self-control problem. As a result, these individuals may end up worse off than without the opportunity to commit, as at least they would have kept their money. For example, Giné, Karlan, and Zinman (2010) find that 66% of smokers who took up a deposit contract for smoking cessation failed to quit smoking. White, Dow, and Ruangrunghiranya (2013) supplemented a deposit contract with incentives and more than half of smokers still failed to quit. Researchers have yet to find a way around the issue of undercommitment.

A final issue is the inflexibility of hard commitments, which are binding by design. This comes at a cost to users. For example, if a person has a commitment savings account for health emergencies, what happens if a non–health emergency arises? Should the person be allowed to withdraw money from the account? It is as yet unclear if complete inflexibility is necessary for the success of health commitment contracts or whether a softer commitment might be just as effective.

Structure of Incentives and Programs

Next, we move to general principles that can diminish the negative impacts of cognitive biases. We believe that researchers and policy makers should attempt to incorporate these principles into programs and policies.

Self-control failures are caused by the temptation to capture immediate rewards and avoid immediate costs. One of the best ways for external incentives to compete with a tempting option is to make them available when the tempting option presents itself. A reward for weight loss will be more effective if offered at a weekly weigh-in than if offered at the end of a yearlong program. Moreover, the tendency to sharply discount any and all future consequences means that smaller immediate rewards can be at least as effective, if not more so, than larger rewards delivered in the future. Thornton (2008) shows that even the smallest rewards can substantially increase the willingness of individuals to learn their HIV status.

Public health practitioners often seek to change behavior over the long term. Rather than providing one big payoff at the end, a well-designed program should provide incremental incentives along the way. Doing so can increase the salience of the incentives and help stave off procrastination. O'Donoghue and Rabin (1999b) argue that optimal incentives for procrastinators typically involve increasing the incentives as time passes. This is precisely the approach taken by behavioral researchers, who offered subjects an escalating reward schedule that paid drug users for abstinence in increasing amounts over time (Higgins et al., 1991; Higgins, Wong, Badger, Haug Ogden, & Dantona, 2000). The approach has been successfully applied to several types of drugs.

The timing of incentives is only one factor of note. Another is the salience of incentives. In order for incentives to motivate, the potential recipients first need to recognize that the incentives are available. The more salient they are, the more likely they will change behavior. Some employers offer wellness programs that include rewards for completing certain activities, like a health risk assessment, or reaching certain goals, like blood pressure below some cutoff. These companies often provide the rewards as a discount on the person's health insurance premium, which only appears on the worker's paystub. A much more salient approach would be to hand cash directly to workers at the time it is earned.

Public health programs of all sorts can maximize their impact by harnessing the power of default options. In "Field Evidence of Self-Control Problems," we discussed the susceptibility of individuals to default options because the time and effort involved in making a choice can lead to procrastination. Default effects are accentuated by failures of attention and memory. We may not remember that we need to update our annual choice of health insurance plan or refill our psychiatric medications. This leads to a bias toward the status quo. Setting smart defaults can dramatically improve the behavior of distracted or present-biased individuals.

Optimal defaults should be set to encourage good health, as in the case of home delivery of chronic medications. Optimal defaults may involve requiring people to make an active choice, rather than simply falling back on the default option. Active choice ensures that the person's underlying preferences are respected and also has the virtue of ensuring that the default options are socially acceptable. Otherwise, the public health community faces the risk of backlash from pushing its priorities on an unwilling general public. In cases where one option is socially beneficial, such as organ donation, active-choice systems may be enhanced by framing the decision to highlight the benefits of the socially preferred option. For example, instead of asking, "Would you like to donate your organs?," we might ask, "Would you like to donate your organs in order to save lives?" (Keller, Harlam, Loewenstein, & Volpp, 2011). Default systems should set deadlines to ensure that individuals select a choice in a timely manner. Optimal defaults should typically avoid complex enrollment rules and procedures, restrictions on choices, and barriers to switching. The designer should aim to make it as easy as possible for individuals to implement their preferred choices.

Sin Taxes

Taxation has been the preferred policy instrument of economists for regulating the consumption of risky health products, such as tobacco and alcohol. The empirical literature has borne out the effectiveness of this approach. Countless studies have shown that individuals respond to the prices of risky health goods (e.g., IARC, 2011). Economists have traditionally argued that sin taxes are appropriate for recouping the external costs that consumers impose on society, that is, the negative externalities. To the extent that consumers impose costs on themselves or their family, economists have traditionally argued that consumers already take those costs into account when choosing to consume the risky product, even if the product is addictive or harmful. According to this view, the government has no role in regulating products that do not produce externalities on net, aside from educating consumers about health risks and restricting the access of minors.[4]

Behavioral economists have enriched the traditional view of sin taxation. They have argued that sin taxes should also incorporate the costs from internalities, such as present bias. Cognitive biases prevent afflicted individuals from following through on their plans, and taxes may be able to help individuals to implement their long-run preferences.

Gruber and Köszegi (2001) apply the β-δ model to estimate the optimal level of tobacco taxes, including the cost of sophisticated present bias to smokers. Assuming a modest degree of present bias of $\beta = 0.9$, the authors calculate an optimal cigarette tax of $1 to $3 per pack to account for internalities from present bias. This estimate only includes the cost of premature death to the smoker. It does not include the costs of secondhand smoke, the long-run costs of low birth weight from mothers who smoke, smoking-related fires, the disutility to the smoker from smoking-related illness, and many other costs. Moreover, this estimate does not apply to naïvely present-biased smokers, for whom the optimal tax would likely be much higher.

Levy (2010) builds on the work of Gruber and Köszegi to calculate the optimal tax on smokers using an empirical estimate of present bias and adding the effect of projection bias to smokers. He estimates that the optimal tax rate would be $8 to $11 per pack, an order of magnitude larger than the current US federal tax rate of roughly $1 per pack. Behavioral economists have only begun to apply these insights to other health goods.

A common concern of sin taxes is that they have the potential to be regressive, disproportionately harming low-income individuals. The potential regressivity of sin taxes becomes more complicated once behavioral factors are considered. Gruber and Köszegi (2004) find that tobacco taxes are substantially less regressive after factoring in that lower income smokers are more sensitive to cigarette prices than are higher income smokers. Cigarette taxes become less regressive as the degree of present bias increases in the population. That is because the self-control benefits of tobacco taxation are largest for the lowest income groups such that on net they are better off after the taxation.

Differential Impact on Vulnerable Populations

While cognitive biases affect all of us, there are good reasons to believe that certain vulnerable populations may be particularly affected. We focus on two vulnerable groups: low-income individuals, and adolescents and young adults. Identifying the groups at greatest risk is important for targeting interventions and, in the case of low-income individuals, for reducing health and economic disparities.

Low-Income Individuals

Low-income individuals may be hit hardest by cognitive biases. Avoiding mental mistakes requires time, effort, knowledge, and, at times, financial resources, all of which are on average more scarce among the poor. The poor face a staggering number of cognitive demands: finding and maintaining work, securing food, and navigating a complex, and frequently hostile, economic environment. With all of these competing demands, low-income individuals often have the least amount of cognitive bandwidth left over to allocate to intertemporal health choices. By virtue of their poverty, these individuals are also least likely to have access to decision aids that might keep cognitive biases in check.

There has been growing interest in the social determinants of cognitive biases. Several studies have established that cognitive performance decreases when a person is mentally taxed (Mani, Mullainathan, Shafir, & Zhao, 2013; Mullainathan & Shafir, 2013; Spears, 2011). The issue is not that the poor make bad choices because they are innately less capable, but rather that anyone who finds himself in a state of cognitive scarcity is prone to making mistakes. Poor people just tend to face severe mental strain on a more routine basis than the rest of us. A challenge for the field of behavioral economics is to develop interventions tailored to low-resource individuals and communities.

Adolescents and Young Adults

Researchers should also take special note of the effect of cognitive biases on adolescents and young adults. Neuroscientists have found that the development of the brain's limbic system continues throughout young adulthood, leading adolescents and young adults to have reduced cognitive control and increased sensitivity to rewards. This may account in part for the greater adoption of risky health behaviors in adolescence and young adulthood.

Many habits form early in life when individuals are least able to counter the pull of cognitive biases. For example, drug addicts typically first start to use in adolescence or young adulthood. These stages of life present critical time periods in which behavioral scientists might be able to intervene to influence the long-term trajectories of people's health. For example, Matthew Rabin (2013) has proposed that researchers experiment with age-based taxation, in which young people face higher tax rates on cigarettes or alcohol than the old.

Conclusion

Economists have traditionally relied on observed choices and behaviors to infer individuals' innate preferences for health and other aspects of their lives. Economists have gone so far as to refer to choices as "revealed preferences." In this chapter, we characterized ways that our intertemporal choices and our preferred plans can diverge. Cognitive errors undermine our plans and lead us to make suboptimal choices about our health.

We focused on a handful of cognitive challenges: self-control problems, misprediction of future preferences, overconfidence, and limited attention and memory. Behavioral researchers have constructed a large body of work exploring each of these concepts. As the field of behavioral economics has grown, interest has spread to new topics of intertemporal choice, and the list of behavioral economic concepts will continue to grow in the coming years. Researchers have only begun to realize the potential of these existing and emerging insights for promoting health.

Notes

1. Paul Samuelson (1937) recognized the restrictiveness of a constant discount function when he introduced discounted utility, although exponential discounting nevertheless became standard economic practice.
2. This property is called a "constant marginal rate of substitution."
3. Other factors contributing to default effects include a lack of an understanding of the choice situation, a perception that the default is an endorsement of a certain choice, the complexity of the choice leading to delay, and inattention to nondefault options.
4. By "on net," we mean that the external costs outweigh the external benefits of the good. Indeed, at current levels of excise taxes in the United States, analyses suggest that smokers are already subsidizing the healthcare costs of nonsmokers, if restricting the analysis to only account for externalities.

References

Acland, D., & Levy, M. R. (2015). Naiveté, projection bias, and habit formation in gym attendance. *Management Science*, *61*(1), 146–160.

Ainslie, G. (1992). *Picoeconomics: The strategic interaction of successive motivational states within the person.* New York, NY: Cambridge University Press.

Albrecht, K., Volz, G., Sutter, M., Laibson, D., & von Cramon, D. (2011). What is for me is not for you: Brain correlates of intertemporal choice for self and other. *Social Cognitive and Affective Neuroscience, 6*(2), 218–225.

Ariely, D., & Wertenbroch, K. (2002). Procrastination, deadlines, and performance: Self-control by precommitment. *Psychological Science, 13*, 219–224.

Armor, D. A., & Taylor, S. E. (1998). Situated optimism: Specific outcome expectancies and self-regulation. *Advances in Experimental Social Psychology, 30*, 309–379.

Badger, G. J., Bickel, W. K., Giordano, L. A., Jacobs, E. A., Loewenstein, G., & Marsch, L. (2007). Altered states: The impact of immediate craving on the valuation of current and future opioids. *Journal of Health Economics, 26*(5), 865–876.

Becker, G. S., Grossman, M., & Murphy, K. M. (1994). An empirical analysis of cigarette addiction. *American Economic Review, 84*(3), 396–418.

Becker, G. S., & Murphy, K. M. (1988). A theory of rational addiction. *Journal of Political Economy, 96*(4), 675–700.

Bénabou, R., & Tirole, J. (2004). Willpower and personal rules. *Journal of Political Economy, 112*(4), 848–886.

Bernheim, B. D., & Rangel, A. (2004). Addiction and cue-triggered decision processes. *American Economic Review, 94*(5), 1558–1590.

Bryan, G., Karlan, D., & Nelson, S. (2010). Commitment devices. *Annual Review of Economics, 2*(1), 671–698.

Camerer, C., Issacharoff, S., Loewenstein, G., O'Donoghue, T., & Rabin, M. (2003). Regulation for conservatives: Behavioral economics and the case for "Asymmetric Paternalism." *University of Pennsylvania Law Review, 151*(3), 1211–1254.

Chabris, C. F., Laibson, D. I., & Schuldt, J. P. (2008). Intertemporal choice. In S. N. Durlauf & L. E. Blume (Eds.), *The New Palgrave dictionary of economics* (2nd ed.). New York, NY: Palgrave Macmillan.

Chapman, G. B., Li, M., Colby, H., & Yoon, H. (2010). Opting in vs. opting out of influenza vaccination. *JAMA, 304*(1), 43–44.

Chetty, R., Looney, A., & Kroft, K. (2009). Salience and taxation: Theory and evidence. *American Economic Review, 99*(4), 1145–1177.

DellaVigna, S. (2009). Psychology and economics. *Journal of Economic Literature, 47*(2), 315–372.

DellaVigna, S., & Malmendier, U. (2006). Paying not to go to the gym. *American Economic Review, 96*(3), 694–719.

Duflo, E., Kremer, M., & Robinson, J. (2011). Nudging farmers to use fertilizer: Theory and experimental evidence from Kenya. *American Economic Review, 101*(6), 2350–2390.

Epstein, S. (1994). Integration of the cognitive and the psychodynamic unconscious. *American Psychologist, 49*(8), 709–724.

Frederick, S, Loewenstein, G., & O'Donoghue, T. (2002). Time discounting and time preference: A critical review. *Journal of Economic Literature, 40*(2), 351–401.

Free, C., Knight, R., Robertson, S., Whittaker, R., Edwards, P., Zhou, W., . . . Roberts, I. (2011). Smoking cessation support delivered via mobile phone text messaging (txt-2stop): A single-blind, randomised trial. *Lancet, 378*, 49–55.

Fong, G. T., Hammond, D., Laux, F. L., Zanna, M. P., Cummings, K. M., Borland, R., & Ross, H. (2004). The near-universal experience of regret among smokers in four countries: Findings from the International Tobacco Control Policy Evaluation Survey. *Nicotine and Tobacco Research, 6*(Suppl. 3), S341–S351.

Fudenberg, D., & Levine, D. K. (2006). A dual-self model of impulse control. *American Economic Review, 96*(5), 1449–1476.

Giné, X., Karlan, D., & Zinman, J. (2010). Put your money where your butt is: A commitment contract for smoking cessation. *American Economic Journal: Applied Economics, 2*(4), 213–235.

Giordano, L. A., Bickel, W. K., Loewenstein, G., Jacobs, E. A., Marsch, L., & Badger, G. J. (2002). Mild opioid deprivation increases the degree that opioid-dependent outpatients discount delayed heroin and money. *Psychopharmacology, 163*, 174–182.

Gruber, J., & Köszegi, B. (2001). Is addiction rational? Theory and evidence. *Quarterly Journal of Economics, 116*(4), 1261–1303.

Gruber, J., & Köszegi, B. (2004). Tax incidence when individuals are time-inconsistent: The case of cigarette excise taxes. *Journal of Public Economics, 88*, 1959–1987.

Gruber, J., & Mullainathan, S. (2005). Do cigarette taxes make smokers happier? *BE Journal of Economic Analysis and Policy, 5*(1).

Gul F., & Pesendorfer W. (2001). Temptation and self-control. *Econometrica, 69*(6), 1403–1435.

Halpern, S. D., Loewenstein, G., Volpp, K. G., Cooney, E., Vranas, K., Quill C. M., ... Bryce, C. (2013). Default options In advance directives influence how patients set goals for end-of-life care. *Health Affairs, 32*(2), 408–417.

Halpern, S. D., Ubel, P. A., & Asch, D. A. (2007). Harnessing the power of default options to improve health care. *New England Journal of Medicine, 357*(13), 1340–1344.

Harris, P. (1996). Sufficient grounds for optimism? The relationship between perceived controllability and optimistic bias. *Journal of Social and Clinical Psychology, 15*, 9–52.

Hastings, J., & Washington, E. (2010). The first of the month effect: Consumer behavior and store responses. *American Economic Journal: Economic Policy, 2*(2), 142–162.

Haynes, A. B., Weiser, T. G., Berry, W. R., Lipsitz, S. R., Breizat, A. H., Dellinger, E. P., ... Gawande, A. A. (2009). A surgical safety checklist to reduce morbidity and mortality in a global population. *New England Journal of Medicine, 360*, 491–499.

Higgins, S. T., Delaney, D. D., Budney, A. J., Bickel, W. K., Hughes, J. R., Foerg, F., & Fenwick, J. W. (1991). A behavioral approach to achieving initial cocaine abstinence. *American Journal of Psychiatry, 148*(9), 1218–1224.

Higgins, S. T., Wong, C. J., Badger, G. J., Haug Ogden, D. E., & Dantona, R. L. (2000). Contingent reinforcement increases cocaine abstinence during outpatient treatment and 1 year of follow-up. *Journal of Consulting and Clinical Psychology, 68*(1), 64–72.

International Agency for Research on Cancer (IARC). (2011). Effectiveness of tax and price policies for tobacco control. Chapter 5; 137–200.

Johnson, E. J., & Goldstein, D. (2003). Do defaults save lives? *Science, 302*(5649), 1338–1339.

Kahneman, D. (2011). *Thinking, fast and slow*. New York, NY: Farrar, Straus, and Giroux.

Kahneman, D., & Tversky, A. (2000). *Choices, values, and frames*. New York, NY: Cambridge University Press.

Kahneman, D., Slovic, P., & Tversky, A. (Eds.). (1982). *Judgment under uncertainty: Heuristics and biases.* Cambridge, UK: Cambridge University Press.

Keller, P. A., Harlam, B., Loewenstein, G., & Volpp, K. G. (2011). Enhanced active choice: A new method to motivate behavior change. *Journal of Consumer Psychology, 21*(4), 376–383.

Khwaja, A., Silverman, D., & Sloan, F. (2007). Time preference, time discounting, and smoking decisions. *Journal of Health Economics, 26*, 927–949.

Kirby, K. N., Petry, N. M., & Bickel, W. K. (1999) Heroin addicts discount delayed rewards at higher rates than non-drug using controls. *Journal of Experimental Psychology: General, 128*, 78–87.

Klabunde, C. N., Brown, M., Ballard-Barbash, R., White, M. C., Thompson, T., Plescia, M., & King, S. C. (2012). Cancer screening—United States, 2010. *Morbidity and Mortality Weekly Report, 61*(3), 41–45.

Laibson, D. (1997). Golden eggs and hyperbolic discounting. *Quarterly Journal of Economics, 112*, 443–477.

Levy, M. R. (2010). *An empirical analysis of biases in cigarette addiction.* Working paper, University of California at Berkeley.

Loewenstein, G. (2005). Hot-cold empathy gaps and medical decision making, *Health Psychology, 24*(4 Suppl.), S49–S56.

Loewenstein, G., & O'Donoghue, T., & Rabin, M. (2003). Projection bias in predicting future utility. *Quarterly Journal of Economics, 118*(4), 1209–1248.

Loewenstein, G., & Prelec, D. (1992). Anomalies in intertemporal choice: Evidence and an interpretation. *Quarterly Journal of Economics, 107*, 573–597.

Malarcher, A., Dube, S., Shaw, L., Babb, S., & Kaufmann, R. (2011). Quitting smoking among adults—United States, 2001–2010. *Morbidity and Mortality Weekly Report, 60*(44), 1513–1519.

Mani, A., Mullainathan, S., Shafir, E., & Zhao, J. (2013). Poverty impedes cognitive function. *Science, 341*, 976–980.

McClure, S. M., Laibson, D. I., Loewenstein, G., & Cohen, J. D. (2004). Separate neural systems value immediate and delayed monetary rewards. *Science, 306*(5695), 503–507.

McLellan, A., Lewis, D. C., O'Brien, C. P., & Kleber, H. D. (2000). Drug dependence, a chronic medical illness: Implications for treatment, insurance, and outcomes evaluation. *Journal of the American Medical Association, 184*(13), 1689–1695.

Metcalfe, J., & Mischel, W. (1999). A hot/cool-system analysis of delay of gratification: Dynamics of willpower. *Psychological Review, 106*(1), 3–19.

Milkman, K. L., Beshears, J., Choi, J. J., Laibson, D., & Madrian, B. C., (2011). Using implementation intentions prompts to enhance influenza vaccination rates. *Proceedings of the National Academy of Sciences USA, 108*, 10415–10420.

Milkman, K. L., Beshears, J., Choi, J. J., Laibson, D., & Madrian, B. C., (2013). Planning prompts as a means of increasing preventive screening rates. *Preventive Medicine, 56*, 92–93.

Mischel, W., Shoda, Y., & Rodriguez, M. L. (1989). Delay of gratification in children. *Science, 244*, 933–938.

Montoy, J. C., Dow, W. H., & Kaplan, B. (2014). *Active-choice and opt-out HIV screening: A randomized controlled trial.* Working paper, University of California at Berkeley.

Mullainathan, S., & Shafir, E. (2013). *Scarcity: Why having too little means so much.* New York, NY: Times Books.

O'Donoghue, T., & Rabin, M. (1999a). Doing it now or later. *American Economic Review, 89*(1), 103–124.

O'Donoghue, T., & Rabin, M. (1999b). Incentives for procrastinators. *Quarterly Journal of Economics, 114*(3), 769–816.

O'Donoghue, T., & Rabin, M. (2001). Choice and procrastination. *Quarterly Journal of Economics, 116*, 121–160.

Orphanides, A., & Zervos, D. (1995). Rational addiction with learning and regret. *Journal of Political Economy, 103*(4), 739–758.

Osterberg, L., & Blaschke, T. (2005). Adherence to medication. *New England Journal of Medicine, 353*(5), 487–497.

Phelps, E. S., & Pollak, R. A. (1968). On second-best national saving and game-equilibrium growth. *The Review of Economic Studies, 35*(2), 185–199.

Promberger, M., Brown, R. C. H., Ashcroft, R. E., & Marteau, T. M. (2011). Acceptability of financial incentives to improve health outcomes in UK and US samples. *Journal of Medical Ethics, 37*(11), 682–687.

Rabin, M. (2013). Healthy habits: Some thoughts on the role of public policy in healthful eating and exercise under limited rationality. In A. Oliver (Ed.), *Behavioural public policy* (pp. 115–139). New York, NY: Cambridge University Press.

Read, D., & van Leeuwen, B. (1998). Predicting hunger: The effects of appetite and delay on choice. *Organizational Behavior and Human Decision Processes, 76*(2), 189–205.

Rodgers A., Corbett T., Bramley D., Riddell, T., Wills, M., Lin R., & Jones, M. (2005). Do u smoke after txt? Results of a randomised trial of smoking cessation using mobile phone text messaging. *Tobacco Control, 14*, 255–261.

Samuelson, P. (1937). A note on measurement of utility. *Review of Economic Studies, 4*, 155–161.

Schelling, T. C. (1980). The intimate contest for self-command. *Public Interest, 60*, 94–118.

Seligman, H. K., Bolger, A. F., Guzman, D., López, A., & Bibbins-Domingo, K. (2014). Exhaustion of food budgets at month's end and hospital admissions for hypoglycemia. *Health Affairs, 33*(1), 116–123.

Sellito, M., Ciaramelli, E., & di Pellegrino, G. (2011). The neurobiology of intertemporal choice: Insight from imaging and lesion studies. *Review of Neuroscience, 22*(5), 565–574.

Shapiro, J. M. (2005). Is there a daily discount rate? Evidence from the food stamp nutrition cycle. *Journal of Public Economics, 89*, 303–325.

Shiffrin, R., & Schneider, W. (1977). Controlled and automatic human information processing. *Psychological Review, 84*(2), 127–190.

Shiv, B., Loewenstein, G., Bechara, A., Damasio, H., & Damasio, A. (2005). Investment behavior and the negative side of emotion. *Pyschological Science, 16*(6), 435–439.

Simon, H. A. (1957). *Models of man, social and rational: Mathematical essays on rational human behavior in a social setting.* New York, NY: John Wiley & Sons.

Sloman, S. A. (1996). The empirical case for two systems of reasoning. *Psychological Bulletin, 119*(1), 3–22.

Slovic, P. (Ed.) (2001). *Smoking: Risk, perception, and policy*. Thousand Oaks, CA: Sage.

Smith, A. (1981). *The theory of moral sentiments* (D. D. Raphael & A. L. Macfie, Eds.) Indianapolis, IN: Liberty Fund. (original work published 1759)

Spears, D. (2011). Economic decision-making in poverty depletes behavioral control. *BE Journal of Economic Analysis and Policy, 11*(1), Article 72.

Strotz, R. H. (1956). Myopia and inconsistency in dynamic utility maximization. *Review of Economic Studies, 23*, 165–180.

Sunstein, C. R., & Thaler, R. H. (2008). *Nudge: Improving decisions about health, wealth, and happiness*. New Haven, CT: Yale University Press.

Thaler, R. H., & Shefrin, H. M. (1981). An economic theory of self-control. *Journal of Political Economy, 89*, 392–406.

Thaler, R. H., & Sunstein, C. R. (2003). Libertarian paternalism. *American Economic Review Papers & Proceedings, 93*(2), 175–179.

Thornton, R. L. (2008). The demand for, and impact of, learning HIV status. *American Economic Review, 98*(5), 1829–1863.

Vervloet, M., Linn, A. J., van Weert, J. C. M., de Bakker, D. H., Bouvy, M. L., & van Dijk, L. (2012). The effectiveness of interventions using electronic reminders to improve adherence to chronic medication: A systematic review of the literature. *Journal of the American Medical Informatics Association, 19*, 696–704.

Viscusi, W. K. (1992). *Smoking: Making the risky decision*. New York, NY: Oxford University Press.

Weinstein, N. D. (1980). Unrealistic optimism about future life events. *Journal of Personality and Social Psychology, 39*(5), 806–820.

Weinstein, N. D. (1987). Unrealistic optimism about susceptibility to health problems: Conclusions from a community-wide sample. *Journal of Behavioral Medicine, 10*(5), 481–500.

Weinstein, N. D., & Klein, W. M. (1995). Resistance of personal risk perceptions to debiasing interventions. *Health Psychology, 14*(2), 132–140.

Wertenbroch, K. (1998). Consumption self-control via purchase quantity rationing of virtue and vice. *Marketing Science, 17*, 317–37.

White, J. S., Dow, W. H., & Rungruanghiranya, S. (2013). Commitment contracts and team incentives: A randomized controlled trial for smoking cessation in Thailand. *American Journal of Preventive Medicine, 45*(5), 533–542.

Wilde, P. E., & Ranney, C. K. (2000). The monthly food stamp cycle: Shopping frequency and food intake decisions in an endogenous switching regression framework. *American Journal of Agricultural Economics, 82*(1), 200–213.

Zhou, X., Nonnemaker, J., Sherrill, B., Gilsenan, A. W., Coste, F., & West, R. (2009). Attempts to quit smoking and relapse: Factors associated with success or failure from the ATTEMPT cohort study. *Addictive Behaviors, 34*, 365–373.

3 | Maintenance of Healthy Behaviors

FORMING AND CHANGING HABITS

DENNIS RÜNGER AND WENDY WOOD

ONCOMMUNICABLE DISEASES (NCDS) ARE THE primary cause of death and disability around the world. There are four main types of NCDs: cardiovascular diseases such as stroke and heart attack, cancers, chronic lung diseases (e.g., asthma, emphysema), and diabetes. The World Health Organization (WHO, 2014) estimates that in 2008, NCDs accounted for 63% of the 57 million global deaths. Men in the WHO European region, for example, are about 13 times more likely to die from NCDs than from communicable diseases. These statistics are sobering, yet there is also room for optimism because most of these deaths are, in fact, preventable. Four lifestyle habits, in particular, put people at risk of developing NCDs: insufficient physical activity, overindulgence in alcohol, tobacco use, and an unhealthful diet (Leventhal, Weinman, Leventhal, & Phillips, 2008). Altering these health-damaging behaviors is a cornerstone to improving the health of the general population.

As we explain in this chapter, changing the habitual behaviors that contribute to NCDs presents particular challenges for intervention science. Given the slow progression of lifestyle-related diseases, short spurts of healthful behaviors, such as going to the gym for a week, are unlikely to have much benefit. Instead, protection against the risks of NCDs comes primarily from the repetition of healthful lifestyle behaviors over time. This is the challenge for behavior change interventions: to make the changes stick. A new, healthy behavior maintains when people continue to perform it, despite occasional relapses, at least a few months beyond the end of an intervention treatment (Fjeldsoe, Neuhaus, Winkler, & Eakin, 2011).

In general, classic behavior change interventions designed to impart information, promote effective goal setting, and heighten self-efficacy have a poor track record of creating enduring change (Artinian et al., 2010; Marteau, Hollands, & Fletcher, 2012). In the short term, such interventions can yield impressive immediate behavior change. After the intervention has ended, however, the new behavior is often performed sporadically or perhaps not at all, as people increasingly revert back to earlier unhealthful habits (Brown et al., 2009; Neve, Morgan, Jones, & Collins, 2010). Behavioral *nudge* interventions that change the structure of available health choices hold greater promise of enduring change within specific decision contexts (Hollands et al., 2013; Johnson et al., 2012). These interventions promote healthy choices by altering the ways that decision tasks are structured and the ways that options are presented in a particular setting. Yet there is little evidence that the effects of such interventions generalize to contexts outside of a given decision architecture.

The present chapter offers a novel approach to maintaining lifestyle interventions by incorporating insights from dual-process models in psychology. These models stipulate that human behavior is controlled by a combination of psychological processes that are, on the one hand, effortful, conscious, and controlled and, on the other hand, effortless, nonconscious, and automatic (Sherman, Gawronski, & Trope, 2014). These dual processes are sometimes referred to in a global way as two separate systems, *System 1* and *System 2* (Kahneman, 2011). As we explain, many classic interventions fail because they do not adequately address the automatic components of everyday behavior in general, and the role of habits in particular. These automatic behavioral responses can promote relapse back into unhealthful lifestyles, despite people's best intentions. Yet habits are not just obstacles to health. They also can be harnessed to promote more healthful behaviors that persist over time. In short, a key objective for health interventions should be to impart new, health-promoting habits that replace existing, health-damaging ones.

In this chapter, we first provide an overview of the psychology of habits, especially how they are triggered automatically by recurring features of the environment. Then we consider the conditions under which habits develop and the implications for habit formation interventions. From a habit perspective, automaticity in performance is key to maintenance of new behaviors given the many demands on people in daily life that limit more thoughtful decision making. A closer look at the brain mechanisms underlying habits and goal-directed actions provides insights into how habit and decision making interact to guide action. Finally, we suggest three types of behavioral intervention that can lead to habit change, including controlling unwanted behaviors, disrupting cues, and activating alternative, healthier actions. The conclusion to the chapter discusses why people are largely unaware of habits in their own behavior.

Habits in Daily Life

William James, a founding figure of American psychology, opined that "all our life, so far as it has definite form, is but a mass of habits" (James, 1921, p. 64). James's intuition about the prevalence of habits accords with results from diary studies of day-to-day living (Wood, Quinn, & Kashy, 2002). In this research, participants were prompted hourly to record what they were doing, thinking, and feeling. About 40% of the behaviors recorded across several days were performed almost daily and usually in the same location. Participants paid little attention to these behaviors and were usually thinking about something other than what they were doing, suggesting they were performed automatically. It seems, then, that much of everyday behavior is structured around automatic, habitual repetition.

Features of Habitual Behavior

A habit is a response pattern that occurs consistently in a particular context. Someone might, for example, pick up a pastry every morning on her way to work or light a cigarette whenever she leaves her office building. To acquire a habit, a behavior needs to be performed repeatedly under recurring circumstances, so that cognitive associations are formed in memory between context cues and the behavior. These associations increase in strength with every repetition of the behavior. Eventually, perceiving the cues alone is sufficient to trigger the associated response. At this point in the learning process, then, a habit has been established. As we will explain, habits are a type of automatic behavior that is activated directly by the context and that does not require a preceding goal or intention to act (Gardner, 2014; Wood & Neal, 2007).

Habits Are Context-Cued Responses

A variety of context cues can trigger habits, ranging from simple elements of the external environment (e.g., physical locations, other people) to internal states such as feelings or sensations. Complex combinations of multiple cues allow for habits with very specific triggering conditions. Consequently, habit responses can be finely attuned to situational features. The sight of a traffic light turning red, for example, triggers a braking response that differs depending on your vehicle. If you are driving a car, you step on the brake pedal, but if you are riding a bicycle, you squeeze the brake levers on your handlebar. A principal goal of psychological research on habit performance is to understand the memory processes that give rise to habit responses. Such knowledge is indispensable for designing interventions that effectively disrupt undesirable habits and establish new, health-promoting habits (van't Riet, Sijtsema, Dagevos, & De Bruijn, 2011).

To understand the cuing processes behind everyday habits, Neal, Wood, Labrecque, and Lally (2012) tested whether perception of context cues could in fact bring to mind the behaviors typically performed in those contexts. Participants included runners with strong habits who ran regularly in the same location and runners with weak habits who ran only sporadically, along with some nonrunners. To test the cognitions that underlie running habits, participants were first asked where they typically ran (or, for nonrunners, where they would run if they ever did). This information was then used in the experimental task. The locations participants mentioned were presented so quickly that they were difficult, if not impossible, to recognize consciously. Then, following each location word was a string of letters. Sometimes the letters formed the target words "running" and "jogging." If the location brought thoughts of running to mind, participants should be very fast to see the target word after being exposed (outside of consciousness) to the place where they typically ran. This in fact happened for runners with strong habits but not for those with weaker habits.

Presumably, seeing one's running shoes or a running partner would have had the same effect for participants whose running habit was triggered by these cues. This study shows that habitual behaviors can become mentally linked with the contexts in which they are typically performed.

In a second study, Neal et al. (2012) evaluated whether people unthinkingly carry out the activated habit. They reasoned that fans who frequently go to sports stadiums have acquired a habit of speaking loudly when there. Like health habits, this response should be activated automatically just by being exposed to the triggering cues. Some participants were shown pictures of the stadiums they visited regularly. The pictures served as backgrounds in a visual search task in which participants had to say aloud the name of items when they found them in the pictures. Indicating the impact of habits on overt behaviors, participants with stronger habits to attend sports stadiums spoke more loudly when naming the items after seeing stadiums than participants with weaker habits.

Many everyday habits consist of a series of actions and involve the manipulation of various objects. Making coffee and making tea are two prototypical examples. Such routine sequential actions can be understood as recurrent perception-action loops (Botvinick & Plaut, 2004): Perceiving certain cues in the environment (e.g., an empty tea cup) triggers an associated action (putting a tea bag into the cup). The action changes the environment, which provides a new set of cues (cup with tea bag in it). These cues, in conjunction with a memory of the previously completed action, elicit the next action in the sequence (pouring hot water).

Botvinick and Plaut (2004) implemented these principles in an artificial neural network that they trained to make coffee and tea. The network comprised three layers of simple processing units. The units of the input layer represent perceived objects. Activation propagates through connections from the input layer to an internal or hidden layer and from there to the output layer. The output layer contains units that correspond to actions for manipulating objects. The hidden layer is equipped with recurrent connections that feed back information about the state of the layer at the previous processing step. Training the network entails teaching it to choose the correct action given the currently perceived state of the environment. Botvinick and Plaut (2004) showed that this network architecture is sufficient to learn the sequential tasks of making coffee and tea.

In summary, context cues directly activate mental representations of habitual responses and influence overt behavior. These cues consist of the current environment and prior actions in a sequence, which together can activate complex sequential habits. Importantly, participants in Neal et al.'s (2012) studies did not intend to be thinking about running or speaking loudly, but thoughts of these actions arose when they perceived the relevant context. Similarly, once Botvinick and Plaut's (2004) artificial neural network had learned to associate objects with the appropriate responses, then the environmental triggers initiated routinized sequential actions. This is a central insight for health interventions—habits are activated in memory and often performed without people intending to do so.

Many everyday health behaviors are likely triggered without intention. In illustration, shortly after a smoking ban was introduced in public places in England, 42% of smokers who regularly visited pubs acknowledged unintentionally starting to light up while there (Orbell & Verplanken, 2010). Although smokers presumably did not want to be fined for smoking illegally, their old habits were still activated by being in a pub. Participants who had a stronger habit of smoking while drinking (assessed before the smoking ban came into effect) were especially likely to produce these accidental *action slips*. In the next section of the chapter, we elaborate on this point, that habits may be performed even when people do not intend to do so.

Habits Do Not Depend on Goals

Some habits are good for us in the sense that they help us to meet important long-term goals, and other habits are bad in the sense that they impede goal pursuit. The psychology behind habit performance is the same for both good and bad habits (Neal, Wood, & Drolet, 2013). That is, the response is cued by associated contexts regardless of whether or not people want to perform it and value the outcomes produced.

People are probably more aware of their own bad habits than good ones. Good habits are essentially transparent to personal introspection. For example, most of us have a habit to brush our teeth before going to bed, which allows us to do so without much thought or effort. You may not even be aware of this habit until you travel to a new location and have to think about brushing (e.g., locating toothbrush, toothpaste, sink). When the habit is not available, you might find yourself deciding, "I'll skip brushing tonight because it's just too much trouble." In contrast to the transparency of good habits, bad habits come into focus because of their serious, deleterious effects that can impede health goals. It makes sense that psychological research has focused primarily on bad habits, and that each of us is probably most aware of the unwanted habits that we are struggling to change.

The idea that habits are not dependent on goals and response outcomes counters most people's understanding of their behavior. We think of behavior as mostly purposeful and goal directed. If a person wakes up with a bothersome sore throat, for example, he or she might make hot tea and then drive to a pharmacy to buy lozenges. If a goal-directed action is successful (the sore throat soothed), it is likely to be repeated. A negative outcome (the throat pain became even worse) decreases the likelihood that the action will be chosen again. By contrast, fully developed habits are largely controlled by antecedent stimuli, which means that they are cued by recurring features of the context (e.g., running locations, sports stadiums, being in a familiar pub), and the consequences of habitual behaviors become relatively unimportant (Dezfouli & Balleine, 2012; Dickinson, Nicholas, & Adams, 1983). This is another way of saying that people perform habits even when they do not intend to do so.

To show that habits are driven by context cues and not by goal outcomes, research has manipulated the value of outcomes for a response. Sensitivity to outcome value has been explored most systematically in research with nonhuman animals. Hungry rats, for example, were trained to press a lever for a drop of sucrose solution (Dezfouli & Balleine, 2012). Some rats received a moderate amount of training, while others were trained extensively and formed habits to press the lever. Subsequently, some rats were allowed to consume as much sucrose as they wanted to, which decreases their desire for the food reward. If the rats were pressing to get the reward, then they should stop when sated. And the moderately trained rats did just this. When sated, they reduced their lever pressing. In contrast, the rats with habits to press the lever continued just as often as their former hungry selves. Their lever-pressing habit was triggered by the sight of the lever, rather than by the goal to obtain a food reward.

In a similar experiment with humans, participants received potato chips as a reward for repeatedly pressing a button when they saw one image, and candy for pressing a different button when shown another image (Tricomi, Balleine, & O'Doherty, 2009). Some participants were trained only for a few minutes, whereas others were trained extensively over 3 days until they had formed a button-pressing habit. Then, to make chips or candy less desirable, participants overate one of these rewards, until it was no longer pleasant. When tested at the task again, moderately trained participants pressed the button less often to the image that was associated with the food that they had overeaten. Participants with habits, however, kept pressing the buttons to both images, regardless of whether they had tired of the associated food reward. Thus, the habitual button-pressing response was dissociated from its consequences.

Everyday health habits also seem to be repeated in a context-cued manner that is insensitive to how much people value the outcome of the behaviors. This was demonstrated most clearly in a field experiment in which moviegoers consumed popcorn while watching trailers in a movie theater (Neal, Wood, Wu, & Kurlander, 2011). Unbeknownst to the patrons, the popcorn was either freshly made or stale, being about a week old. When participants were later asked how much they liked the popcorn, they were clear—the stale, spongy popcorn was rated at the bottom of the scale. The interesting question in this study was whether this preference influenced eating. The answer was yes, but only for participants who typically did not eat popcorn when in the cinema and so were not driven by habits. They ate what they liked, and those given a bag of fresh popcorn ate more than those given stale popcorn. By contrast, moviegoers with strong popcorn-eating habits ate the same amount of popcorn in both conditions, regardless of how palatable it was. Although they said the stale popcorn was awful, they acted on their habit to eat it anyway.

The outcome insensitivity of habitual behaviors explains, in part, why unhealthy habits tend to persist even when they have a negative impact on well-being. That is, the habit is triggered by context cues independently of current goals and intentions. It follows that interventions that merely change health-related goals and convince people, for example, to eat more healthfully or to exercise more, do not impact the mechanisms that generate habitual responses. Therefore, as long as cues in the performance context remain the same, unwanted habits continue to be triggered, often despite our best intentions.

How Habits Are Formed

As we described, the basic process of habit formation, that is, repeating a behavior frequently in a stable context, enables people to learn associations between context cues and the behavior. Eventually, perceiving those features is sufficient to bring the associated response to mind. Given the nature of habit formation, people are more likely to develop some types of health habits than others. Specifically, habits are more likely to form for activities that people perform often in stable contexts, such as exercising and drinking milk, but are less likely for activities they perform infrequently or under varying conditions, such as getting mammograms or flu shots (Ouellette & Wood, 1998; Webb & Sheeran, 2006). In this section of the chapter, we take a closer look at the conditions under which habits are most likely to develop.

Forming Habits Through Unintentional Processes

In many instances, habits are acquired unintentionally, simply as a result of experiencing covariations between actions and contexts in daily life. If someone often eats ice cream on the sofa while watching TV but rarely otherwise, then they are likely to learn associations between that context and indulging in sweets. These covariations arise as people pursue goals in daily life. Typically, a goal can be achieved through various means, that is, different actions can be taken that lead to the same outcome—a principle called *equifinality*. If we want to improve our physical fitness, for example, we can lift weights at the gym, train for a marathon, or ride a bike to work. In many instances, however, the behavioral options to satisfy a goal are somewhat limited. When getting breakfast before work, it is difficult to eat at home unless we plan ahead, purchase breakfast items, and bring them home. More convenient might be stopping at a fast-food restaurant on the drive to work. Given time and other constraints on the choices available to us, we are likely to repeat the same course of action to meet daily goals.

The breakfast example illustrates that on many occasions, habit formation itself is not an intentional learning process. Unless we are trying to learn a new perceptual-motor skill such as playing tennis or driving a car with a manual transmission, we rarely intentionally memorize or rehearse an action or action sequence. Rather, we select a course of action because we want to achieve a goal, and we choose the same actions again under the same circumstances because they were successful in the past and because alternative actions may not be available. In this case, linking context cues and responses in memory is an incidental by-product of goal-directed action.

Research in cognitive psychology has shown that people can learn complex sequential action patterns without intending to do so. Typically, a task is used that contains a hidden regularity that participants do not know about, such as pressing the same sequence of response buttons over and over. With practice, speed and accuracy of responses increase, indicating that participants have learned about the sequential regularity. However, they often find it difficult, if not impossible, to describe the pattern verbally (Frensch & Rünger, 2003; Rünger & Frensch, 2010). That is, although their behavior demonstrates sequence knowledge, participants cannot describe what they are doing—a phenomenon you might recognize if you have tried to describe to a child how to tie shoelaces. You can easily show the child how, but the description is difficult. Especially for well-learned, habitual behaviors, we are often unaware of the cues that trigger performance. This poses a challenge for health interventions because, as we discuss next, an important aspect of altering health-damaging habits is to identify and control or change the environmental triggers of unwanted behaviors.

Finally, habits can also be acquired unintentionally through observing and imitating social models. Chartrand and Bargh (1999) coined the term *chameleon effect* for the unconscious tendency to imitate facial expressions, body posture, and mannerisms during social interactions. The term was inspired by the Woody Allen movie *Zelig* in which Allen plays a character who involuntarily adopts the physical characteristics, mannerisms, and values of the people around him. Importantly, like any other response, a mimicked behavior can become habitual if it is repeated frequently in a stable context, so that the behavior becomes associated with features of the context.

Few studies have investigated social learning with respect to health-related behaviors. In two observational studies of stair/escalator choices at airports, stair use was about twice as high when another person was already on the stairs and thus served as a natural model compared with when the stairs were empty (Adams, Hovell, Irvin, & Sallis, 2006; Webb, Eves, & Smith, 2011). To the best of our knowledge, no study has investigated mimicry in the context of habit formation. We speculate that many health-related habits depend on this type of social learning. For example, it is estimated that only 19% of the world population washes their hands with soap after contact with stool, even though hand washing is an effective means for reducing the spread of diarrhea and other illnesses (Freeman et al., 2014). More likely than not, hand-washing habits, in particular the frequency of hand washing, are influenced by observing and mimicking others.

In summary, people often form habits unintentionally as they go about pursuing goals in daily life. When habits are acquired in this way, people are likely unaware of the specific sequences involved in habit performance and the factors that cue a particular habitual response. This lack of awareness poses particular challenges for health interventions designed to change habits. When people are not aware of the factors that activate a habit, they may not be successful at controlling or changing these cues.

Interventions to Form Healthy Habits

As we explained when introducing this chapter, many behavior change interventions have focused on the short term and have not addressed the psychological processes by which people maintain new healthful behaviors over time (Marteau et al., 2012). Yet a new wave of interventions is being developed in recent years that emphasizes the formation of healthful habits. In essence, these programs encourage the repetition of healthy actions sufficiently often in stable contexts so that habits can form. They build on Lally, Van Jaarsveld, Potts, and Wardle's (2010) foundational research in which participants chose a healthful behavior to perform daily in a recurring context (e.g., taking a walk right after breakfast). Overall, behaviors became more automatic with practice, although participants differed markedly in the number of days it took until they felt that the behavior had become second nature and that they performed it without thinking.

The importance of stable contexts for habit formation was demonstrated in an intervention to promote use of dental floss (Judah, Gardner, & Aunger, 2013). After learning the benefits of flossing, participants formed plans to floss immediately before brushing their teeth or they planned to floss immediately after brushing—so as to use an existing behavior, brushing, to cue the new behavior, flossing. Then participants reported each day on their floss use. Everyone increased flossing during the 28-day study, regardless of the type of plan. However, participants who used tooth brushing to cue flossing were significantly more likely to continue flossing up to 8 months after the study had ended. The benefits of using other routines to cue health behaviors has also been noted in medication adherence. For example, a common aid to remember to take birth-control pills is tying them to some routine event such as waking up (Stawarz, Cox, & Blandford, 2014). In general, these studies show that habit formation depends on stable contexts. Recurring context cues, including prior behaviors in a sequence, become associated with the habit response in mind and automatically activate its performance.

A number of innovative interventions build on these components of habit formation by instantiating repetition of actions in stable contexts. In illustration, McGowan et al.'s (2013) healthy eating program for parents of young children emphasized consistency, routine, and situational prompts for serving fruits and vegetables, healthy snacks, and healthy drinks. At the end of the 8-week study, parents in the intervention group reported that all three feeding behaviors had become more automatic. Furthermore, to the extent that these behaviors had become automatic for parents, their children ate more fruits and vegetables, healthy snacks, and drank more water. Also illustrating a habit formation approach, *Transforming Your Life* (TYL) is a weight-loss program aimed at establishing and strengthening healthy habits and disrupting unhealthy ones (Carels et al., 2011). An important component of the program is creating a food and exercise environment that increases healthy eating and physical activity and encourages automatic responding to health cues. In two different trials that compared long-term weight loss between the 3-month TYL program and other weight-loss programs, the habit-based program yielded comparable or better maintenance during the 6-month no-treatment follow-up period (Carels et al., 2011, 2014).

Incentives for Habit Formation

Given that rewards influence the frequency with which people perform goal-directed behaviors, they are important for habit formation. Much public policy is based on the idea that people can be discouraged to act by financial penalties, such as taxes on alcohol and cigarettes, and encouraged to act by financial incentives, such as government subsidies for healthy foods (An, 2012). Yet rewards also may have unintended effects on people's judgments, such as reducing personal motivation to act in healthful ways once the rewards are removed (Gneezy, Meier, & Rey-Biel, 2011; Marteau, Ashcroft, & Oliver, 2009).

Reward programs designed to increase performance of a behavior may also promote habit formation, primarily when the rewards are experienced in particular ways. For habits to form, responses need to become tied to features of performance contexts and not to the rewarding outcomes (Wood & Neal, 2009). If people continue to be motivated by salient rewards, then behavior will continue to be goal directed instead of being activated by context features.

In the terminology of learning theory, habits develop when the experienced instrumental contingency is low between a behavior and its rewarding outcomes—that is, the rewards are not highly salient motivators of performance (Dezfouli & Balleine, 2012; Dickinson et al., 1983). Specifically, habit formation is most likely when rewards are given on *interval schedules*, meaning that the reward is received only after a certain time has elapsed. With these schedules, changes in response rate during the time interval do not affect changes in the amount of reward delivered. Rewards low in experienced contingency promote initial performance and context–response learning such that, when habits have formed, the reward is not represented in the context-response associations in memory (Knowlton & Yin, 2006). In contrast, with *ratio schedules*, each response is followed by a reward with a certain probability. Consequently, more responses lead to more reward. This reinforcement schedule tends to produce goal-directed behavior: If the reward is omitted, then the behavior typically ceases.

Interventions that provide rewards on interval schedules thus should be most successful at generating long-term maintenance of healthy behaviors. Unfortunately, little research has tested this idea. Burns et al. (2012) reviewed the amount of weight lost in 27 health interventions that rewarded losses with material incentives following various reward schedules. In these studies, weight loss was generally short-lived regardless of reward schedule, and only a few interventions in the review tested long-term effects. Some suggestion of habit formation using an interval-type schedule was provided in Charness and Gneezy's (2009) study of gym attendance. College student participants who received $100 to go to the gym eight times during the month-long study showed a continued heightened attendance rate for 7 weeks following the intervention. Because the reward was for an overall attendance goal, it was not likely to be highly salient during any one trip to the gym. However, Acland

and Levy's (2013) replication revealed only modest long-term gains in gym attendance after the incentive ended. Thus, intervention research has yet to demonstrate the types of incentive programs that can best promote habit formation in everyday life.

In summary, lifestyle changes such as starting a daily exercise regime or switching from a meat-heavy to a vegetarian diet often begin with the intention to replace unwanted habits with new habits that are more conducive to health and well-being. However, habits also take root unintentionally, because repeating a behavior frequently in the same context is sufficient to form a habit. Interventions to form new habits emphasize these two central components: repeated action in recurring contexts. For such interventions, rewards might be given on interval schedules so that the reward can increase performance without being a highly salient motivator. With such reward schedules, people can learn context-response associations that cue the behavior automatically and promote behavior maintenance.

Automaticity Is Key to Behavior Maintenance

Following a successful behavioral intervention, participants likely are of two minds: Along with new intentions and high efficacy to adhere to healthy plans, they also may have old unhealthy habits. Short-term interventions can change people's beliefs and help them set goals, but they are less effective at changing unwanted habits. This point was made clearly by Webb and Sheeran's (2006) meta-analysis of 47 intervention studies that examined whether changes in intentions were translated into subsequent changes in behavior. The majority of interventions tried to change health behaviors (e.g., condom use, sun protection) by providing information, enhancing skills, and promoting goal setting. The results showed that changes in intention engendered changes in behavior except when the behavior was likely to be habitual in that it could be performed often in recurring contexts (e.g., seatbelt use). Changing intentions had only limited impact on these behaviors, presumably because people practiced them into habits, and these old habits continued to be cued by exposure to everyday performance contexts.

To understand why habits do not shift with shifts in goals and intentions, it is helpful to think about habit formation. Habits develop gradually as context-response associations are formed and strengthened over time. The slow, incremental nature of habit learning is functional because such learning is protected from being unduly distorted by short-term changes in behavior that can occur as people act in a nonhabitual, goal-directed manner. Unfortunately, this resistance to change is true not only for desirable habits but also for undesirable ones. Habitual behavior is supported by strong, stable mental representations, making forgetting or unlearning of habits difficult. In this regard, habits are like sensorimotor skills (e.g., riding a bicycle, playing tennis) that can be retained despite decades of nonuse. Even the largely effective *implementation intentions*, or if-then plans to act on intentions at particular times and places (Gollwitzer & Sheeran, 2006), are not very successful at controlling strong habits. For example, only adolescent smokers with weak smoking habits, but not those with strong habits, were able to use implementation intentions to avoid smoking in situations that typically triggered their smoking habit (Webb, Sheeran, & Luszczynska, 2009).

The upshot of the stability of habit memories is that people may have multiple, conflicting guides for how to act. They might consciously intend to lose weight or maintain a recent weight loss yet have old habits for overeating and constant snacking. When the multiple memory systems that guide action do not correspond, people's best intentions can get lost in the interplay between the slow-to-change habit system and their current desires and decisions. This section of the chapter explains why habits often predominate over goals and intentions in guiding action.

The trade-off between goal-directed and habitual action is not a simple dichotomy. Up until now, we have oversimplified these as separate modes of action involving strong habits or thoughtful decisions. However, any one action likely draws to varying extents on habits and other memory systems. Habit strength itself is a continuum that reflects the learned covariation between context cues and a response, with each experience incrementally adding to or detracting from the strength of a habit. Thus, it makes sense to think of actions not as habitual versus nonhabitual but as having different amounts of habit strength. In addition, unlike button-press tasks in psychological experiments, everyday behaviors are often complex, extend in time, and have multiple components. Going to the gym probably involves some decision making (e.g., lift weights today or go to spin class?) along with some habitual routines (e.g., getting dressed in gym clothes). Thus, some components of a single behavior might be thoughtful and others habitual.

Factors That Promote Habitual Behavior

Several factors influence whether people rely more on habits or on thoughtful decisions at any given moment in daily life. In general, when people are stressed, overwhelmed, and hurried, they are less motivated and less able to make deliberate decisions and therefore rely more on their old habits. This switch to habits might be adaptive because it reduces hesitation and delays in responding, along with saving cognitive resources to better cope with the demands of the situation (Schwabe & Wolf, 2013). We first discuss how habit strength, distraction, lowered willpower, and stress influence the interplay between decision making and more automatic responses, and then we consider the implications for designing health interventions that will have persisting impact over time.

Habit Strength

The stronger a habit becomes, the more likely it is to dominate behavior control to the exclusion of goals and intentions. This is the conclusion of several studies that evaluated whether habits or behavioral intentions are better predictors of future behavior. For example, Ji and Wood's (2007) participants initially reported on their intentions to buy fast food, watch news on TV, and take the bus during the next week. Then they reported once per day for the next 7 days whether they performed each behavior. The results showed that people with weak habits acted on their intentions, but not those with strong habits—they just kept repeating the habit regardless of what they had intended. Nearly identical results were reported for drinking milk, eating snack food, and riding bicycles (Danner, Aarts, & Vries, 2008; de Bruijn, Kremers, Singh, van den Putte, & van Mechelen, 2009). Thus, when habits are strong, people tend to repeat what they have done in the past even if they intend to do otherwise.

Absentmindedness and Distraction

Following the idea that habits predominate when people cannot easily deliberate, research on *action slips*, or unintended actions, suggests that people slip up mostly when they are distracted or not attending to what they are doing (Norman, 1981). William James (1890) relayed an anecdote from a friend who would go to his bedroom to dress for dinner, take off all of his clothes, and, when thinking about the day, might inadvertently get into bed because a bedtime routine was triggered by the bedroom, late hour, and undressing. In experience-sampling studies of everyday behaviors, such *habit intrusions* make up about 40% of all everyday action slips (Reason, 1992). Thus, when people are distracted or thinking about something other than what they are doing, they are likely to fall back on old habits.

Willpower

Although strong habits tend to prevail over intentions in the long run, people usually can inhibit an unwanted habit if they intend to do so and they monitor their behavior closely, but the act of inhibition is cognitively effortful and requires willpower. Unfortunately, our ability to exert this kind of self-control is limited. According to the strength model of self-control (Baumeister & Heatherton, 1996; Baumeister, Tice, & Muraven, 2000), volitional acts such as exerting self-control draw on a limited resource. Exerting the volition to act drains this resource and impairs subsequent efforts at self-control. The term *ego depletion* describes the state of the self when self-control resources are diminished. From this perspective, self-control is similar to a muscle that becomes fatigued with exertion and replenishes with rest.

When people are in a state of depletion, they may fall back on performing an unwanted habit because they are unable to override the response and to initiate an alternative action (Hagger, Wood, Stiff, & Chatzisarantis, 2010). In this way, lowered self-control can increase performance of unhealthy habits. For example, a study of social drinkers found that on days with more self-control demands, participants drank more, were more intoxicated, and were more likely to violate a self-imposed limit on alcohol consumption (Muraven, Collins, Shiffman, & Paty, 2005). Also, smokers who were asked to resist eating tempting sweets were more likely to smoke during a subsequent 10-minute break than smokers who were trying to refrain from eating a plate of vegetables (Shmueli & Prochaska, 2009). Finally, male social drinkers whose capacity for self-control was taxed by having to avoid thinking about a white bear subsequently consumed more alcohol during a taste test of Budweiser and Beck's beer (Muraven, Collins, & Neinhaus, 2002). Thus, when self-control is lowered by volitional acts, people tend to fall back into habits and other automatic action patterns.

Stress

The experience of stress also promotes habitual responding at the expense of goal-directed actions (Schwabe & Wolf, 2013). In an experimental demonstration, participants learned to choose cues that could yield food rewards, with one cue for chocolate milk and another for orange juice. After training at the task, participants filled themselves with one of the foods. Then, some participants placed their right hand into ice water for 3 minutes—a stressful, painful, and unpleasant experience. When participants were tested again, stressed participants responded habitually and chose the cue associated with the food they had just eaten, despite reporting that the overeaten food was now unpleasant. When not stressed, participants were able to avoid the food that was now undesirable, indicating that their responses were goal directed.

This pattern in which stress decreases decision making and increases reliance on habits is also evident with stress induced pharmacologically (i.e., by administering a synthetic glucocorticoid plus an adrenoreceptor antagonist; Schwabe, Tegenthoff, Höffken, & Wolf, 2012). Before the learning phase of the choice task, participants were administered the stressor or a placebo. When tested after overconsuming one of the food rewards, participants in the placebo group responded in goal-directed ways, choosing the cue associated with the desired (uneaten) reward. By contrast, the stressed participants continued to respond habitually, choosing the cue to the overeaten food as frequently as the cue to the valued food. Thus, physical stress, and presumably social stressors as well, reduce decision-making capabilities and orient people to respond habitually, even when they do not desire the habit outcome.

In this section, we reviewed a number of factors that influence whether goals and intentions or response habits emerge as the driving forces of behavior. As such, they also contribute to the success and failure of health interventions. Depending on how stressed or distracted a person is, he or she will be more or less able to override an unhealthful habit. For example, making new, healthier food choices in the grocery store is cognitively more effortful than sticking to a routine of heading straight to the frozen section to fetch a pizza. In this example, it would be advisable to shop for groceries on the weekend, rather than after a busy day at work in a state of ego depletion.

The Neural Basis of Goal-Directed and Habitual Action

We have described different factors that can bias people toward responding in a habitual or in a goal-directed manner. Ultimately, the goal is to understand the causal mechanisms that are responsible for such shifts in the control of behavior. Stress, for example, has been shown to promote habitual responding, but it could do so in at least two ways: by strengthening the habit response system or by impeding goal-directed responding. One way to disentangle the impact of different memory systems is to identify—and to manipulate directly—the brain processes that give rise to the observable behavior.

The transition from goal-directed action to habitual responding is attributed to learning-related shifts of neural activity in cortical brain areas and in the basal ganglia (Graybiel, 2008; Knowlton & Yin, 2006). The basal ganglia are a set of subcortical nuclei that contribute to movement, cognition, and emotion, and that play important roles in neurodegenerative disorders such as Parkinson's disease and Huntington's disease. They interact with the cortex in so-called cortico-basal ganglia loops (Alexander, DeLong, & Strick, 1986; Middleton & Strick, 2002). Animal research has shown that the shift from goal-directed to stimulus-driven, habitual responding is mediated primarily by two cortico-basal ganglia loops. The *associative loop* supports working memory functions and goal-directed actions. The *sensorimotor loop* is generally regarded as the neural substrate of automatic, habitual behaviors (Graybiel, 2008; Knowlton & Yin, 2006). Rats, for example, do not acquire a lever-pressing habit when the sensorimotor portion of the striatum, the input structure to the basal ganglia, is surgically lesioned prior to learning to press a lever for sucrose. Even after extended training, these rats responded to outcome devaluation by pressing the lever less frequently, indicating goal-directed responding (Yin, Knowlton, & Balleine, 2004).

Rats and humans rely more on habits when the neural circuits responsible for goal-directed action are disrupted. After a moderate amount of training in a lever-pressing task, rats avoided pressing a lever after the associated reward was devalued, indicating that their responses were goal directed. In contrast, when a specific region of the basal ganglia that participates in the *associative loop*, the posterior dorsomedial striatum, was inactivated pharmacologically, lever pressing was unaffected by reward value; the rats acted on their habits (Yin, Ostlund, Knowlton, & Balleine, 2005). In the stress study by Schwabe et al. (2012) that we mentioned earlier, neuroimaging data helped to explain why pharmacologically stressed participants responded habitually whereas unstressed, control participants did not: The stress manipulation selectively affected two brain areas in the network for goal-directed action, the orbitofrontal and medial prefrontal cortex, rendering participants insensitive to changes in outcome value.

Thus, when the neural mechanisms associated with goals were disrupted, participants fell back on their habits.

If different memory systems acquire a behavior in parallel and are vying for behavioral control, it may be necessary to coordinate their activity to ensure that the memory system that produces the behavior most reliably and effectively dominates (Hikosaka, Nakamura, & Sakai, 2002). Smith and Graybiel (2013a, 2013b) recently showed that the infralimbic cortex (IL) in rats has such a controlling influence over memory systems for habitual and goal-directed actions. Using optogenetics, they were able to switch on and off a maze-running habit. In their study, rats with genetically engineered IL neurons were trained to navigate a maze for reward until the behavior became habitual. By delivering light through the device that was used to record the activity of IL neurons, it was possible to reduce the activity of these cells. When the light was turned on, the acquired habit was blocked and the rats acted in a goal-directed manner (i.e., they avoided running into a maze arm with a devalued reward). Switching off the light would reinstate normal brain activity almost instantly, and the rats would resume their maze-running habit (i.e., run to valued and devalued rewards equally often).

Neuroscience research is constantly expanding our knowledge of the neurobiology of habits and goal-directed behavior. In the not-too-distant future, it may be possible to develop health interventions that target directly the brain mechanisms that give rise to a variety of health-harming behaviors. Today, neurosurgical interventions such as deep brain stimulation (DBS) are used to treat the most severe cases of neurological disorders that do not respond to conventional treatments. After the success of DBS in treating movement-related disorders such as Parkinson's disease, the neurosurgical intervention is now being investigated for severe, treatment-resistant cases of psychiatric disorders (Mayberg & Holtzheimer, 2011). With DBS it was possible, for example, to dramatically reduce the compulsive behavior and rituals of a patient who had been suffering from severe obsessive-compulsive disorder for more than 20 years (Nuttin, Cosyns, Demeulemeester, Gybels, & Meyerson, 1999). Although invasive interventions like DBS will most likely never be used to change lifestyle habits, it does not require much imagination to envision pharmacological interventions that, for example, attenuate the activity of habit-related neural circuits or strengthen the neural pathways for goal-directed action. At present, however, lifestyle changes are most likely accomplished with the help of behavioral interventions.

Behavioral Interventions to Change a Habit

The ability to form habits enables us to perform many recurring tasks efficiently, freeing up cognitive resources, for example, to plan ahead or to reflect on our own behavior. Unfortunately, because habits can be—and often are—acquired unintentionally, behaviors that are damaging to our health and well-being become routinized when they are repeated frequently in the same context. Moreover, goals can change over time, and people may no longer want to perform a habit that used to be consistent with their goals. In fact, many health interventions are designed to do just this—convince people to adopt new health goals and understand the importance of changing existing unhealthy patterns.

In this section, we review research on the psychology of habit change and describe the attributes of interventions likely to be successful at changing habits. Although people cannot easily forget habit memories or overwrite them with new goals and intentions, the influence of habits on behavior can be broken. First, we describe how people might exert self-control in order to block the mechanisms that trigger performance, including inhibiting the cued response and thinking of alternative responses. Second, we describe how habits can be broken when changes in the performance context remove the cues that trigger habitual responding (Verplanken & Wood, 2006). Finally, we describe interventions that increase the accessibility of the desired response when people are ready to act and in this way provide a ready alternative to the habit in mind.

Self-Control Strategies for Changing Habits

To bring into focus the characteristics of habits that render them resistant to change, it is helpful to distinguish between unwanted habits and temptations. A temptation is a desire that people try to resist because it conflicts with their goals (e.g., wanting to eat a piece of cake while on a weight-loss diet). In perhaps the most famous research in this area, Walter Mischel at Stanford University tested the ability of 3- to 6-year-old children to resist temptation and delay gratification (Metcalfe & Mischel, 1999). Some children were presented with a desirable food item (e.g., a marshmallow or a pretzel stick) and faced the following dilemma: After the experimenter left the room, the child could summon him with a bell to get the treat or wait until the experimenter returned and receive two of the same treat. On average, the children held out for less than 3 minutes before ringing the bell.

Only about 30% were able to resist the temptation until the experimenter returned after about 15 minutes.

Temptations arise from hot, emotional stimuli that activate visceral factors such as hunger, thirst, and sexual desire (Loewenstein, 1996). Habits, in contrast, are typically triggered by affectively neutral context cues. These two types of automatic responding thus may require very different types of self-control strategies. These different strategies were evident in experience sampling studies in which participants reported several times a day on how they tried to control unwanted responses (Quinn, Pascoe, Wood, & Neal, 2010). Approximately 12% of the unwanted behaviors they were trying to control were habits, given that they were frequently performed in the same location, and 38% were temptations, given that participants reported that they would derive immediate pleasure from the unwanted response. What were the most effective self-control strategies for inhibiting habits and resisting temptations?

Overall, participants reported only moderate success in controlling either type of unwanted response, but somewhat different strategies were effective with each. For strong temptations, the most effective approach was stimulus control, which involved removing the tempting stimulus or leaving the situation altogether. Illustrating this strategy, some of the children in Mischel's experiments spontaneously covered their eyes to resist the treat during the delay period, and when the treats were out of sight altogether, they waited the longest to bring back the experimenter (Metcalfe & Mischel, 1999). Habits, in contrast, are context-cued responses that may be acquired unintentionally, so that people are unaware of the effect of context cues on their behavior. Thus, they are not likely to be able to identify and control the stimulus. Instead, a strategy involving vigilant monitoring of the behavior to make sure it was not inadvertently cued proved to be most effective in daily life for controlling unwanted habits (Quinn et al., 2010). Through monitoring their responses, people could control their tendency to act habitually.

In summary, even with the most suitable self-control strategy, vigilant monitoring, people in daily life are likely to be only moderately successful in inhibiting unwanted habit responses. Moreover, it is uncertain whether behavior inhibition is sustainable over the long term. The limits of self-control become painfully apparent in relapse statistics for a wide range of addictive behaviors. For example, the majority of smokers who attempt to quit without treatment relapse within the first 8 days, and only 3%–5% are still abstinent after 6 months

(Hughes, Keely, & Naud, 2004). Research on thought suppression and behavioral inhibition has shown that these forms of self-regulation can yield paradoxical and counterproductive effects such as negative affect, postsuppression rebound of a target thought, preoccupied thinking about an inhibited response, and even an eventual increase in an unwanted behavior (Wenzlaff & Wegner, 2000). Thus, monitoring and inhibition are not likely to be effective intervention strategies but instead may represent short-term means of controlling habit performance.

Disrupting Contexts to Change Habits

Habits also can be broken by changing cues in the performance context. Context change is a powerful ally in changing habits because it frees people to establish new patterns of behavior in the absence of competing habit cues (Verplanken & Wood, 2006). People naturally experience changes in everyday performance contexts when, for example, they move to new locations, start new jobs, and join new groups of friends. According to the *habit discontinuity* hypothesis, when contexts change in this way, people no longer rely on habit cues to action, and they consider what to do in a more deliberative manner (Verplanken, Walker, Davis, & Jurasek, 2008).

In a test of habit discontinuity, college students transferring to a new university reported before and after the transfer on the habit strength of behaviors such as exercising and watching TV, along with their intentions to perform each behavior (Wood, Tam, & Witt, 2005). When the performance context for each behavior at the new university was similar to the old one (e.g., a gym in the apartment building), habitual behaviors persisted at the new university irrespective of what students intended to do. When contexts changed, however, students' behaviors came under intentional control, and they exercised and watched TV only to the extent that they intended to perform these actions. Also supporting habit discontinuity, a study of British driving habits found that participants who had recently moved residence (and thus disrupted driving cues) but not those who stayed put were guided by their environmental values to drive their cars less often (Verplanken et al., 2008).

In summary, the memory trace of a habit is difficult to unlearn, but its influence can be broken. Breaking habits becomes easier when contexts shift so that the old performance cues no longer activate the unwanted habitual response.

Interventions to Heighten the Cognitive Accessibility
of Healthy Behaviors

Another potential route for changing habits involves heightening the salience of a healthy response. With both the old habit as well as a healthy alternative in mind, people who are highly motivated to change might be able automatically to act in healthful ways.

Increasing the accessibility of the healthy option is the logic behind *implementation intentions* (Gollwitzer & Sheeran, 2006). These if-then action plans, much like habits, promote performance at particular times and in specific contexts. Research has shown that implementation intentions that link specific situations to desired responses (e.g., "When I feel the urge to eat candy, I will have a piece of fruit instead") are more effective in promoting healthy behaviors than more generic intentions (e.g., "I will eat more healthily;" Orbell & Sheeran, 2000; Sheeran & Orbell, 1999). Furthermore, such intentions might be useful in habit change. In one intervention, Adriaanse, Gollwitzer, de Ridder, de Wit, and Kroese (2011) had participants form an intention to perform a healthy behavior in the context that typically activated an unhealthy one (e.g., "While watching TV tonight, I will eat celery"). Tying implementation plans to habit cues in this way increased the ability to bring healthy behaviors to mind. The increased accessibility of the healthy action actually rivaled that of the unwanted habit. However, implementation intentions will not always be effective at altering habits. Unlike habit automaticity, these intentions depend on people's broader goals. For example, college students carried out their implementation intentions to study at particular places and times only if they wanted to study to get good grades (Sheeran, Webb, & Gollwitzer, 2005). Furthermore, as we pointed out earlier with respect to habitual smokers, implementation intentions are less useful at changing strong habits, perhaps because of the very high accessibility of such responses (Webb & Sheeran, 2006).

Another potential way to increase the cognitive accessibility of a healthy option is *point-of-choice prompts*. These interventions might involve signs or other reminders of specific healthful actions in a situation where people usually respond in unhealthy ways. This approach has been tested most frequently with interventions to promote stair climbing over elevator and escalator use in public settings. Several reviews of this research concluded that prompts to take the stairs have modest but consistent success, with the majority of studies reporting significant increases in stair climbing (e.g., Nocon, Müller-Riemenschneider, Nitzschke, &

Willich, 2010; Soler et al., 2010). Demonstrating how point-of-choice prompts can promote new responses that counter old habits, Tobias (2009) evaluated a campaign in Cuba to promote waste separation for recycling. Following distribution of the message "Please classify and separate! Glass—Aluminum—Paper—Cardboard—Plastic," which was designed to be displayed at the location where waste was collected, participants reported daily how much waste they separated. Although the reminder became less effective over time, this decrease was counteracted for participants who recycled sufficiently often to form a habit. Thus, the increased accessibility of a recycling habit appeared to compensate for the tendency to attend less to the reminder to recycle over time.

The real power of accessible responses should become apparent when people are distracted, overwhelmed, or stressed and unable to think carefully about what they want to do. Then, they should automatically carry out the response in mind. Illustrating this process, Salmon, Fennis, de Ridder, Adriaanse, and de Vet (2014) provided participants with information that a majority of others had chosen a healthful food (e.g., rice crackers) over a more desirable but less healthful one (e.g., chocolate bar). When their self-control was lowered because they had just performed a task requiring self-control, participants were more likely to adopt the option chosen by most others.

In summary, interventions that increase the accessibility of alternatives to unwanted habits can promote healthy responding. Forming implementation intentions and providing point-of-choice prompts are examples of such interventions. People are most likely to carry out the accessible healthful actions when competing habits are weaker and when self-control is lowered so that they are unable to think carefully about what they want to do.

Conclusion

In this chapter, we noted that many health behavior interventions fail to generate long-term change because they do not address the automatic triggers that can promote relapse to unhealthful habits despite people's best intentions. After an intervention has ended, new health behaviors may be performed sporadically or perhaps not at all, as people increasingly revert back to existing habits.

To address the challenges of maintaining healthy behaviors, we recommended that interventions incorporate insights from dual-process models in psychology, especially the habitual, automatic components of everyday behavior. Because habits are guided by slowly accruing memories built on experienced covariation between context cues and responses, they do not readily change along with intentions and beliefs. We highlighted a new generation of behavior change interventions designed to create enduring change by addressing the habit system. Such interventions build new, healthy habits through repeated actions in stable contexts and change old, unhealthy ones through controlling, disrupting, or providing accessible action alternatives to habit cues. In short, we argue that key objectives for health interventions should involve the habit system so as to harness automatic responding in the service of health goals.

The benefits of engaging habits arise from the large swath of everyday behavior activated by context-response associations. However, this mechanism guiding action is at odds with most people's intuitive notion that our actions are largely goal directed. To understand this discrepancy, readers should bear in mind that people learn habits while they pursue everyday goals. Even though control is eventually delegated to the stimulus environment, the repeated behavior is often congruent with general goals. As long as habits do not contravene goals and intentions, people probably do not pay much attention to their habits or reflect on possible causes of their actions.

Another reason for the common compatibility of habits and goals is that people are likely to rationalize their habits and strive to generate explanations for their behavior that seem reasonable and logical (Wood & Neal, 2007). Most smokers, for example, have no shortage of arguments in defense of their smoking habit (e.g., it relaxes them, heightens the pleasure from a cup of coffee). These arguments, however, may sound less convincing to smokers after they manage to quit and no longer feel pressured to justify the health-damaging habit. In this way, people reconcile their goals and attitudes to be consistent with their behaviors.

In summary, few of us are aware of the habit memories that guide our actions, sometimes in ways that conflict with goals and intentions. However, these memories can sabotage healthy behavior choices and lead people to revert back into old habits. Thus, health interventions that change only the more thoughtful aspects of behavior can leave people with the best of intentions but few tools to implement them in the face of strong habits. Maintenance of change is best secured through healthy habits as well as healthy intentions.

Acknowledgments

The authors would like to thank Peggy Lin for her comments on an earlier draft of this chapter. Preparation of this chapter was supported by a grant from the John Templeton Foundation. The opinions expressed in this publication are those of the authors and do not necessarily reflect the views of the Foundation.

References

Acland, D., & Levy, M. (2013). Naiveté, projection bias, and habit formation in gym attendance. Working paper series. *Social Science Research Network*. Retrieved 07/01/2014, from https://gspp.berkeley.edu/research/working-paper-series/naivete-projection-bias-and-habit-formation-in-gym-attendance

Adams, M. A., Hovell, M. F., Irvin, V., & Sallis, J. F. (2006). Promoting stair use by modeling: An experimental application of the Behavioral Ecological Model. *American Journal of Health Promotion, 21*(2), 101–109. doi:10.4278/0890-1171-21.2.101

Adriaanse, M. A., Gollwitzer, P. M., de Ridder, D. T. D., de Wit, J. B. F., & Kroese, F. M. (2011). Breaking habits with implementation intentions: A test of underlying processes. *Personality and Social Psychology Bulletin, 37*(4), 502–513. doi:10.1177/0146167211399102

Alexander, G. E., DeLong, M. R., & Strick, P. L. (1986). Parallel organization of functionally segregated circuits linking basal ganglia and cortex. *Annual Review of Neuroscience, 9*(1), 357–381. doi:10.1146/annurev.ne.09.030186.002041

An, R. (2012). Effectiveness of subsidies in promoting healthy food purchases and consumption: A review of field experiments. *Public Health Nutrition, 16*(7), 1215–1228. doi:10.1017/S1368980012004715

Artinian, N. T., Fletcher, G. F., Mozaffarian, D., Kris-Etherton, P., Van Horn, L., Lichtenstein, A. H., ... Burke, L. E. (2010). Interventions to promote physical activity and dietary lifestyle changes for cardiovascular risk factor reduction in adults: A scientific statement from the American Heart Association. *Circulation, 122*(4), 406–441. doi:10.1161/CIR.0b013e3181e8edf1

Baumeister, R. F., & Heatherton, T. F. (1996). Self-regulation failure: An overview. *Psychological Inquiry, 7*(1), 1–15. doi:10.1207/s15327965pli0701_1

Baumeister, R. F., Tice, D. M., & Muraven, M. (2000). Ego depletion: A resource model of volition, self-regulation, and controlled processing. *Social Cognition, 18*(2), 130–150. doi:10.1521/soco.2000.18.2.130

Botvinick, M. M., & Plaut, D. C. (2004). Doing without schema hierarchies: A recurrent connectionist approach to normal and impaired routine sequential action. *Psychological Review, 111*(2), 395–429. doi:10.1037/0033-295X.111.2.395

Brown, T., Avenell, A., Edmunds, L. D., Moore, H., Whittaker, V., Avery, L., & Summberbell, C. (2009). Systematic review of long-term lifestyle interventions to prevent weight gain and morbidity in adults. *Obesity Reviews, 10*(6), 627–638. doi:10.1111/j.1467-789X.2009.00641.x

Burns, R. J., Donovan, A. S., Ackermann, R. T., Finch, E. A., Rothman, A. J., & Jeffery, R. W. (2012). A theoretically grounded systematic review of material incentives for weight loss: Implications for interventions. *Annals of Behavioral Medicine, 44*(3), 375–388. doi:10.1007/s12160-012-9403-4

Carels, R. A., Burmeister, J. M., Koball, A. M., Oehlhof, M. W., Hinman, N., LeRoy, M., . . . Gumble, A. (2014). A randomized trial comparing two approaches to weight loss: Differences in weight loss maintenance. *Journal of Health Psychology, 19*(2), 296–311. doi:10.1177/1359105312470156

Carels, R. A., Young, K. M., Koball, A., Gumble, A., Darby, L. A., Wagner Oehlhof, M., . . . Hinman, N. (2011). Transforming your life: An environmental modification approach to weight loss. *Journal of Health Psychology, 16*(3), 430–438. doi:10.1177/1359105310380986

Charness, G., & Gneezy, U. (2009). Incentives to exercise. *Econometrica, 77*(3), 909–931. doi:10.3982/ECTA7416

Chartrand, T. L., & Bargh, J. A. (1999). The chameleon effect: The perception-behavior link and social interaction. *Journal of Personality and Social Psychology, 76*(6), 893–910.

Danner, U. N., Aarts, H., & Vries, N. K. (2008). Habit vs. intention in the prediction of future behaviour: The role of frequency, context stability and mental accessibility of past behaviour. *British Journal of Social Psychology, 47*(Pt 2), 245–265. doi:10.1348/014466607X230876

de Bruijn, G-J., Kremers, S. P. J., Singh, A., van den Putte, B., & van Mechelen, W. (2009). Adult active transportation: Adding habit strength to the theory of planned behavior. *American Journal of Preventive Medicine, 36*(3), 189–194. doi:10.1016/j.amepre.2008.10.019

Dezfouli, A., & Balleine, B. W. (2012). Habits, action sequences and reinforcement learning. *European Journal of Neuroscience, 35*(7), 1036–1051. doi:10.1111/j.1460-9568.2012.08050.x

Dickinson, A., Nicholas, D. J., & Adams, C. D. (1983). The effect of the instrumental training contingency on susceptibility to reinforcer devaluation. *Quarterly Journal of Experimental Psychology Section B: Comparative and Physiological Psychology, 35*(1), 35–51. doi:10.1080/14640748308400912

Fjeldsoe, B., Neuhaus, M., Winkler, E., & Eakin, E. (2011). Systematic review of maintenance of behavior change following physical activity and dietary interventions. *Health Psychology, 30*(1), 99–109. doi:10.1037/a0021974

Freeman, M. C., Stocks, M. E., Cumming, O., Jeandron, A., Higgins, J. P. T., Wolf, J., . . . Curtis, V. (2014). Hygiene and health: Systematic review of handwashing practices worldwide and update of health effects. *Tropical Medicine and International Health, 19*(8), 906–916. doi:10.1111/tmi.12339

Frensch, P. A., & Rünger, D. (2003). Implicit learning. *Current Directions in Psychological Science, 12*(1), 13–18. doi:10.1111/1467-8721.01213

Gardner, B. (2014). A review and analysis of the use of 'habit' in understanding, predicting and influencing health-related behaviour. *Health Psychology Review.* Epub ahead of print. doi:10.1080/17437199.2013.876238

Gollwitzer, P. M., & Sheeran, P. (2006). Implementation intentions and goal achievement: A meta-analysis of effects and processes. *Advances in Experimental Social Psychology, 38*, 69–119.

Gneezy, U., Meier, S., & Rey-Biel, P. (2011). When and why incentives (don't) work to modify behavior. *Journal of Economic Perspectives, 25*(4), 1–21. doi:10.1257/jep.25.4.1

Graybiel, A. M. (2008). Habits, rituals, and the evaluative brain. *Annual Review of Neuroscience, 31*(1), 359–387. doi:10.1146/annurev.neuro.29.051605.112851

Hagger, M. S., Wood, C., Stiff, C., & Chatzisarantis, N. L. D. (2010). Ego depletion and the strength model of self-control: A meta-analysis. *Psychological Bulletin, 136*(4), 495–525. doi:10.1037/a0019486

Hikosaka, O., Nakamura, K., & Sakai, K. (2002). Central mechanisms of motor skill learning. *Current Opinion in Neurobiology, 12*, 217–222. doi:10.1016/S0959-4388(02)00307-0

Hollands, G. J., Shemilt, I., Marteau, T. M., Jebb, S. A., Kelly, M. P., Nakamura, R., ... Ogilvie, D. (2013). Altering micro-environments to change population health behaviour: Towards an evidence base for choice architecture interventions. *BMC Public Health, 13*(1), 1218. doi:10.1186/1471-2458-13-1218

Hughes, J. R., Keely, J., & Naud, S. (2004). Shape of the relapse curve and long-term abstinence among untreated smokers. *Addiction (Abingdon, England), 99*(1), 29–38.

James, W. (1890). *The principles of psychology* (Vol. 1). New York: Holt.

James, W. (1921). *Talks to teachers on psychology: and to students on some of life's ideals.* New York: Henry Holt.

Ji, M. S., & Wood, W. (2007). Purchase and consumption habits: Not necessarily what you intend. *Journal of Consumer Psychology, 17*(4), 261.

Johnson, E. J., Shu, S. B., Dellaert, B. G. C., Fox, C., Goldstein, D. G., Häubl, G., ... Weber, E. U. (2012). Beyond nudges: Tools of a choice architecture. *Marketing Letters, 23*(2), 487–504. doi:10.1007/s11002-012-9186-1

Judah, G., Gardner, B., & Aunger, R. (2013). Forming a flossing habit: An exploratory study of the psychological determinants of habit formation. *British Journal of Health Psychology, 18*(2), 338–353. doi:10.1111/j.2044-8287.2012.02086.x

Kahneman, D. (2011). *Thinking, fast and slow.* New York: Macmillan.

Knowlton, B. J., & Yin, H. H. (2006). The role of the basal ganglia in habit formation. *Nature Reviews Neuroscience, 7*(6), 464–476. doi:10.1038/nrn1919

Lally, P., Van Jaarsveld, C., Potts, H. W. W., & Wardle, J. (2010). How are habits formed: Modelling habit formation in the real world. *European Journal of Neuroscience, 40*, 998–1009. doi:10.1002/ejsp.674

Leventhal, H., Weinman, J., Leventhal, E. A., & Phillips, L. A. (2008). Health psychology: The search for pathways between behavior and health. *Annual Review of Psychology, 59*, 477–505. doi:10.1146/annurev.psych.59.103006.093643

Loewenstein, G. (1996). Out of control: Visceral influences on behavior. *Organizational Behavior and Human Decision Processes, 65*(3), 272–292. doi:10.1006/obhd.1996.0028

Marteau, T., Ashcroft, R., & Oliver, A. (2009). Using financial incentives to achieve healthy behaviour. *British Medical Journal, 338*, 983–985. doi:10.1136/bmj.b1415

Marteau, T. M., Hollands, G. J., & Fletcher, P. C. (2012). Changing human behavior to prevent disease: The importance of targeting automatic processes. *Science, 337*(6101), 1492–1495. doi:10.1126/science.1226918

Mayberg, H. S., & Holtzheimer, P. E. (2011). Deep brain stimulation for psychiatric disorders. *Annual Review of Neuroscience, 34*, 289–307. doi:10.1146/annurev-neuro-061010-113638

McGowan, L., Cooke, L. J., Gardner, B., Beeken, R. J., Croker, H., & Wardle, J. (2013). Healthy feeding habits: Efficacy results from a cluster-randomized, controlled exploratory trial of a novel, habit-based intervention with parents. *American Journal of Clinical Nutrition, 98*(3), 769–777. doi:10.3945/ajcn.112.052159

Metcalfe, J., & Mischel, W. (1999). A hot/cool-system analysis of delay of gratification: Dynamics of willpower. *Psychological Review, 106*(1), 3–19. doi:10.1037/0033-295X.106.1.3

Middleton, F. A., & Strick, P. L. (2002). Basal-ganglia "projections" to the prefrontal cortex of the primate. *Cerebral Cortex, 12*(9), 926–935. doi:10.1093/cercor/12.9.926

Muraven, M., Collins, R. L., & Neinhaus, K. (2002). Self-control and alcohol restraint: An initial application of the self-control strength model. *Psychology of Addictive Behaviors, 16*(2), 113–120. doi:10.1037//0893-164X.16.2.113

Muraven, M., Collins, R. L., Shiffman, S., & Paty, J. A. (2005). Daily fluctuations in self-control demands and alcohol intake. *Psychology of Addictive Behaviors, 19*(2), 140–147. doi:10.1037/0893-164X.19.2.140

Neal, D. T., Wood, W., & Drolet, A. (2013). How do people adhere to goals when willpower is low? The profits (and pitfalls) of strong habits. *Journal of Personality and Social Psychology, 104*(6), 959–975.

Neal, D. T., Wood, W., Labrecque, J., & Lally, P. (2012). How do habits guide behavior? Perceived and actual triggers of habits in daily life. *Journal of Experimental Social Psychology, 48*, 492–498.

Neal, D. T., Wood, W., Wu, M., & Kurlander, D. (2011). The pull of the past: When do habits persist despite conflict with motives? *Personality and Social Psychology Bulletin, 37*(11), 1428–1437. doi:10.1177/0146167211419863

Neve, M., Morgan, P. J., Jones, P. R., & Collins, C. E. (2010). Effectiveness of web-based interventions in achieving weight loss and weight loss maintenance in overweight and obese adults: A systematic review with meta-analysis. *Obesity Reviews, 11*(4), 306–321. doi:10.1111/j.1467-789X.2009.00646.x

Nocon, M., Müller-Riemenschneider, F., Nitzschke, K., & Willich, S. N. (2010). Review article: Increasing physical activity with point-of-choice prompts—a systematic review. *Scandinavian Journal of Public Health, 38*(6), 633–638. doi:10.1177/1403494810375865

Norman, D. A. (1981). Categorization of action slips. *Psychological Review, 88*(1), 1–15. doi:10.1037/0033-295X.88.1.1

Nuttin, B., Cosyns, P., Demeulemeester, H., Gybels, J., & Meyerson, B. (1999). Electrical stimulation in anterior limbs of internal capsules in patients with obsessive-compulsive disorder. *Lancet, 354*(9189), 1526. doi:10.1016/S0140-6736(99)02376-4

Orbell, S., & Sheeran, P. (2000). Motivational and volitional processes in action initiation: A field study of the role of implementation intentions. *Journal of Applied Social Psychology, 30*(4), 780–797. doi:10.1111/j.1559-1816.2000.tb02823.x

Orbell, S., & Verplanken, B. (2010). The automatic component of habit in health behavior: Habit as cue-contingent automaticity. *Health Psychology, 29*(4), 374–383. doi:10.1037/a0019596

Ouellette, J. A., & Wood, W. (1998). Habit and intention in everyday life: The multiple processes by which past behavior predicts future behavior. *Psychological Bulletin, 124*(1), 54. doi:10.1037//0033-2909.124.1.54

Quinn, J. M., Pascoe, A., Wood, W., & Neal, D. T. (2010). Can't control yourself? Monitor those bad habits. *Personality and Social Psychology Bulletin, 36*(4), 499–511. doi:10.1177/0146167209360665

Reason, J. T. (1992). Cognitive underspecification. In B. J. Baars (Ed.), *Experimental slips and human error* (pp. 71–91). Boston, MA: Springer.

Rünger, D., & Frensch, P. A. (2010). Defining consciousness in the context of incidental sequence learning: Theoretical considerations and empirical implications. *Psychological Research, 74*(2), 121–137. doi:10.1007/s00426-008-0225-8

Salmon, S. J., Fennis, B. M., de Ridder, D. T. D., Adriaanse, M. A., & de Vet, E. (2014). Health on impulse: When low self-control promotes healthy food choices. *Health Psychology, 33*(2), 103–109. doi:10.1037/a0031785

Schwabe, L., Tegenthoff, M., Höffken, O., & Wolf, O. T. (2012). Simultaneous glucocorticoid and noradrenergic activity disrupts the neural basis of goal-directed action in the human brain. *Journal of Neuroscience, 32*(30), 10146–10155. doi:10.1523/JNEUROSCI.1304-12.2012

Schwabe, L., & Wolf, O. T. (2013). Stress and multiple memory systems: From 'thinking' to 'doing'. *Trends in Cognitive Sciences, 17*(2), 60–68. doi:10.1016/j.tics.2012.12.001

Sheeran, P., & Orbell, S. (1999). Implementation intentions and repeated behaviour: Augmenting the predictive validity of the theory of planned behaviour. *European Journal of Neuroscience, 29*, 349–369.

Sheeran, P., Webb, T. L., & Gollwitzer, P. M. (2005). The interplay between goal intentions and implementation intentions. *Personality and Social Psychology Bulletin, 31*(1), 87–98. doi:10.1177/0146167204271308

Sherman, J. W., Gawronski, B., & Trope, Y. (Eds.). (2014). *Dual-process theories of the social mind*. New York: Guilford Press.

Shmueli, D., & Prochaska, J. J. (2009). Resisting tempting foods and smoking behavior: Implications from a self-control theory perspective. *Health Psychology, 28*(3), 300–306. doi:10.1037/a0013826

Smith, K. S., & Graybiel, A. M. (2013a). A dual operator view of habitual behavior reflecting cortical and striatal dynamics. *Neuron, 79*(2), 361–374. doi:10.1016/j.neuron.2013.05.038

Smith, K. S., & Graybiel, A. M. (2013b). Using optogenetics to study habits. *Brain Research, 1511*, 102–114. doi:10.1016/j.brainres.2013.01.008

Soler, R. E., Leeks, K. D., Buchanan, L. R., Brownson, R. C., Heath, G. W., & Hopkins, D. H. (2010). Point-of-decision prompts to increase stair use. *American Journal of Preventive Medicine, 38*(2S), S292–S300. doi:10.1016/j.amepre.2009.10.028

Stawarz, K., Cox, A. L., & Blandford, A. (2014). Personalized routine support for tackling medication non-adherence. Retrieved 06/01/2014, from http://usabilitypanda.com/publications/StawarzCoXBlandford2014_personalized-routines.pdf

Tobias, R. (2009). Changing behavior by memory aids: A social psychological model of prospective memory and habit development tested with dynamic field data. *Psychological Review, 116*(2), 408–438. doi:10.1037/a0015512

Tricomi, E., Balleine, B. W., & O'Doherty, J. P. (2009). A specific role for posterior dorsolateral striatum in human habit learning. *European Journal of Neuroscience*, *29*(11), 2225–2232. doi:10.1111/j.1460-9568.2009.06796.x

van't Riet, J., Sijtsema, S. J., Dagevos, H., & De Bruijn, G-J. (2011). The importance of habits in eating behaviour. An overview and recommendations for future research. *Appetite*, *57*, 585–596. doi:10.1016/j.appet.2011.07.010

Verplanken, B., & Wood, W. (2006). Interventions to break and create consumer habits. *Journal of Public Policy and Marketing*, *25*(1), 90–103. doi:10.1509/jppm.25.1.90

Verplanken, B., Walker, I., Davis, A., & Jurasek, M. (2008). Context change and travel mode choice: Combining the habit discontinuity and self-activation hypotheses. *Journal of Environmental Psychology*, *28*(2), 121–127. doi:10.1016/j.jenvp.2007.10.005

Webb, O. J., Eves, F. F., & Smith, L. (2011). Investigating behavioural mimicry in the context of stair/escalator choice. *British Journal of Health Psychology*, *16*(2), 373–385. doi:10.1348/135910710X510395

Webb, T. L., & Sheeran, P. (2006). Does changing behavioral intentions engender behavior change? A meta-analysis of the experimental evidence. *Psychological Bulletin*, *132*(2), 249–268. doi:10.1037/0033-2909.132.2.249

Webb, T. L., Sheeran, P., & Luszczynska, A. (2009). Planning to break unwanted habits: Habit strength moderates implementation intention effects on behaviour change. *British Journal of Social Psychology*, *48*(Pt 3), 507–523. doi:10.1348/014466608X370591

Wenzlaff, R. M., & Wegner, D. M. (2000). Thought suppression. *Annual Review of Psychology*, *51*(1), 59–91. doi:10.1146/annurev.psych.51.1.59

Wood, W., & Neal, D. T. (2007). A new look at habits and the habit-goal interface. *Psychological Review*, *114*(4), 843–863. doi:10.1037/0033-295X.114.4.843

Wood, W., & Neal, D. T. (2009). The habitual consumer. *Journal of Consumer Psychology*, *19*(4), 579–592. doi:10.1016/j.jcps.2009.08.003

Wood, W., Quinn, J. M., & Kashy, D. A. (2002). Habits in everyday life: Thought, emotion, and action. *Journal of Personality and Social Psychology*, *83*(6), 1281. doi:10.1037//0022-3514.83.6.1281

Wood, W., Tam, L., & Witt, M. G. (2005). Changing circumstances, disrupting habits. *Journal of Personality and Social Psychology*, *88*(6), 918–933. doi:10.1037/0022-3514.88.6.918

World Health Organization. (2014). *Deaths from NCDs*. Retrieved February 2015, from http://www.who.int/gho/ncd/mortality_morbidity/ncd_total/en/

Yin, H. H., Knowlton, B. J., & Balleine, B. W. (2004). Lesions of dorsolateral striatum preserve outcome expectancy but disrupt habit formation in instrumental learning. *European Journal of Neuroscience*, *19*, 181–189. doi:10.1046/j.1460-9568.2003.03095.x

Yin, H. H., Ostlund, S. B., Knowlton, B. J., & Balleine, B. W. (2005). The role of the dorsomedial striatum in instrumental conditioning. *European Journal of Neuroscience*, *22*(2), 513–523. doi:10.1111/j.1460-9568.2005.04218.x

4 | Emotions and Health Decision Making

EXTENDING THE APPRAISAL TENDENCY FRAMEWORK TO IMPROVE HEALTH AND HEALTHCARE

REBECCA FERRER, WILLIAM KLEIN, JENNIFER LERNER, VALERIE REYNA, AND DACHER KELTNER

N AN ERA OF UNPRECEDENTED focus on health policy and behavioral prevention of disease (e.g., Barry & Edgman-Levitan, 2012),[1] understanding the relevance of behavioral science to health is critical. The decisions that people make about their health and the health of others significantly affect the quality, trajectory, and length of human life. Given that many causes of mortality and reduced quality of life, such as heart disease, diabetes, and cancer, can be prevented with behavioral modifications (Fisher et al., 2002; Ford, Zhao, Tsai, & Li, 2011; Khaw et al., 2008; Pearson et al., 2002; Stefanek et al., 2009), recent findings from the field of behavioral science specifying how emotion alters judgments and decision making (Lerner et al., 2015) may offer a key to better outcomes.[2] Specifically, contrary to the popular view that emotions generally contaminate rational decision making, converging evidence indicates that they actually can improve decisions (e.g., Damasio, 1994; Lerner & Keltner, 2000, 2001; Loewenstein & Lerner, 2003).

The field of behavioral economics has begun to make important connections between behavioral science and systems-level interventions. Behavioral economic principles are beginning to be incorporated into health policies and interventions at a variety of levels (see Thaler & Sunstein, 2008). These policies have achieved varied success (see Marteau, Ogilvie, Suhrcke, & Kelly, 2011) but are currently limited to leveraging basic research on economic decision making and have not yet capitalized on research demonstrating that emotion influences decisions.

In the health domain, research suggests that global affective states—feeling good or bad—contribute to unhealthy behaviors such as smoking (e.g., Addicott, Gray, & Todd, 2009; Perkins et al., 2008), alcohol consumption (e.g., Kelly, Masterman, & Young, 2011; Ostafin & Brooks, 2011), and overeating (e.g., Loxton, Dawe, & Cahill, 2011). Emotions also contribute to health-related risk perceptions (Peters, Lipkus, & Diefenbach, 2006) and health decisions made in response to numeric information (Peters et al., 2009). However, less systematic attention has been paid to discrete emotions such as anger, fear, sadness, or disgust (and positive discrete emotions such as gratitude or pride), despite evidence in other domains demonstrating that emotions of the same valence (e.g., anger and fear) can yield dramatically different decisions and behaviors (e.g., Lerner & Keltner, 2000, 2001).

Integral emotions—those that are normatively relevant to a decision because they are elicited by a component of the decision or would be influenced by an outcome of the decision—can predict health decisions (see DeSteno, Gross, & Kubzansky, 2013).[3] For example, worry about a health threat may trigger preventive behavior (e.g., Hay, McCaul, & Magnan, 2006). From a functional perspective that views the purpose of emotions as means to motivate fulfillment of goals (see Keltner & Gross, 1999), integral emotions may produce adaptive decisions because they highlight threats, motivate mitigating actions, or signal that a goal has been achieved. However, these are not the only affective influences on judgment and decision making; consumer and decision scientists have also focused on incidental emotions—those elicited by a person, situation, or stimuli not normatively relevant to the decision—and found that they can also influence unrelated decisions (Loewenstein & Lerner, 2003; Loewenstein, Weber, Hsee, & Welch, 2001). For example, sadness elicited by a prior event has been found to influence eating behavior (Garg & Lerner, 2013). The influence of incidental emotions can linger, even when decision makers face substantial incentives to avoid bias (e.g., Lerner, Small, & Loewenstein, 2004) and after the emotion experience itself has ceased (Andrade & Ariely, 2009; Schwarz & Clore, 1983).

Sometimes the influence of incidental emotions may be overwhelmed by integral emotions; for example, a patient's amusement over a film may dissipate when she receives a disease diagnosis. However, many complex emotions may contribute to affective experiences at any given time (see Wilson & Gilbert, 2003, for a discussion), and incidental emotions may be equal contributors even when integral emotion is powerful, particularly when the incidental emotion is felt intensely or is the result of a very personally relevant event. Thus, the same cancer patient could feel fear at a diagnosis, but not forget—or stop feeling—the anger she feels over a previous argument with her spouse. Objectively, this incidental anger should not factor into a treatment decision, as it is not normatively relevant to the decision (e.g., Han, Keltner, & Lerner, 2007). However, that anger is still meaningful and salient, and may carry over to influence her subsequent cancer treatment decisions. Thus, it is imperative to consider the influence of both incidental and integral emotions on health judgment and decision making.

Health-related interventions could capitalize on this basic knowledge of the role of emotion in decision making. Currently, behavioral economics interventions for population-level health behaviors and decisions tend to take a one-size-fits-all approach. For example, some countries have successfully leveraged basic knowledge about human decision making and defaults to improve organ donation rates by creating conventions where choices to donate are "opt-out" rather than "opt-in" (Johnson & Goldstein, 2003; van Dalen & Henkens, 2014). This suggests that leveraging defaults may be a promising direction for other behavioral economics health interventions. However, emerging evidence cautions against treating defaults as a panacea; in one instance, an opt-out colorectal cancer screening intervention actually *decreased* screening rates (Narula, Ramprasad, Ruggs, & Hebl, 2013).

Contextual factors such as emotion may explain the varying success or failure of defaults and other behavioral economics interventions. As it turns out, individuals lean more toward the default choice when a decision is emotionally laden (Luce, 1998), as is presumably the case with organ-donation decisions. Moreover, emotions such as anger may reduce (or reverse) reliance on defaults (Garg, Inman, & Mittal, 2005), suggesting the possibility that implementing a default that angers individuals—such as imposing a default option on a behavior that people are extremely resistant to—may backfire. Other examples of behavioral economics interventions that have failed or induced unhealthy behaviors (e.g., Chernev, 2011; Wansink & Chandon, 2006) underscore the importance of understanding contextual factors such as emotion that could predispose success or failure.

Connecting Emotion Research With Health Decisions

The appraisal tendency framework (ATF; Han et al., 2007; Lerner & Keltner, 2000; 2001; Lerner & Tiedens, 2006) is useful for clarifying and predicting how specific, discrete emotions systematically improve or degrade health-related decisions and interventions. The ATF can identify (1) individual differences in the tendency to respond to situations with certain discrete emotions (Ambady & Gray, 2002; Lerner & Keltner, 2001) and (2) certain health situations that routinely evoke a particular discrete emotion (such as cancer and fear; e.g., Holland, 2003).

We note that the influence of emotion on particular decision-making tendencies depends on the properties of a decision (Lerner & Tiedens, 2006). For example, the fact that anger increases risk taking may lead to increased benefits when the option associated with the most likely benefit is also uncertain, ambiguous, or risky (Ferrer, Maclay, Rim, Litvak, & Lerner, unpublished data), as is the case with some treatments for cancer or other diseases. As such, emotions can facilitate or hinder decision making—or augment or degrade intervention efforts—depending on the circumstances (Reyna, Nelson, Han, & Pignone, in press). Thus, rather than predicting that a specific emotion is always beneficial or deleterious, the ATF may pinpoint how specific emotions interact with certain types of health decisions, thereby shedding light on decisions that would benefit or be hindered by particular emotions.

Our review focuses largely on research on incidental emotions because such research involves highly controlled paradigms and experimental inductions, allowing us to draw causal conclusions about the general influence of discrete emotions on judgment and decision-making patterns. Notably, some studies have targeted discrete integral emotions (e.g., fear or worry) in a health context, but they typically have not isolated the influence of such emotions on subsequent judgment and decision making. Rather, these inductions often occur in the context of health behavior change interventions that are designed to intervene on many other constructs and processes (e.g., Portnoy, Ferrer, Bergman, & Klein, 2013; Witte & Allen, 2000). When inductions take this inclusive approach, it is not possible to infer mechanism (Suls, Luger, & Martin, 2010).[4] Thus, such studies cannot fully identify systematic ways that particular emotions can influence patterns of health-related decision making. For this reason, these studies are beyond the scope of this review. Because theory (Han et al., 2007; Keltner & Gross, 1999; Lerner, Han, & Keltner, 2007) and research (Isen & Erez, 2007; Lerner, Gonzalez, Small, & Fischhoff, 2003) suggest that that the pattern of judgment and decision making arising from an emotion will be similar regardless of whether it is integral or incidental, studies of incidental emotion allow us to infer patterns of the general influence of discrete emotions, both incidental and integral, on health-related decision making.

In this chapter, we consider the effects of emotion on four general categories of judgments and thought processes relevant to health decisions: risk perception, valuation and reward seeking, interpersonal attribution, and depth of information processing. We discuss ways in which emotions may improve or degrade health decisions through their influence on these judgments and thought processes in two health decision domains: choices about health promotion and prevention behaviors (e.g., choices about food, tobacco, physical activity) and medical decisions (e.g., decisions about preventive care and treatment). We then discuss broad policy implications of these areas.

We define decision making broadly, extending beyond single-event decisions (e.g., cancer screening) to include decisions and choices that contribute to behavioral patterns or maintenance (e.g., decisions to quit smoking or food choices as contributors to a pattern of adhering to smoking-cessation or weight-loss programs), given that similar underlying psychological, affective, and decisional processes contribute to a diverse array of decisions (e.g., Reyna, 2008). Although maintenance choices are made over time and can require frequent decision making (Rothman, Baldwin, & Hertel, 2004), behavioral patterns or maintenance initiated by a single decision (e.g., whether to enter a smoking-cessation program) can be influenced by emotion. Moreover, frequently experienced emotions (e.g., those repeatedly triggered by a volatile relationship, a frustrating job, or a satisfying friendship) can systematically influence repeated decisions that contribute to patterns of behavioral maintenance.

The Appraisal Tendency Framework

The appraisal tendency framework (ATF) provides a useful theoretical foundation for understanding how emotions influence health-related decisions. The ATF assumes that specific emotions give rise to corresponding cognitive and motivational processes that are related to the target of the emotion (i.e., the situation, person, or other stimulus that elicited the emotion), which account for the effects of each emotion upon judgment and decision making. In contrast to theories that predict how broad mood states (positive or negative) may influence judgment and decision making (e.g., Bower, 1991; Forgas, 2003; Isen, 1993), the ATF offers specific predictions for how discrete emotions will influence judgment and decision making (see Tables 4.1 and 4.2).

TABLE 4.1 Appraisal Dimensions, Core Appraisal Themes, and Content/Process Effects of Negatively Valenced Emotions

	ANGER	DISGUST	SADNESS	SHAME	GUILT	FEAR
Appraisal dimensions						
Certainty	High	High	Medium	Medium	Medium	Low
Personal control	High	High	Low	High	High	Low
Other/situational responsibility	High	Medium	High	Medium	Low	Medium
Attentional activity	Medium	Low	Low	Medium	Low	Medium
Anticipated effort	Medium	Medium	Low	Medium	Medium	High
Core appraisal theme	Being slighted or demeaned[a]	Taking in or standing too close to an indigestible object or idea[a]	Feeling irrevocable loss[a]	Failing to live up to an ego ideal[a]	Disobeying a moral imperative[a]	Facing existential threats[a]
Content effects						
Risk perceptions	*Perceive low risk*	*Perceive low risk*	—	*Perceive low risk*	*Perceive low risk*	Perceive high risk
Valuation and choice	*High valuation and reward seeking*	Low valuation and disposal	High valuation and reward seeking	*High valuation and reward seeking*	—	*Low valuation and disposal*
Interpersonal attribution	Decrease trust and cooperation, increase blame	—	Decrease trust and cooperation, increase blame	—	Increase trust and cooperation, decrease blame	—
Information processing effects	Employ heuristic processing	*Employ heuristic processing*	—	—	—	Employ systematic processing
	Perceive low "unknown risk" and "dread risk"	*Perceive low "unknown risk"*	Seek rewards even in presence of risk	*Perceive low "dread risk," seek rewards even in presence of risk*	*Perceive low "dread risk"*	Perceive high "unknown risk" and "dread risk"

[a]Adapted from Lazarus (1991), p. 826.
NOTE: Italics denote untested prediction.

TABLE 4.2 Appraisal Dimensions, Core Appraisal Themes, and Action Tendencies of Positively Valenced Emotions

	HAPPINESS	PRIDE	RELIEF	GRATITUDE	HOPE	SURPRISE
Appraisal dimensions						
Certainty	High	High	Medium	Medium	Low	Low
Personal control	Medium	High	Medium	Low	Medium	Medium
Other/situational responsibility	Medium	Low	Medium	High	High	High
Attentional activity	Medium	Medium	Low	Medium	High	Medium
Anticipated effort	Low	Low	Low	Low	High	Medium
Core appraisal theme	Making acceptable progress toward achieving a goal[a]	Feeling self or social worth advancing due to being credited with a highly valued object or accomplishment[a]	Achieving a goal after expecting the worst	Crediting another with an altruistic gift[a]	Fearing the worst but yearning for better[a]	Unexpectedly having a positive outcome
Content effects						
Risk perceptions	Perceive low "unknown risk"	Perceive low "unknown risk" and "dread risk"	Perceive low "unknown risk" and "dread risk"	Perceive high "dread risk"	Perceive high "unknown risk"	Perceive high "unknown risk"
Valuation and choice	—	—	—	—	High valuation and reward seeking	—
Interpersonal attribution	—	Decrease trust and cooperation, increase blame	—	Increase trust and cooperation, decrease blame	Increase trust and cooperation, decrease blame	Increase trust and cooperation, decrease punitive judgments
Information processing effects	Employ heuristic processing	Employ heuristic processing	—	—	Employ systematic processing	Employ systematic processing

[a]Adapted from Lazarus (1991), p. 826.
NOTE: Italics denote untested prediction

Emotion theorists have argued that a range of cognitive *appraisal dimensions*, or categorical dimensions characterizing cognitive tendencies associated with emotion, usefully differentiate emotional experience. In one empirical examination of appraisal dimensions, Smith and Ellsworth (1985) identified six dimensions that categorize patterns of thinking associated with different emotions: *pleasantness/valence* (whether the emotion is pleasant); *certainty* (whether the emotion was elicited by a predictable stimulus); *personal control* (whether emotion was elicited by something under one's personal control); *other or situational responsibility* (whether the emotion was elicited by a stimulus controlled by another person or a situation); *attentional activity* (whether the emotion was elicited by a stimulus that demands attention); and *anticipated effort* (the amount of effort an individual anticipates will be necessary to deal with the emotion or its elicitor).

According to the ATF, patterns of cognitive appraisals along these dimensions provide a basis for comparing and contrasting discrete emotions. For example, certainty and control are the central dimensions that separate anger from fear. Anger is associated with appraisals of certainty about an event and individual control for negative events. Fear, by contrast, is associated with appraisals of uncertainty about what happened and situational control for negative events. Despite its positive valence, happiness, like anger, is associated with an elevated sense of certainty and individual control (Smith & Ellsworth, 1985; Weiner, 1986). Therefore, happiness, at least in one respect, resembles anger more so than fear.

Each emotion is also accompanied by a core *appraisal theme* (Lazarus, 1991), which is a mental schema associated with the emotion that summarize the specific harms or benefits associated with the target or elicitor of the emotion. Emotion-specific core appraisal themes affect the likelihood of specific courses of action (Frijda, 1986; Lazarus, 1991; Scherer, 1988). For example, sadness is accompanied by a core appraisal theme or mental schema of loss; anger involves a core appraisal theme of being slighted or demeaned (Lazarus, 1991). The ATF proposes that these appraisal themes systematically trigger a predisposition toward specific *action tendencies*, behavioral patterns aimed at overcoming obstacles or meeting goals made salient by the emotion and its core appraisal theme (Frijda, 1986). These action tendencies are triggered when the appraisal dimensions associated with an emotion are also relevant to a particular judgment or decision. For example, fear is associated with high uncertainty and reflects core appraisal themes of being threatened; thus, it is relevant to judgments about risk and triggers risk-avoidant behavior (see also Rivers, Reyna, &

Mills, 2008). Sadness, by contrast, is characterized by appraisals of experiencing irrevocable loss (Lazarus, 1991) and thus accompanies the action tendency to change one's circumstances, perhaps by seeking rewards (Lerner et al., 2004).

In sum, the ATF predicts that each emotion has motivational properties that fuel carryover to subsequent judgments and decisions. The form of that carryover is termed *appraisal tendencies*—where the *appraisal dimension* and *appraisal theme* are together activated by the properties of a situation to shape behavioral *action tendencies* that predispose certain judgments, decisions, and actions. Although tailored to help the individual respond to the event that evoked an emotion, appraisal tendencies persist beyond the eliciting situation and affect both the content and depth of thought. Broadly speaking, appraisal tendency influences on judgment and decision making can be divided into two categories: *content effects* and *depth-of-processing effects*.

Content Effects

The ATF specifies action tendencies that affect the actual content of thoughts related to a decision (Lerner & Keltner, 2000, 2001). Consider the effects of sadness and anger on judgments of blame. Sadness both co-occurs with appraisals of situational control in the immediate situation and also triggers appraisal tendencies to perceive situational control even in new situations. Anger, by contrast, co-occurs with appraisals of individual control and triggers appraisal tendencies to perceive individual control. Consequently, sad people will attribute blame to situational factors, and angry people will attribute blame to other individuals.

Here, we summarize three categories of judgments or thought patterns that are particularly relevant to health decisions: risk perception and preference; valuation and reward seeking; and interpersonal attributions such as stereotyping, trust, and blame. These content effects systematically predispose advantageous or disadvantageous health decision making, depending on the context.

Risk Perception

Risk perceptions, or judgments about the likelihood of a given outcome, are influenced by emotions (Lerner & Keltner, 2000, 2001; Loewenstein & Lerner, 2003; Loewenstein et al., 2001; Slovic, Finucane, Peters, & MacGregor, 2002). Given that many health-related decisions are made under the threat of disease (e.g., smoking under threat of lung cancer and cardiovascular disease) and involve factors that influence risk perceptions, such as dread and lack of control, research on emotion and risk perceptions is exceptionally pertinent (see Rothman, Kelly, Hertel, & Salovey, 2003). Emotions associated with certainty and control appraisals are directly relevant to risk (Lerner & Keltner, 2001), given that uncertainty about and lack of control over a threat affect risk perception (Slovic, 1987).

More specifically, converging evidence suggests that fear, anger, and happiness can systematically influence risk perceptions. Compared to happiness (Johnson & Tversky, 1983) and anger (Lerner & Keltner, 2001), fear triggers more pessimistic risk judgments and risk-averse choices. Researchers have applied these findings in attempts to determine when persuasive messages will be most well received. Individuals respond differently to risk information when it is framed in terms of losses or gains (Kahneman & Tversky, 2000), an effect that can be amplified or attenuated by emotional states (e.g., DeSteno, Petty, Rucker, Wegener, & Braverman, 2004; Wegener, Petty, & Klein, 1994). For example, loss-framed messages have been found to be more persuasive for sad individuals, whereas happy individuals are more persuaded by gain-framed messages (Keller, Lipkus, & Rimer, 2003; Wegener et al., 1994). Policy makers may be able to leverage these findings when crafting public health messages. Although most research on risk perception focuses on fear, anger, and happiness, other emotions associated with certainty and control, such as pride and surprise, may also yield systematic influences on decisions under uncertainty (see Table 4.1 for predictions).

Valuation and Reward Seeking

A second category of thought processes relevant to the content of health decisions involves the way people estimate the value of different choice options, and the general tendency toward reward-seeking behaviors that favor more highly valued options. These effects are particularly relevant to intertemporal choices, or decisions that require us to weigh smaller, immediate benefits against larger, delayed benefits. Valuation and reward seeking in intertemporal choice are relevant to many health-related behaviors (Critchfield & Kollins, 2001). For example, drinking alcohol, eating nonnutritious foods, and smoking cigarettes are behaviors that result in immediate hedonic gratification, but avoiding these behaviors can bring a substantial delayed benefit: preventing disease and improving quality of life in older age.

Consistent with ATF predictions, research has shown that sadness increases valuation of reward (and reward seeking), compared to anxiety (Raghunathan & Pham, 1999), happiness (Chuang & Lin, 2007), and disgust (Cryder, Lerner, Gross, & Dahl, 2008; Han et al., 2010; Lerner et al., 2004). Because of increased valuation of reward, sad individuals are willing to forgo greater future rewards to receive immediate gratification (Lerner, Li, & Weber, 2013). Additionally, although individuals tend to forgo delayed benefits to receive less substantial but immediate benefits (intertemporal choice bias), happy individuals are less willing than individuals in a neutral emotional state to forgo greater future monetary rewards in exchange for receiving lesser rewards more quickly (Ifcher & Zarghamee, 2011). Most research on valuation and reward seeking focuses on sadness, disgust, and happiness, but other emotions with core appraisal themes related to valuation (e.g., envy, hope) are potential avenues for future research (see Table 4.1).

Interpersonal Attribution

Emotions can systematically influence interpersonal attributions such as trust, blame, and stereotyping. Attributions influence physicians' perceptions of patients and patients' responsiveness to physicians. Interpersonal attributions may also play a role in health-related behaviors, such as overeating or smoking, particularly given that many such behaviors are influenced by interactions with peers and others (Conner & Norman, 1996).

Because of increased certainty appraisals and subsequent reliance on heuristics, anger increases stereotyping compared to sadness (Bodenhausen, Sheppard, & Kramer, 1994a; DeSteno, Dasgupta, Bartlett, & Cajdric, 2004) or fear (Tiedens & Linton, 2001). Anger also increases perceived accountability because of its core appraisal theme of being slighted or demeaned (Lerner, Goldberg, & Tetlock, 1998). Happiness and gratitude, associated with the appraisal that others are in control, increase trust as compared to sadness. Anger, however, lowers trust ratings compared to sadness, again because it is associated with an appraisal of being slighted and demeaned, which does not engender trust (Dunn & Schweitzer, 2005).[5] Moreover, gratitude not only increases trust but, relative to anger, also makes individuals more likely to accept advice (Dunn & Schweitzer, 2005). Other emotions that may affect interpersonal attributions are pride, envy, and shame (see Table 4.1).

Depth-of-Processing Effects

The ATF also predicts the depth with which decision makers process information (Lerner & Tiedens, 2006). Evidence suggests there may be two distinct styles of cognitively processing information: System 1 (heuristic-intuitive) and System 2 (systematic-deliberative)—differentiated by the depth with which information is processed (e.g., Chaiken, Liberman, & Eagly, 1989; Petty & Cacioppo, 1986; but see Reyna, 2012)—and that our emotions influence depth of processing (Lerner & Tiedens, 2006). For example, emotions that have a high certainty appraisal, such as anger and happiness, are associated with heuristic processing (System 1), because certainty leads to less motivation to systematically process or be vigilant toward details (Bodenhausen et al., 1994a; Tiedens & Linton, 2001; Weary & Jacobson, 1997).[6] Emotions such as fear and relief, which are endemic in medical decisions, are also associated with depth-of-processing effects (see Table 4.1).

Depth-of-processing effects are highly relevant to decisions about health, which typically require individuals to process a great deal of information regarding the risks and benefits of a procedure, screening, or treatment. Further, health communications involve conveying complex information about health risks and preventive behaviors, and the depth with which information is processed could affect how persuasive it is to them. For example, given that individuals tend to be defensive against threatening information (Kunda, 1987), they may be motivated to process the information contained in a health message more heuristically if it is personally threatening.

Heuristic (System 1) processing can also lead to decision biases, even (and here, most prominently) among experts (Reyna, Chick, Corbin, & Hsia, 2014). Emotion-triggered heuristic processing may be beneficial (e.g., when an individual uses heuristic cues to correctly identify evidence-based evidence for engaging in healthy behaviors) or deleterious (e.g., when a patient only skims an informed consent form when participating in a clinical trial), depending on the decision and decision maker. Indeed, research suggests that anger-facilitated heuristic processing can be beneficial if those heuristic cues are valid (Moon & Mackie, 2007), even improving the degree to which information is correctly extracted and maintained from complex documents such as medical informed consents (Ferrer et al., in press).

Notably, depth-of-processing effects can co-occur and interact with content effects; depth of processing can influence how risk information is processed, how information about intertemporal choice is processed, and how that available information is processed into attributions. For example, increased stereotyping in an interpersonal setting involves elevated reliance on heuristic information processing strategies (e.g., Bodenhausen et al., 1994a; DeSteno, Dasgupta, et al., 2004).

Decisions About Health Promotion and Disease Prevention Behaviors

Guided by the ATF, the effects of information content and depth of processing can be used to identify ways that emotion may systematically benefit or hinder choices about health promotion and disease prevention behaviors. Given that many health behaviors are undertaken to reduce the risk of disease, emotion has the potential to shape decisions about these behaviors through its influence on risk perception. Valuation and reward seeking can be directly related to health behaviors. Many products currently on the market could be classified as healthful (e.g., gym memberships) or unhealthful (e.g., fast food), and emotions influence purchasing behavior. We also know that emotion effects on valuation influence intertemporal choice, or tendencies to seek immediate rewards despite long-term health benefit (e.g., consumption of unhealthy foods, inactivity, smoking, alcohol consumption). The influence of emotion on interpersonal attribution may also play a prominent role in health behaviors, particularly when those behaviors are motivated in part by social norms or take place in a social context. Finally, emotion-driven depth of processing can be relevant to health communications and other health behavior interventions designed to target knowledge. Here, we review research to date that addresses these issues, and we consider potential gaps in the field.

Risk Perception and Communication

Emotion influences risk perceptions for diseases that could be prevented through healthy behaviors (e.g., Johnson & Tversky, 1983; Lerner & Keltner, 2001). Further, research on emotion and health message framing has demonstrated that fearful individuals are more persuaded by loss-framed messages about the consequences of failing to eat fruits and vegetables (given that fear promotes loss-averse behaviors), whereas angry individuals are more persuaded by gain-framed messages about the benefits of consumption (given that anger promotes approach behaviors and behavioral control), demonstrated by an increase of self-reported intake

2 weeks after the message was presented (Gerend & Maner, 2011). Thus, emotions such as anger should hinder health decisions under risk framed as losses, whereas fear should benefit these types of decisions.

Valuation and Reward Seeking

Sadness, associated with high valuation and reward seeking, increases the consumption of hedonic foods, whereas disgust, associated with trading away or disposal, decreases consumption of these types of foods (Garg & Lerner, 2013). Individuals induced to a sad emotional state also consume higher amounts of hedonic foods than those induced to feel happy (Garg, Wansink, & Inman, 2007; Wansink, Cheney, & Chan, 2003). Given the high caloric and poor nutritional content in hedonic foods, food consumption is one domain in which sadness could contribute to less healthy decision making, whereas disgust or happiness could improve it. This knowledge could lead to ATF theory-based interventions to develop emotion regulation skills to decouple the link between sadness and high-calorie eating.

It is likely that emotion could systematically influence other health behaviors that involve reward seeking and intertemporal choice. It seems likely that sadness and disgust would influence health decisions like smoking, inactivity, and alcohol consumption, all involving intertemporal choice; sadness should increase willingness to risk later health outcomes in service of immediate gratification associated with negative health behaviors, whereas disgust may demotivate these behaviors. The effect of sadness may be exacerbated in adolescents and young adults, where achieving immediate pleasure is a highly prioritized goal (Reyna & Farley, 2006).

Disgust has already been leveraged in smoking policy, in that many cigarette warning labels target disgust (Hammond, Fong, McDonald, Brown, & Cameron, 2004). Although disgust in these labels may be integrally related to smoking, some warning labels in other countries have been effective to the degree that they elicit disgust even when the disgusting images have seemingly no relevance to smoking (Hammond et al., 2004). Extending this hypothesis, sadness could increase smoking, which has potentially important implications, given that some antismoking advertisements may elicit sadness rather than fear by depicting a dying person.

Interpersonal Attribution

Individuals may be more motivated to engage in interpersonally relevant healthy behaviors (e.g., those involving social normative influence, such as smoking) if they are experiencing pride, an emotion involving attributions about the self in comparison to attributions about others. Supporting this hypothesis, research has demonstrated that pride increases perseverance on effortful and hedonically negative tasks (Williams & DeSteno, 2008). Han and colleagues (2007) hypothesize that pride may reduce binge drinking, because it may reduce social normative influences (Conner & Norman, 1996) by decreasing self-other similarity. Indeed, research suggests that individuals may differentiate themselves from peers by engaging in behavior they think is desirable but *not* normative, such as reducing alcohol consumption as a function of believing that other students drink excessively (Ferrer, Dillard, & Klein, 2011); pride would likely strengthen these effects. These effects may also generalize to related behaviors, such as exercise, healthy nutrition, safer sex, and abstention from cigarette smoking. As such, pride seems an important emotion to leverage in interventions. Moreover, positioning interventions and communications in contexts where pride is facilitated by an outside source (e.g., sporting events or graduations) may increase their effectiveness.

Medical Decision Making

Both healthy individuals and those with illness or disease are faced with many decisions in a clinical encounter. All patients make decisions about preventive care and screening. Patients with illness or disease also face decisions about diagnostic procedures and treatments, as well as later decisions about adherence to treatment. These decisions, ideally, involve understanding information about risks and benefits, and negotiating those risks and benefits in the context of personal preference, values, and priorities. For this reason, depth of processing and risk perception are intimately related to medical decision making.

Moreover, medical decisions are often highly interpersonal. Clinical encounters can also involve weighing multiple treatment or preventive options, relevant to valuation and reward seeking. The decision maker has a team of providers and a network of invested family members, friends, and colleagues, extending the traditional conceptualization of a simpler dyadic patient–provider interaction. This network can actively contribute to decisions, and as such, interpersonal attributions are crucial determinants of the decision process and outcome. As with health decisions, the ATF may be leveraged to make predictions about which emotions may systematically influence particular medical decisions, allowing for a broad picture of which types of emotions help and hinder specific types of medical decisions.

Risk Perception and Communication

Because emotion influences perceptions related to disease risk (e.g., Lerner & Keltner, 2001; Peters, Burraston, & Mertz, 2004), anger and happiness should decrease, and fear increase, perceived susceptibility to disease risk in the context of medical decision making. Consistent with this prediction, basic research has demonstrated that mammography messages framed in terms of gains are more persuasive for happy, compared to sad, individuals (Keller et al., 2003; Wegener et al., 1994).

In practice, risks in medical decision making are relatively complex. Screening decisions involve weighing the risk of not detecting disease early when it is potentially easier to treat versus the risk of a false positive or of finding disease that would not be fatal (e.g., finding cancer in someone who will likely die of another cause before cancer could progress). Similarly, not undergoing genetic testing means a missed opportunity to address modifiable risk factors among those at high risk (e.g., more frequent mammograms or prophylactic mastectomy to reduce breast cancer risk), whereas testing means a risk of physical or psychological consequences associated with a positive result (e.g., dread associated with having the gene for Huntington's disease). Treatment decisions also carry risks that are difficult to equate and weigh—risks of drug side effects versus risks of the consequences of failure to adhere (e.g., disease progression or death). Emotions relevant to risk perception may influence these types of decisions differently depending on which risks are salient (e.g., risk of cancer vs. risk of side effects). Often, these trade-offs involve weighing overall risk and benefit rather than systematically integrating such information into the decision (Reyna, 2008, 2012).

In situations in which choosing a risky option is advantageous (e.g., a risky but high-reward treatment in absence of other options), the ATF would predict that anger would facilitate risk taking, whereas fear would hinder it. Similarly, in situations where the risk of a false-positive screening or detecting disease is salient and *not* screening is rendered a risk-averse behavior, anger would be more beneficial than fear. In contrast, in situations where choosing a risky option is not recommended (e.g., a risky treatment when other effective treatment options are available) or the risk of disease is salient in the context of a screening decision, fear should facilitate decision making, whereas anger should hinder it.

Valuation and Reward Seeking

Different types of treatment and preventive care can be subject not only to financial valuation but also to valuation of the treatment itself—that is, the features of the treatment, including potential benefit and fit with personal priorities and values. Thus, emotions that influence choices involving valuation, such as sadness and disgust, are relevant. Sadness decreases susceptibility to the status quo bias, compared to anger (Garg et al., 2005), ostensibly because sadness may trigger the action tendency of seeking a reward to fill a loss—essentially, an extension of demonstrated tendencies to trade away a current product for a new one (e.g., Lerner et al., 2004). This may have implications for treatment-related trade-offs between the status quo (e.g., living with disability) and undertaking treatment (e.g., having surgery). Similarly, some types of screening, such as colorectal cancer screening, can be done using multiple methods that involve trade-offs between invasiveness and accuracy (e.g., fecal occult blood test vs. colonoscopy); emotion may influence the ways in which these types of options are weighed and the decisions made in these contexts.

In decisions that involve choosing between types of treatment or screening, sadness may hinder decision making when the status quo is recommended, and optimize decision making when there is not a status-quo option. Extending this research, disgust could bias decisions toward refusing *any* treatment; as such, disgust could be anticipated to hinder treatment decision making (see Reyna et al., in press).

Interpersonal Attribution

Evidence on emotion and attribution suggests that emotions can systematically improve or degrade patient–provider interactions. Anger increases stereotyping (compared to sadness and fear; Bodenhausen et al., 1994a; DeSteno, Dasgupta, et al., 2004; Tiedens & Linton, 2001) and attributions of accountability (Lerner et al., 1998). Anger also decreases trust, whereas happiness and gratitude increase it (compared to sadness). Gratitude also increases advice taking (Dunn & Schweitzer, 2005). Thus, angry patients may be least likely to trust a physician and accept advice (e.g., adhere to recommended treatment) due to increased trust; however, a competing prediction would be that angry patients may be more likely to rely on the expertise of the physician as a heuristic. Patients experiencing gratitude or happiness should be most poised to make the best decisions in situations where the course of action is fairly straightforward, given high levels of trust and increased reliance on expertise, which could lead to adherence to physician recommendations. Conversely, sadness or fear would enhance decision making when recommendations are ambiguous and depend on personal values and priorities.

Emotions experienced by the provider during a clinical encounter can also bias patient decisions. This has implications for clinical encounters involving a patient with a condition that can be attributed to behavioral causes (e.g., lung cancer attributed to smoking or diabetes related to poor eating behaviors). Although healthcare providers are trained to avoid conveying blame to patients (e.g., Cegala & Broz, 2003), a provider may be more likely to attribute responsibility to a patient if the provider enters the clinical encounter in an angry state, which has the potential to lead to lower quality of care, poorer outcomes, and less satisfaction in the clinical encounter for those patients. Emotion also influences perspective taking; shame decreases perspective-taking ability compared to guilt, perhaps because shame is more self-focused (Yang, Yang, & Chiou, 2010). Hence, guilt should enhance, and shame attenuate, a provider's ability to empathize with a patient's situation or best understand the type of care or treatment plan for a given patient.

Depth of Processing

Given the tendency to process information more heuristically (System 1) and less systematically (System 2) depending on emotional state (Bodenhausen, Kramer, & Susser, 1994b; Mackie & Worth, 1989, 1991; Schwarz & Bless, 1991; Schwarz, Bless, & Bohner, 1991; Tiedens & Linton, 2001), individuals in emotional states that predispose processing styles influence health-related information in a clinical encounter. Although heuristic processing can be adaptive, in that it allows individuals to integrate more perceptual and cognitive information than would be possible with systematic processing, it can also lead to cognitive biases (Tversky & Kahneman, 1974), which can be detrimental when a decision is important. Thus, predisposition toward heuristic or systematic processing could have significant implications for health-related judgment and decision making, in that it could lead to less careful scrutiny of risks and benefits in informed consent, biasing treatment decisions. Indeed, research shows that emotion can induce heuristic information processing, particularly among men (although note that anger-induced heuristic processing can actually improve understanding and retention of information, as previously discussed; Ferrer et al., in press).

Clinical decision making offers an interesting context for examining the systematic influence of emotions in an ecologically valid context. For example, some clinical care decisions, such as colorectal cancer screening, can evoke disgust, which could systematically bias individuals in unrelated or tenuously related follow-up decisions. If screening is made salient immediately prior to a treatment decision, and disgust is elicited, it could lead to lower uptake of or adherence to that treatment given that disgust promotes disposal or pushing away. Similarly, Han et al. (2010) speculate that a cancer patient nauseated by chemotherapy might be too inclined to switch therapies, motivated by the disgust appraisal and disposal action tendency, rather than by intolerance for the nausea itself.

Policy Implications

Given the empirically and theoretically supported influence of emotion on health judgment and decision making, it is critical that research on this topic be considered in public policy. Advances in shaping health policy have recently benefited from behavioral economics (e.g., Johnson et al., 2012; Thaler & Sunstein, 2008), and incorporating emotion research into policy development may further these advances. In an era of rising healthcare costs, changing healthcare policy, and increased regulation of health-related products (e.g., tobacco products), research on emotion, judgment, and decision making needs to be incorporated into policy development. Because of the importance of these connections combined with the dearth of available research, we consider here possibilities for future research.

Importantly, research on emotion offers insights not only for policy development but also for understanding judgment and decision making among those who are contributing to policy. Research suggests that differences in political ideology may be due largely in part to individuals' moral judgments (Graham, Haidt, & Nosek, 2009), and that moral judgments have a strong affective component (Haidt, 2001). As such, policy decision making, particularly as it relates to policies that involve moral foundations, such as universal healthcare, are likely influenced by emotions.

Risk Perception

Many policy-level decisions are informed by expert risk evaluations. For example, experts within the Food and Drug Administration (FDA) inform decisions to approve various drugs based on evidence of efficacy and safety. Similarly, healthcare policy can be informed by decisions made by the U.S. Preventive Services Task Force (USPSTF), a government-appointed expert panel that makes recommendations for screening and other medical guidelines, based on thorough analysis of risks and benefits. Although previously summarized research demonstrates that discrete emotions influence risk perception and judgment under uncertainty, existing research has examined such judgments in the general population. Little is known about the role of emotion in expert risk judgments. For example, expert risk perceptions may be vulnerable to influence by fear or anger, with beneficial or deleterious consequences to the degree that policies are intended to be risk averse (or vice versa).

Emotion research may also hold the key to effectively implementing regulatory policy. The FDA's regulatory authority over tobacco[7] prohibits any use of terminology to imply tobacco products are lower risk, given that these claims are unsubstantiated (i.e., there is no evidence to suggest that smoking light cigarettes is less risky than smoking other types of cigarettes). Identifying explicit terminology (e.g., the use of "light," "low," and "moderate" as cigarette product descriptors) is relatively simple, but implicit strategies for conveying low risk are more difficult to identify. Research on emotion could help to identify advertisements that leverage visual or linguistic features to elicit emotions associated with certainty (e.g., happiness) that decrease risk perception.

Valuation and Reward Seeking

The FDA's regulatory authority over tobacco products also includes a mandate for graphic warning labels on cigarette packages. Research on emotion, valuation, and choice can lend insight into graphic labels that would be particularly effective (e.g., disgust, reducing valuation and subsequent consumption) versus counterproductive (e.g., sadness increasing valuation and subsequent consumption).

Research on emotion's role in intertemporal choice has lessons for policies facilitating behavioral prevention by identifying which communications and interventions have the most potential for effectiveness, as well as which modes of dissemination would work best. This could maximize government investments such as ongoing healthcare reform efforts in the United States[8] that include a $15 billion fund for prevention and public health programs. Health communications supported under this fund could be strategically matched with television programming that elicits emotions that would potentiate the effectiveness of advertisements (Garg et al., 2007). For example, messages promoting physical activity could be strategically placed to follow a pride-invoking scene (e.g., a scene in which a character reaches his or her full potential professionally or athletically). Conversely, such public health messaging may be less effective when disseminated during television programs that elicit sadness, given that reward-seeking action tendencies (e.g., Garg & Lerner, 2013) could override any health behavior intentions generated by health messaging.

Depth of Processing

Given that emotion influences depth of processing, emotion research could be leveraged to better communicate health recommendations and policy to the public. For example, better communication strategies for screening guidelines could decrease suspicious reactions to USPSTF recommendations (e.g., recommendations against screening tests such as prostate-specific antigen tests), which could have downstream implications for how the guidelines are implemented in policy. Particular visual cues (e.g., pictures used to prime affective states) could be embedded in such information to trigger emotions associated with improved processing, or such information could be strategically communicated in television programming known to elicit these emotions (e.g., sadness, triggering System 2 processing). Naturally, given the concern for decision autonomy, consumers should be informed about the use of such cues.

Evidence supports the possibility that emotion influences healthcare policy decisions, particularly as they relate to universal healthcare mandates. Sadness increases (and anger decreases) welfare given to hypothetical recipients (Small & Lerner, 2008), an effect driven by depth of processing; that is, thinking more in depth about the hypothetical welfare recipient triggered an increased willingness to lend aid in sad compared to angry participants. Thus, sadness and anger experienced by policy makers would be expected to influence healthcare reform policy decisions, such that sad (compared to angry) policy makers could be more likely to vote for policies mandating universal healthcare coverage policies.

Broad Future Directions

Broad research questions related to emotion and health-related decision making span prevention and promotion choices, as well as medical decision making. This research has the potential to inform health-related research and policy moving forward. A significant example of such a research question involves examining what happens when integral and incidental emotions conflict (e.g., when an individual enters an anxiety-provoking medical decision-making situation after feeling envious of someone in the waiting room), or when emotions are experienced in concert (e.g., sadness and fear; see Larsen, McGraw, Mellers, & Cacioppo, 2004; Peters et al., 2004). In instances in which mixed emotions arise, *both* emotional states may influence behavior concurrently or interactively (Lerner & Tiedens, 2006). However, there is a dearth of research on mixed emotions—such as sadness and anger as a result of a cancer diagnosis, or the meta-emotional state of being happy about the ability to express sadness (i.e., "to have a good cry"; Ersner-Hershfield, Mikels, Sullivan, & Carstensen, 2008). Preliminary research has suggested that inducing a contradictory emotion subsequent to an earlier induction is difficult (i.e., sadness blunted subsequent anger and vice versa: Winterich et al., 2010). Moreover, research is necessary to examine how emotions interact with other social psychological or self-related constructs to influence health behavior. For example, fear and anger may reduce the effectiveness of health interventions that rely on bolstering self-integrity (Ferrer, Koblitz, Klein, & Graff, in preparation). Additional research on the influence of blended emotions on health judgment and decision making is necessary.

In a separate line of inquiry, research is necessary to examine how emotions contribute to habitual or repeated behaviors (e.g., eating choices, smoking, medication adherence). Health behavior offers many promising avenues for extending the ATF to examine complex, real-world behavioral decisions potentially influenced by emotion. Further, ecologically valid health-related decision-making research could examine whether emotions influence familiar decisions in the same way they do novel decisions. Examining repeated choice would also allow for a better understanding of habituation to emotional influences themselves (e.g., repeated disgusting images on cigarette warning labels).

Another question concerns developmental differences in the influence of emotion. Research has demonstrated that individuals rely on affective processes increasingly in later stages of life (Peters, Diefenbach, Hess, & Vastfjall, 2008, Peters, Hess, Vastfjall, & Auman, 2007), potentially due to age-related deficits in the deliberative system that motivate increased reliance on affect and a learned reliance on affective or intuitive processing, which may be more efficient and advanced than deliberative processing (Peters et al., 2007, 2008; Reyna & Brainerd, 2011). Another line of research indicates that emotional influences on judgment and decision making may also be particularly salient in adolescence (Rivers et al., 2008; Steinberg, 2008), suggesting that the trajectory of emotional influence on decisions may take a U-shaped pattern, where influences are strongest earlier and later in life. Although research in these areas has focused largely on integral affective influences, it stands to reason that age may moderate the effects of emotion predicted by the ATF, such that emotion effects on judgment and decision making are stronger in adolescence and older age. Research is necessary to examine this possibility, especially in light of research on prefrontal changes and disinhibition in adolescence and old age. This research is particularly important in a health context, as risky behaviors and related health consequences are common in adolescence, and diseases are increasingly prevalent as individuals age.

A final broad future direction concerns leveraging knowledge about emotion and health decision making to facilitate personalized recommendations about health behaviors, screenings, or treatments. That is, health decisions can also be guided under a decision architecture that takes into account an individual's emotional profile (e.g., developmental influences, individual differences, and state emotions) currently contributing to an individual's emotional state and the likely patterns of judgment and decision making that will arise in that context. Knowing whether a person is fearful, angry, sad, or disgusted (or some combination of these) in a medical context, and understanding judgment and decision-making implications for such emotion states, has tremendous potential to improve outcomes by allowing healthcare providers the potential to tailor discussions about health behaviors, screenings, or treatments based on patients' emotional state. This may be particularly important in pain or symptom management, where affective beliefs substantially differentiate how patients approach key decisions (e.g., Falzer et al., 2013).

Taken together, this research synthesis indicates that systematic research on emotions and health-decision making can improve health and healthcare. The ATF provides a useful framework to systematically identify ways that specific emotions interact with the situation to engage decision processes that would improve or degrade decisions. This research has implications for understanding and motivating healthy behaviors and improving process of care and medical decisions, with currently undertapped future translational potential for improving quality, trajectory, and length of life.

Notes

1. See also http://www.pcori.org/about-us/landing/
2. We define emotion as a relatively brief affective reaction to a specific person, situation, or sensory stimuli (see Keltner & Lerner, 2010). Unlike moods, which tend to be viewed as less intense positive or negative affective states that are sustained over some period of time, we use the term *emotion* to refer to discrete categories of feeling state that differ not only in terms of valence but also on a variety of other cognitive appraisal dimensions (e.g., Smith & Ellsworth, 1985). Our use of emotion is closely related to the concept of an "emotion schema" (Izard, 2007).
3. Research has also examined how health behaviors might influence emotions, such as with exercise and positive affective outcomes (e.g., Hall, Ekkekakis, & Petruzzelo, 2002).
4. Although health researchers have advocated for small-scale experiments that isolate and control constructs in isolation (Suls et al., 2010), in practice this has not occurred with emotion inductions.
5. Guilt and pride had no influence, perhaps because they are not associated with the other-control dimension.
6. Research has also shown that generalized positive affect facilitates flexible thinking (Fredrickson, 2001; Isen, 2001), including by physicians (Estrada, Isen, & Young, 1997). These findings are somewhat contradictory to findings that happiness triggers heuristic processing (Bodenhausen et al., 1994a). There are several potential reasons for this discrepancy, including the possibility that positive affect inductions trigger discrete affective states other than happiness (e.g., gratitude). Indeed, in certain contexts, discrete positive emotion states (hope and pride) are associated with higher and lower levels of fluid processing, respectively (Cavanaugh Cutright, Luce, & Bettman, 2011). A complex discussion of these discrepant results is beyond the scope of this chapter.
7. See http://www.fda.gov/tobaccoproducts/default.htm
8. see http://www.healthcare.gov/

References

Addicott, A. K., Gray, J. J., & Todd, B. L. (2009). Mood, dietary restraint, and women's smoking and eating urges. *Women and Health, 49*, 310–320.

Ambady, N., & Gray, H. M. (2002). On being sad and mistaken: Mood effects on the accuracy of thin-slice judgments. *Journal of Personality and Social Psychology, 83*(4), 947.

Andrade, E. B., & Ariely, D. (2009). The enduring impact of transient emotions on decision making. *Organizational Behavior and Human Decision Processes, 109*, 1–8.

Barry, M. J., & Edgman-Levitan, S. (2012). Shared decision making—the pinnacle of patient-centered care. *New England Journal of Medicine, 366*(9), 780–781.

Bodenhausen, B. V., Kramer, G. P., & Susser, K. (1994b). Happiness and stereotypic thinking in social judgment. *Journal of Personality and Social Psychology, 66*, 621–632.

Bodenhausen, G. V., Sheppard, L. A., & Kramer, G. P. (1994a). Negative affect and social judgment: The differential impact of anger and sadness. *European Journal of Social Psychology, 24*, 45–62.

Bower, G. H. (1991). Mood congruity of social judgments. In J. P. Forgas (Ed.), *Emotion and social judgments* (pp. 31–53). Elmsford, NY: Pergamon Press.

Cavanaugh, L. A., Cutright, K. M., Luce, M. F., & Bettman, J. R. (2011). Hope, pride, and processing during optimal and nonoptimal times of day. *Emotion, 11*, 38.

Cegala, D. J., & Broz, S. L. (2003). Provider and patient communication skills training. In T. L. Thompson, A. M. Dorseym, K. I. Miller, & R. Parrott (Eds.), *Handbook of health communication*. London: Erlbaum.

Chaiken, S., Liberman, A., & Eagly, A. H. (1989). Heuristic and systematic information processing within and beyond the persuasion context. In J. S. Uleman & J. A. Bargh (Eds.), *Unintended thought* (pp. 212–252). New York: Guilford Press.

Chernev, A. (2011). The dieter's paradox. *Journal of Consumer Psychology, 21*(2), 178–183.

Chuang, S-C., & Lin, H-M. (2007). The effect of induced positive and negative emotion and openness-to-feeling in student's consumer decision making. *Journal of Business Psychology, 22*, 65–78.

Conner, M., & Norman, P. (1996). *Predicting health behaviour: Research and practice with social cognition models*. Maidenhead, UK: Open University Press.

Critchfield, T. S., & Kollins, S. H. (2001). Temporal discounting: Basic research and the analysis of socially important behavior. *Journal of Applied Behavior Analysis, 34*, 101–122.

Cryder, C. E., Lerner, J. S., Gross, J. J., & Dahl, R. E. (2008). Misery is not miserly: Sad and self-focused individuals spend more. *Psychological Science, 19*, 525–530.

Damasio, A. (1994). *Descartes error: Emotion, rationality and the human brain.* New York: Putnam.

DeSteno, D., Gross, J. J., & Kubzansky, L. (2013). Affective science and health: The importance of emotion and emotion regulation. *Health Psychology, 32*(5), 474.

DeSteno, D., Dasgupta, N., Bartlett, M. Y., & Cajdric, A. (2004b). Prejudice from thin air: The effect of emotion on automatic intergroup attitudes. *Psychological Science, 15*, 319–342.

DeSteno, D., Petty, R. E., Rucker, D. D., Wegener, D. T., & Braverman, J. (2004). Discrete emotions and persuasion: The role of emotion-induced expectancies. *Journal of Personality and Social Psychology, 86*(1), 43–56.

Dunn, J., & Schweitzer, M. (2005). Feeling and believing: The influence of emotion on trust. *Journal of Personality and Social Psychology, 6*, 736–748.

Ersner-Hershfield, H., Mikels, J. A., Sullivan, S. J., & Carstensen, L. L. (2008). Poignancy: Mixed emotional experience in the face of meaningful endings. *Journal of Personality and Social Psychology, 94*, 158–167.

Estrada, C. A., Isen, A. M., & Young, M. J. (1997). Positive affect facilitates integration of information and decreases anchoring in reasoning among physicians. *Organizational Behavior and Human Decision Processes, 72*(1), 117–135.

Falzer, P. R., Leventhal, H. L., Peters, E., Fried, T. R., Kerns, R., Michalski, M., & Fraenkel, L. (2013). The practitioner proposes a treatment change and the patient declines: What to do next? *Pain Practice, 13*, 215–226.

Ferrer, R. A., Dillard, A. J., & Klein, W. M. P. (2011). Projection, conformity and deviance regulation: A prospective study of alcohol use. *Psychology and Health, 27,* 688–703.

Ferrer, R. A., Stanley, J., Graff, K., Goodman, N., Nelson, W., Salazar, S., & Klein, W. M. P. (in press). The influence of emotion on the informed consent process in cancer clinical trials. *Journal of Behavioral Decision-Making.*

Fisher, E. B., Walker, E. A., Bostrom, A., Fischhoff, B., Haire-Joshu, D., & Johnson, S. B. (2002). Behavioral science research in the prevention of diabetes: Status and opportunities. *Diabetes Care, 25,* 599–606.

Ford, E. S., Zhao, G., Tsai, J., & Li, C. (2011). Low-risk lifestyle behaviors and all-cause mortality: Findings from the National Health and Nutrition Examination Survey III Mortality Study. *American Journal of Public Health, 101,* 1922–1929.

Forgas, J. P. (2003). Affective influences on attitudes and judgments. In R. Davidson, K. Scherer, & H. Goldsmith (Eds.), *Handbook of affective sciences* (pp. 596–618). New York: Oxford University Press.

Fredrickson, B. L. (2001). The role of positive emotions in positive psychology: The broaden-and-build theory of positive emotions. *American Psychologist, 56,* 218.

Frijda, N. H. (1986). *The emotions.* Cambridge, UK: Cambridge University Press.

Garg, N., Inman, J., & Mittal, V. (2005). Incidental and task-related affect: A re-inquiry and extension of the influence of affect on choice. *Journal of Consumer Research, 32,* 154–159.

Garg, N., & Lerner, J. S. (2013). Sadness and consumption. *Journal of Consumer Psychology, 23*(1), 106–113.

Garg, N., Wansink, B., & Inman, J. J. (2007). The influence of incidental affect on consumers' food intake. *Journal of Marketing, 71,* 194–206.

Gerend, M. A., & Maner, J. K. (2011). Fear, anger, fruits, and veggies: Interactive effects of emotion and message framing on health behaviors. *Health Psychology, 30,* 420–423.

Graham, J., Haidt, J., & Nosek, B. A. (2009). Liberals and conservatives rely on different sets of moral foundations. *Journal of Personality and Social Psychology, 96*(5), 1029.

Haidt, J. (2001). The emotional dog and its rational tail: a social intuitionist approach to moral judgment. *Psychological Review, 108*(4), 814.

Hall, E. E., Ekkekakis, P., & Petruzzello, S. J. (2002). The affective beneficence of vigorous exercise revisited. *British Journal of Health Psychology, 7,* 47–66.

Hammond, D., Fong, G. T., McDonald, P. W., Brown, S., & Cameron, R. (2004). Graphic Canadian cigarette warning labels and adverse outcomes: Evidence from Canadian smokers. *American Journal of Public Health, 94,* 1442–1445.

Han, S., Lerner, J. S., & Keltner, D. (2007). Feelings and consumer decision making: The Appraisal-Tendency Framework. *Journal of Consumer Psychology, 17,* 158–168.

Han, S., Lerner, J. S., & Zeckhauser, R. (2010). *Disgust promotes disposal: Souring the status quo.* Faculty Research Working Paper Series, RWP10-021. Boston: John F. Kennedy School of Government, Harvard University.

Hay, J. L., McCaul, K. D., & Magnan, R. E. (2006). Does worry about breast cancer predict screening behaviors? A meta-analysis of the prospective evidence. *Preventative Medicine, 42,* 401–408.

Holland, J. C. (2003). Psychological care of patients: Psycho-oncology's contribution. *Journal of Clinical Oncology, 21,* 253s–265s.

Ifcher, J., & Zarghamee, H. (2011). Happiness and time preference: The effect of positive affect in a random-assignment experiment. *American Economic Review, 101,* 3109–3129.

Isen, A. M. (1993). Positive affect and decision making. In M. Lewis & J. Haviland (Eds.), *Handbook of emotions,* (pp. 261–277). New York: Guilford Press.

Isen, A. M. (2001). An influence of positive affect on decision making in complex situations: Theoretical issues with practical implications. *Journal of Consumer Psychology, 11,* 75–85.

Isen, A. M., & Erez, A. (2007). Some measurement issues in the study of affect. In Ong, A. D., and Manfred, H. M. (Eds.), *Oxford handbook of methods in positive psychology* (pp. 250–265). New York: Oxford University Press.

Izard, C. E. (2007). Basic emotions, natural kinds, emotion schemas, and a new paradigm. *Perspectives on Psychological Science, 2,* 260–280.

Johnson, E. J., & Goldstein, D. (2003). Do defaults save lives? *Science,* 1338–1339.

Johnson, E. J., & Tversky, A. (1983). Affect, generalization, and the perception of risk. *Journal of Personality and Social Psychology, 45,* 20–31.

Johnson, E. J., Shu, S. B., Dellaert, B. G., Fox, C., Goldstein, D. G., Häubl, G., ... & Weber, E. U. (2012). Beyond nudges: Tools of a choice architecture. *Marketing Letters, 23*(2), 487–504.

Kahneman, D., & Tversky, A. (2000). *Choices, values, and frames.* New York: Cambridge University Press.

Keller, P. A., Lipkus, I. M., & Rimer, B. K. (2003). Affect, framing, and persuasion. *Journal of Marketing Research, 40,* 56–64.

Kelly, A. B., Masterman, P. W., & Young, R. M. (2011). Negative mood, implicit alcohol-related memory, and alcohol use in young adults: The moderating effect of alcohol expectancy. *Addictive Behaviors, 36,* 148–151.

Keltner, D., & Gross, J. J. (1999). Functional accounts of emotions. *Cognition and Emotion, 13*(5), 467–480.

Keltner, D., & Lerner, J. S. (2010). Emotion. In D. T. Gilbert, S. T. Fiske, & G. Lindzey (Eds.), *The handbook of social psychology* (pp. 317–352). New York: Wiley.

Khaw, K-T., Wareham, N., Bingham, S., Welch, A., Luben, R., & Day, N. (2008). Combined impact of health behaviours and mortality in men and women: The EPIC-Norfolk Prospective Population Study. *PLoS Medicine, 5,* e12.

Kunda, Z. (1987). Motivated inference: Self-serving generation and evaluation of casual theories. *Journal of Personality and Social Psychology, 53,* 636–647.

Larsen, J. T., McGraw, A. P., Mellers, B. A., & Cacioppo, J. T. (2004). The agony of victory and the thrill of defeat: Mixed emotional reactions to disappointing wins and relieving losses. *Psychological Science, 15,* 325–330.

Lazarus, R. S. (1991). Progress on a cognitive-motivational-relational theory of emotion. *American Psychologist, 46,* 819–834.

Lerner, J. S., Goldberg, J. H., & Tetlock, P. E. (1998). Sober second thought: The effects of accountability, anger, and authoritarianism on attributions of responsibility. *Personality and Social Psychology Bulletin, 24,* 563–574.

Lerner, J. S., Gonzalez, R. M., Small, D. A., & Fischhoff, B. (2003). Effects of fear and anger on perceived risks of terrorism: A national field experiment. *Psychological science, 14*(2), 144–150.

Lerner, J. S., Han, S., & Keltner, D. (2007). Feelings and consumer decision making: Extending the Appraisal-Tendency Framework. *Journal of Consumer Psychology, 17*(3), 181–187.

Lerner, J. S., & Keltner, D. (2000). Beyond valence: Toward a model of emotion-specific influences on judgment and choice. *Cognition and Emotion, 14*, 473–493.

Lerner, J. S., & Keltner, D. (2001). Fear, anger, and risk. *Journal of Personality and Social Psychology, 81*, 146–159.

Lerner, J., Li, Y., & Weber, E. (2013). The financial cost of sadness. *Psychological Science, 21*(1), 72–79.

Lerner, J. S., Li, Y., Valdesolo, P., & Kassam, K. (2015). Emotion and decision making. *Annual Review of Psychology, 66*, 799–823.

Lerner, J. S., Small, D. A., & Loewenstein, G. F. (2004). Heart strings and purse strings: Carry-over effects of emotions on economic transactions. *Psychological Science, 15*, 337–341.

Lerner, J. S., & Tiedens, L. Z. (2006). Portrait of the angry decision maker: How appraisal tendencies shape anger's influence on cognition. *Journal of Behavioral Decision Making, 19*, 115–137.

Loewenstein, G. F., & Lerner, J. S. (2003). The role of affect in decision making. In R. Davidson, K. Scherer, & H. Goldsmith (Eds.), *Handbook of affective science* (pp. 619–642). New York: Oxford University Press.

Loewenstein, G. F., Weber, E. U., Hsee, C. K., & Welch, N. (2001). Risk as feelings. *Psychological Bulletin, 127*, 267–286.

Loxton, N. J., Dawe, S., & Cahill, A. (2011). Does negative mood drive the urge to eat? The contribution of negative mood, exposure to food cues and eating style. *Appetite, 56*, 368–374.

Luce, M. F. (1998). Choosing to avoid: Coping with negatively emotion-laden consumer decisions. *Journal of Consumer Research, 24*(4), 409–433.

Mackie, D. M., & Worth, L. T. (1989). Processing deficits and the mediation of positive affect in persuasion. *Journal of Personality and Social Psychology, 57*, 27–40.

Mackie, D. M., & Worth, L. T. (1991). Feeling good, but not thinking straight: The impact of positive mood on persuasion In J. P. Forgas (Ed.), *Emotion and social judgments* (pp. 201–219). Elmsford, NY: Pergamon Press.

Marteau, T. M., Ogilvie, D., Roland, M., Suhrcke, M., & Kelly, M. P. (2011). Judging nudging: Can nudging improve population health? *British Medical Journal, 342*, d228.

Moons, W. G., & Mackie, D. M. (2007). Thinking straight while seeing red: The influence of anger on information processing. *Personality and Social Psychology Bulletin.*

Narula, T., Ramprasad, C., Ruggs, E. N., & Hebl, M. R. (2013). Increasing colonoscopies? A psychological perspective on opting in versus opting out. *Health Psychology, 33*(11), 1426–1429.

Ostafin, B. D., & Brooks, J. J. (2011). Drinking for relief: Negative affect increases automatic alcohol motivation in coping-motivated drinkers. *Motivation and Emotion, 35*, 285–295.

Pearson, T. A., Blair, S. N., Daniels, S. R., Eckel, R. H., Fair, J. M., ... Taubert, K. A. (2002). AHA guidelines for primary prevention of cardiovascular disease and stroke: 2002 update. *Circulation*, *106*, 388–391.

Perkins, K. A., Ciccocioppo, M., Conklin, C. A., Milanek, M., Grottenthaler, A., & Sayette, M. A. (2008). Mood influences on acute smoking responses are independent of nicotine intake and dose expectancy. *Journal of Abnormal Psychology*, *117*, 79–93.

Peters, E., Burraston, B., & Mertz, C. K. (2004). An emotion-based model of stigma susceptibility: Appraisals, affective reactivity, and worldviews in the generation of a stigma response. *Risk Analysis*, *24*, 1349–1367.

Peters, E., Dieckmann, N. F., Västfjäll, D., Mertz, C. K., Slovic, P., & Hibbard, J. (2009). Bringing meaning to numbers: The impact of evaluative categories on decisions. *Journal of Experimental Psychology: Applied*, *15*, 3, 213–227.

Peters, E., Hess, T. M., Vastfjall, D., & Auman, C. (2007). Adult age differences in dual information processes: Implications for the role of affective and deliberative processes in older adults' decision-making. *Perspectives on Psychological Science*, *2*, 1–23.

Peters, E., Lipkus, I., & Diefenbach, M. A. (2006). The functions of affect in health communications and in the construction of health preferences. *Journal of Communication*, *56*, S140–S162.

Peters, W., Diefenbach, M. A., Hess, T. M., & Vastfjall, D. (2008). Age differences in dual information-processing modes: Implications for cancer decision-making. *Cancer*, *113*, 3556–3567.

Petty, R. E., & Cacioppo, J. T. (1986). The elaboration likelihood model of persuasion. *Advances in Experimental Social Psychology*, *19*, 123–205.

Portnoy, D. B., Ferrer, R. A., Bergman, H. E., & Klein, W. M. (2013). Changing deliberative and affective responses to health risk: A meta-analysis. *Health Psychology Review*, *8*(3), 296–318.

Raghunathan, R., & Pham, M. T. (1999). All negative moods are not equal: Motivational influences of anxiety and sadness on decision making. *Organizational Behavior and Human Decision Processes*, *79*, 56–77.

Reyna, V. F. (2008). A theory of medical decision making and health: Fuzzy-trace theory. *Medical Decision Making*, *28*(6), 850–865. doi:10.1177/0272989X08327066

Reyna, V. F. (2012). A new intuitionism: Meaning, memory, and development in fuzzy-trace theory. *Judgment and Decision Making*, *7*(3), 332–359.

Reyna, V. F., & Brainerd, C. J. (2011). Dual processes in decision making and developmental neuroscience: A fuzzy-trace model. *Developmental Review*, *31*, 180–206.

Reyna, V. F., Chick, C. F., Corbin, J. C., & Hsia, A. N. (2014). Developmental reversals in risky decision-making: Intelligence agents show larger decision biases than college students. *Psychological Science*, *25*(1), 76–84.

Reyna, V. F., & Farley, F. (2006). Risk and rationality in adolescent decision-making: Implications for theory, practice, and public policy. *Psychological Science in the Public Interest*, *7*, 1–44.

Reyna, V. F., Nelson. W. L., Han, P. K., & Pignone, M. P. (2015). Decision making and cancer. *American Psychologist*, *70*(2), 105.

Rivers, S. E., Reyna, V. F., & Mills, B. A. (2008). Risk taking under the influence: A fuzzy-trace theory of emotion in adolescence. *Developmental Review, 28,* 107–144.

Rothman, A. J., Baldwin, A. S., & Hertel, A. W. (2004). Self-regulation and behavior change: Disentangling behavioral initiation and behavioral maintenance.

Rothman, A. J., Kelly, K. M., Hertel, A. W., & Salovey, P. (2003). Message frames and illness representations: Implications for interventions to promote and sustain healthy behavior.

Scherer, K. R. (1988). Criteria for emotion-antecedent appraisal: A review. In V. Hamilton, G. H. Bower, & N. H. Frijda (Eds.), *Cognitive perspectives on emotion and motivation* (pp. 89–126). New York: Kluwer Academic/Plenum Publishers.

Schwarz, N., & Bless, H. (1991). Happy and mindless, but sad and smart? The impact of affective states on analytic reasoning. In J. P. Forgas (Ed.), *Emotion and social judgments* (pp. 55–71). Elmsford, NY: Pergamon Press.

Schwarz, N., Bless, H., & Bohner, G. (1991). Mood and persuasion: Affective states influence the processing of persuasive communications. *Advances in Experimental Social Psychology, 24,* 161–199.

Schwarz, N., & Clore, G. L. (1983). Mood, misattribution, and judgments of well-being: Informative and directive functions of affective states. *Journal of Personality and Social Psychology, 45,* 513.

Slovic, P. (1987). Perception of risk. *Science, 236,* 280–285.

Slovic, P., Finucane, M. L., Peters, E., & MacGregor, D. G. (2002). Rational actors or rational fools: Implications of the affect heuristic for behavioral economics. *Journal of Socio-Economics, 31,* 329–342.

Small, D. A., & Lerner, J. S. (2008). Emotional policy: Personal sadness and anger shape judgments about a welfare case. *Political Psychology, 29*(2), 149–168.

Smith, C. A., & Ellsworth, P. C. (1985). Patterns of cognitive appraisal in emotion. *Journal of Personality and Social Psychology, 48,* 813–838.

Steinberg, L. (2008). A social neuroscience perspective on adolescent risk-taking. *Developmental Review, 28,* 78–106.

Stefanek, M. E., Andrykowski, M. A., Lerman, C., Manne, S., Glanz, K., on behalf of the AACR Behavioral Sciences Task Force. (2009). Behavioral oncology and the war on cancer: Partnering with biomedicine. *Cancer Research, 69,* 7151–7156.

Suls, J. M., Luger, T., & Martin, R. (2010). The biopsychosocial model and the use of theory in health psychology. In J. M. Suls, K. W. Davidson, & R. M. Kaplan (Eds.), *Handbook of health psychology and behavioral medicine* (pp. 15–27). New York: Guilford Press.

Tiedens, L. Z., & Linton, S. (2001). Judgment under emotional certainty and uncertainty: the effects of specific emotions on information processing. *Journal of Personality and Social Psychology, 81,* 973–988.

Thaler, R. H., & Sunstein, C. R. (2008). *Nudge.* Yale University Press.

Tversky, A., & Kahneman, D. (1974). Judgment under uncertainty: Heuristics and biases. *Science, 185,* 1124–1131.

van Dalen, H. P., & Henkens, K. (2014). Comparing the effects of defaults in organ donation systems. *Social Science and Medicine, 106,* 137–142.

Wansink, B., & Chandon, P. (2006). Can "low-fat" nutrition labels lead to obesity?. *Journal of Marketing Research, 43*(4), 605–617.

Wansink, B., Cheney, M. M., & Chan, N. (2003). Exploring comfort food preferences across age and gender. *Physiology and Behavior, 79*(4–5), 739–747.

Weary, G., & Jacobson, J. A. (1997). Causal uncertainty beliefs and diagnostic information seeking. *Journal of Personality and Social Psychology, 73*, 839–848.

Weiner, B. (1986). *An attributional theory of motivation and emotion.* New York: Springer-Verlag.

Wegener, D. T., Petty, R. E., & Klein, D. J. (1994). Effects of mood on high elaboration attitude change: The mediating role of likelihood judgments. *European Journal of Social Psychology, 24*, 25–43.

Williams, L. A., & DeSteno, D. (2008). Pride and perseverance: The motivational role of pride. *Journal of Personality and Social Psychology, 94*, 1007–1017.

Wilson, T. D., & Gilbert, D. T. (2003). Affective forecasting. *Advances in Experimental Social Psychology, 35*, 345–411.

Winterich, K. P., Han, S., & Lerner, J. S. (2010). Now that I'm sad, it's hard to be mad: Examining emotion-state transitions. *Personality and Social Psychology Bulletin, 36*, 1467–1483.

Witte, K., & Allen, M. (2000). A meta-analysis of fear appeals: Implications for effective public health campaigns. *Health Education and Behavior, 27*(5), 591–615.

Yang, M-L., Yang, C-C., & Chiou, W-B. (2010). When guilt leads to other orientation and shame leads to egocentric self-focus: Effects of differential priming of negative affects on perspective taking. *Social Behavior and Personality, 38*, 605–614.

5 | Social Norms, Beliefs, and Health

BRENT MCFERRAN

THE EFFECTS OF SOCIAL NORMS—how others act in a given situation—are powerful and have been shown to influence a range of behaviors. Research has found that a host of health behaviors are affected by norms, including exercise behaviors (e.g., John & Norton, 2012), smoking (e.g., Christakis & Fowler, 2008), alcohol and drug usage (e.g., Graham, Marks, & Hansen, 1991), wearing helmets while cycling or skiing, wearing seatbelts, and risky sex (see Sunstein, 1996). Yet most people are largely unaware of the impact these social influences have on their behavior, frequently reporting they have little or no impact, when their actual behavior suggests otherwise (Nolan, Schultz, Cialdini, Goldstein, & Griskevicius, 2008).

In this chapter, I focus on the role social norms play in contributing to one of the world's greatest public health problems: obesity. Although high rates of obesity persist in much of the Western world, many developing nations are quickly catching up (Ng et al., 2014; WHO, 2013). Obesity is a multidetermined problem, but an increase in human caloric consumption has been identified as the primary culprit, and social forces may be playing an important role in shaping dietary decisions. The influence of social forces on eating behavior can take many forms: a person can be influenced by the food choices of others, cultural cuisines (e.g., high-calorie, nutrient-poor foods) can spread from one culture to another, what is perceived as a "normal" body weight is shaped by cultural norms and context, and beliefs about what causes obesity are socially transmitted. This chapter begins by providing an overview of social norms research and sources of influence at a broad level. I then narrow the scope to focus on food consumption and weight gain. Throughout, I discuss how social norms are contributing to society's weight gain, as well as where some of these norms (and beliefs that underlie these norms) may originate.

Social Norms

Norms are, broadly speaking, how others act in a given situation. Research on social norms consistently shows that the behaviors of others in a group strongly influence our own behavior. In perhaps its simplest form this is called "social proof" (sometimes used synonymously with informational social influence, or descriptive norms). This refers to our tendency to look to the behavior of others to determine the appropriate course of judgment or action in a given situation. We interpret the behavior of others as providing information on what should be done in a given situation, and we often act in accordance. Documentation of such effects goes back to at least the 1930s (Sherif, 1936). Because the actions of a majority group shape people's perception of what the "norm" is (e.g., Cialdini & Trost, 1998; Goldstein, Cialdini, & Griskevicius, 2008), our behavior often follows suit. For example, if we are in a group setting and observe that everyone is choosing an obviously wrong answer (Asch, 1956) or littering (Cialdini, 2003), we frequently behave in accordance with the norm that has been established (e.g., also choosing the wrong answer or littering). In social proof, no explicit feedback is needed regarding the social (dis)approval of a given behavior to affect others' behavior—simply the observation of this behavior. The power of social proof underlies a whole host of phenomena, from the wisdom of crowds (i.e., group decisions can often be relied upon to be more accurate than those of individuals; see Surowiecki, 2004) to the usage of laugh tracks (i.e., "canned" background laughter) in television. The purpose of the latter is to increase viewers' enjoyment with the program; if they hear others laughing, it serves as a cue that the viewer should as well, or at the very least it cues that the content is funny to others.

Norms take other forms beyond simply descriptive ones. Cialdini, Reno, and Callgren (1990) lay out two types of norms: descriptive norms (what most others do) and injunctive norms (what most others view as "good" or "bad"). An example of the latter would be a disapproving glare from others for using foul language around children. The descriptive/injunctive distinction is important because invoking different types of norms can have different effects. For many, simply being told that you drink much more than the average person (a descriptive norm) is motivating for cutting back. This social effect has been shown to be particularly strong if the group is somewhat large (versus small, Latane, 1981), similar to us (Goldstein et al., 2008), or one in which we feel close to (or aspire to be like). The more appealing or important a group is to an individual, the more powerful the norms to conform to their behavior can be, a finding with support dating back over 60 years (Festinger, Schachter, & Back, 1950).

Although norms can encourage healthier behaviors, they can also have what is called a boomerang effect. For example, one potential effect of being told you are "below average" (a descriptive norm) on an undesirable behavior (e.g., frequent drinking) could be an increased engagement in that very behavior (e.g., Schultz, Nolan, Cialdini, Goldstein, & Griskevicius, 2007, see also White & Simpson, 2013). Broadly, social norms can shift a person's choices towards the group average, or what is sometimes called the "magnetic middle," which at an individual level can be good or bad. In one example of the boomerang effect, Schultz and colleagues (2007) found that telling people (via a message hung on their doorknobs) they used less energy than their neighbor caused them to subsequently increase their energy usage. This is similar to a related phenomenon, termed *moral licensing*, where feeling that one is doing well in one domain (or acting morally) can cause one to feel "licensed" to make poorer (or immoral) subsequent decisions because of previous virtuous choices (see Khan & Dhar, 2006; Monin & Miller, 2001; Mazar & Zhong, 2010). To then counter the energy usage boomerang effect, Schultz and colleagues (2007) layered an injunctive norm on top of the descriptive one (using a handwritten :) or :(on a subsequent note hung to their door), suggesting (dis)approval for high(low) usage compared to one's peers. The simple addition of a smiley face (an injunctive norm) attenuated the increased usage shown by those who were merely told that they were using less power than their neighbors (a descriptive norm).

Although social norms can be powerful influencers, it is important to remember when designing public health interventions that our behavior does not strongly follow the norms set by those we dislike or with whom we do not aspire to be associated (McFerran, Dahl, Fitzsimons, & Morales, 2010a, 2010b; White & Dahl, 2006, 2007). For instance, when undergraduates were told that a disliked reference group (online gamers) eat junk food frequently, participants' actual junk food consumption declined (Berger & Rand, 2008). In another study (John & Norton, 2013), providing public information about the amount others around them exercised decreased some people's actual exercise behavior, suggestive of the fact that participants were merely looking for an excuse *not* to exercise. Seeing other low exercisers may have licensed them to do just that.

There is also a disconnect that sometimes exists between a person's belief about what is normal or appropriate (the norm) and people's public behavior. An individual's (typically private) attitudes sometimes do not match his or her (generally public) behavior, a state known as pluralistic ignorance. We also tend to assume that social norms are more universal than they are (Prentice & Miller, 1993), and that people's attitudes and beliefs are more homogeneous than is true in reality (e.g., everyone binge drinks, or everyone thinks it is acceptable). One reason why norms have a strong effect is that over time, this disconnect is often resolved by internalizing the norm, and bringing attitudes, norms, and one's own behaviors into consistency. Prentice and Miller (1993) showed this in the context of binge drinking, with the norm exerting an effect on students' drinking behavior—meaning that drinking increased because of a (false) belief that it was normative and desirable to do so. In a related study, Schroeder and Prentice (1998) attempted to combat this effect through messaging. Incoming freshman students were exposed to a video and discussion sessions on alcohol. The discussion either centered on how an individual can make responsible choices (individual-oriented condition) or on pluralistic ignorance and its implications (peer-oriented condition). Four to six months later, students' self-reported drinking was assessed, with those in the peer-oriented condition reporting lower consumption levels, likely because the strength of the drinking norm was reduced in that condition from the treatment.

Social Norms in Food Choice

Although examples of the power of norms are plentiful, they are highly poignant in the domain of food. It has been argued that social influences are a "major, if not the preeminent, influence on eating behavior" (Johnston, 2002, p. 21; see also de Castro, 1994; Goldman, Herman, & Polivy, 1991). There are several sources of social influence in food. First, the presence of others can affect our eating behavior by conveying a norm or making certain norms salient. Second, there are norms set by other peoples' actual choices that affect our own, which are perhaps the strongest norms. Third, the portions offered by those serving us set norms. Fourth, societal norms for different body types can affect our consumption choices. Finally, there are normative beliefs about what causes obesity, which in turn influence behavior. In what follows, I review work in all of these areas.

The Presence of Others

Given we eat most meals in the company of others, research on social norms and eating behavior has centered on understanding how others' presence affects our own food choices. Although the studies presented next examine, largely in experimental settings, how others affect our consumption, there is also evidence that social influences affect food choices and preferences that may precede actual consumption. For example, choices made by parents early on can shape children's food preferences later in life (Birch & Fisher, 1998). Similarly, partners' dietary preferences and requirements almost inevitably affect the other party. If one lives with a vegetarian, the other will likely find himself or herself eating meat less often. Such effects aside, even when the food selection has already been made, social influences play a considerable role in shaping eating behavior.

Social influences can have either a facilitating or attenuating effect on eating behavior, depending on various contextual factors (see Herman, Roth, & Polivy 2003 for a review). Several studies have shown that eating with others (vs. alone) leads to an increase in consumption, called "social facilitation" (e.g., de Castro, 1990, 1994; see also Conger, Conger, Costanzo, Wright, & Matter, 1980; Johnston, 2002; Rosenthal & Marx, 1979). One explanation for this finding is that, with others, the duration of the meal is longer. Not surprisingly, people dine more slowly with others than when eating by themselves, which translates into an increase in consumption. For example, de Castro finds that people eat about 35% more calories if they eat with just one other person, and nearly twice as much in a group of seven or more (de Castro 1990, 1994; de Castro & de Castro, 1989). This facilitation effect is even stronger with friends and family than with other companions. However, there is also research showing the opposite (Herman et al., 2003). In eating, as in other life domains, we aim to project an impression or adhere to social norms (Leary & Kowalski, 1990; Roth, Herman, Polivy, & Pliner, 2001). In many Western cultures, making a good impression might mean eating less, rather than more, when in the company of others. It may be more socially inappropriate to order dessert when no one else does than to pass when others order. This behavior is also often seen among those with eating disorders who frequently binge when they are by themselves and then eat minimally in the company of others (Herman & Polivy, 1980). Further, binge eating itself is influenced by social norms. Crandall (1988) found that among sorority members, an individual's binge eating could be predicted by that of her peers, an effect that got stronger as the peer groups became more cohesive. He argues that like many other behaviors, the spread of binge eating over time can be linked to social forces.

Food Norms Set by the Choices of Others

A second social force is the norm set by those with whom we are eating. If others eat more, we do as well. If everyone orders an appetizer, we are much more likely to do so ourselves, even if we are not particularly hungry. This has been demonstrated in a large number of experiments known as modeling or mimicry studies. In the general paradigm, a confederate and a single subject participate in a study "together." The confederate's food choice is directly manipulated in a manner that the subject notices, such as by having him or her select food first in full view of the subject. The researchers then assess the subsequent choice of the subject (see Herman et al., 2003). These studies consistently show that the norm set by the confederate has a powerful effect on the participant's food choices, in both directions: When the confederate chose and/or ate a large portion, participants were more likely to choose and/or eat more than they otherwise would if alone, and they ate less if the confederate opted for a smaller portion. Further, the norms set by others are so powerful that the confederate does not even have to be physically present. A few studies (e.g., Roth et al., 2001) have used a "remote confederate paradigm," where it is merely suggested (on a piece of paper visible to participants) what others took in previous sessions, to the same effect. In short, the initial choice of the confederate sets an "anchor," which the participant subsequently uses to inform his or her choice. Further, participants rarely report being aware of this source of social influence.

Groups (rather than individuals) may also set norms, and these norms are probably more powerful than individuals, as social pressure increases with group size to some degree. As the group size increases, no one wants to stand out, and people increasingly conform to the group average (Bell & Pliner, 2003). Accordingly, Wansink (2006) recommends that if you are a light eater, you should eat by yourself, and if you eat heavily, you should seek out a group. I would add that if one is concerned about overeating in the presence of others, ordering before others do in a social setting means you set the norm (or anchor) for others to follow.

One's society or culture is perhaps the broadest type of group influence. As immigrants move to places with higher rates of obesity, they tend to gain weight (Goel, McCarthy, Phillips, & Wee, 2004), suggesting that they are adopting the dietary norms prevalent in their environment, and this effect is stronger among those who have a stronger motivation to fit in. One study (Guendelman, Cheryan, & Monin, 2011) showed that pressure felt by immigrants to fit in led them to report a more "American" (and higher calorie) food as their favorite, as well as to select and consume more of these foods when their identity as an American was threatened. Such a finding is consistent with a social identity (Oyserman, Fryberg, & Yoder, 2007) model of health, as food choice is a signal of one's identity to the self and others (Barthes, 1997). Similarly, underprivileged consumers chose smaller sized snacks when they believed that being fit was a status symbol. However, the effect was reversed when being overweight was perceived as a signal of status (Dubois, Rucker, & Galinsky, 2012). Finally, there are other norms, such as eating all of the food one puts on his or her plate, or buying large portions in bulk, which can vary by regions or households but clearly affect intake (Wansink, 2006; Wansink, Payne, & Chandon, 2007). These norms are powerful and can even supersede human physiology; for instance, people who select larger portions tend to eat more than those given small portions, a fact that holds true even when the food does not taste good or consumers are not hungry (Wansink, 2006).

The Body Type of Others

A third source of social influence in food choice is the body type of the other person (or people) consuming alongside us. The modeling or mimicry studies often do not manipulate this factor, assuming the norm is set by the food choice of the other person, irrespective of his or her body type. However, some research suggests the body type of others exerts its own independent (or interactive) influence. Generally there are two types of studies: ones that examine the effect of another person's body type on our food choices when that person is not eating with us, the other examines the effect of eating with others whose body types and food portion sizes are both manipulated. Campbell and Mohr (2011)'s work is one example of the former. They show that priming people with images of overweight consumers (but not obese ones) has been shown to lead to an increase in quantity consumed. Although using different methods, Christakis and Fowler (2007; but see Cohen-Cole & Fletcher, 2008, for a rebuttal) found that a person's chance of becoming obese significantly increased when a close other (e.g., friend, sibling, spouse) became obese. This suggests that social forces or norms regarding body types might lead to a social contagion of weight gain. In a different paradigm, McFerran et al. (2010b) sought to answer the question of whether the body type of a server influences diners' food consumption. We also examined the role of recommendations made by this person (i.e., an indulgent choice or something very healthy). To test this, we used an obesity prosthesis so the same confederate played both a normal-weight and an obese individual. All participants were female. We found opposite effects for dieters and nondieters. Although nondieters ate more when the confederate was thin, dieters ate more snacks when the confederate was heavy. A second study examined only dieters and found that when cookies were recommended by the server, participants chose cookies more often when the server was heavy than when she was thin, but when carrots were recommended, they selected cookies with a greater frequency when she was thin than when she was heavy. Instead of shunning the recommendation of the obese server, dieters were *more* persuaded by her recommendation, choosing both the healthy and the unhealthy snack more often when it was recommended to them. Together, these show that people's food choices (and even body masses) may be shaped not only by what others, eat but also by the body type of others who are merely physically present or in our social network (see also McFerran, Dahl, Fitzsimons, & Morales, 2011).

A final set of studies examines others' choices and their body types simultaneously. Johnston (2002) manipulated both the body type of the confederate and her portion size choice and found the typical modeling effect: People ate more as the confederate's portion size increased. However, the effect was somewhat attenuated when the other was obese: People refrained from indulging when seeing an obese person do so. McFerran et al. (2010a) did something similar: We had the confederate (portraying either a thin or heavy patron, again using an obesity prosthesis) first take a food selection (small or large), and then we measured what the participant subsequently took and ate. There was also a control condition where participants were alone. We replicated the modeling finding that after seeing a large portion (i.e., a high anchor) chosen by the other, people adjusted their consumption downward from the high-quantity anchor to a greater degree when the confederate was obese than when she was thin. However, we also found that rather than further decrease consumption when seeing an obese person choose a small portion, participants increased their portion choice, meaning they adjusted upward from a low anchor when the confederate was obese more than when she was thin. In other words, participants consistently followed the anchor that the confederate set more closely when she was thin than when she was heavy. We argued that these results could be explained parsimoniously based on anchoring and adjustment (Wansink, Kent, & Hoch, 1998): People anchor on the quantities others around them select, but these portions are adjusted according to the body type of the other consumer. A final study showed the adjustment from the anchor was more pronounced for consumers low versus high in appearance self-esteem (Heatherton & Polivy, 1991) and is attenuated when cognitive processing resources are constrained. Together, these studies suggest that social norms regarding portion sizes can strongly impact the food we consume, and that body types of others do matter.

Social Norms and Body Types

There are also strong social norms regarding body types, which can be broken down into descriptive (what most people's actual bodies look like) and injunctive (what most people view as acceptable or ideal). It is clear that these two types of norms are frequently in conflict.

In a descriptive sense, it has been widely reported that the average population in almost all Western countries is getting heavier. In fact, in the United States, over two thirds of adults are either overweight or obese (CDC, 2004), literally making being overweight normal or "average" in the statistical sense. Indeed, the normality of being overweight has been noted many places, including a recent *Huffington Post* report entitled "Is Overweight the New Normal Weight?" (Upton, 2011). In the descriptive sense of norms, being overweight or obese is normative, but that does not necessarily mean it is "desirable" or even "socially acceptable." Those terms are injunctive, meaning they place a value judgment on the behavior, labeling it as "good" or "bad" in some way. There is some support for the idea that the perceived normality of obesity has also increased. One study (Dumas, Sciacca, Decolongon, Rodriguez, & Giardina, 2011) has shown that approximately half of mothers with overweight children erroneously perceive their children as being of normal weight. A 2010 Harris Interactive/HealthDay poll with 2,418 US-based adults found that 30% of overweight people think they are actually normal size, 70% of obese people feel they are merely overweight, and 39% of morbidly obese people think they are overweight but not obese (Harris Interactive, 2010). Research on descriptive norms suggests the situation may worsen because such perceptions can exacerbate the problem. As overweight bodies become more common, it is the person of normal weight who appears not to fit in (which could cause him or her to eat more). In turn, those who are overweight are now, statistically speaking, "normal" and therefore might have a reduced desire to lose weight. Further research on this is needed.

Body type norms can also be shaped by media exposure. There is wide concern that advertising images convey a different and concerning norm: namely, that it is desirable to be very thin. Academics have noted that exposure to thin and "unrealistic" (including digitally altered) images in the media can be detrimental to body image, body-esteem, and both physical and mental health (e.g., Clay, Vignoles, & Dittmar, 2005; Halliwell & Dittmar, 2005; Martin & Kennedy, 1993; Myers & Biocca, 1992; Stice & Shaw 1994; for a review, see Groesz, Levine, & Murnen, 2002). The American Medical Association also recently released a statement emphasizing the importance of advertisers acting responsibly when advertising to youth because digitally altering images (e.g., by slimming the model) can "contribute to unrealistic expectations of appropriate body image" (AMA, 2011, http://www.ama-assn.org/ama/pub/news/news/a11-new-policies.page).

In addition to the (largely descriptive) norms set up by the images themselves, there are explicit statements with divergent messages by producers of fashion images. These statements use injunctive norms to suggest being overweight is either socially unacceptable or acceptable. Statements like "beautiful at any size" suggest that it is acceptable to be overweight. Although there are documented negative effects of overly thin models on their viewers, such models remain the (descriptive) norm. However, some marketers have bucked this trend in recent years. Several firms have launched campaigns that use larger models, arguing that they are more representative of the "average" woman. Perhaps the most well-known example is Dove's "Real Beauty" campaign, in which overweight and obese models were featured with the tagline, "real women with real curves." Similarly, The Body Shop's "Love Your Body" campaign featured the image of an overweight Barbie doll and the tagline, "there are 3 billion women who don't look like supermodels and only 8 who do." Some interpret these campaigns as celebrating the normality of overweight bodies. These ads in effect suggest another (injunctive) norm: Suggesting the models are more "normal," "real," or "authentic" conveys a value judgment about what a normal body looks like (or should look like). Beyond advertising, Debanhams (a large UK department store chain) now features (US) size 14 mannequins in department stores, as does Åhléns, the largest department store chain in Sweden. Several mainstream magazines (e.g., *Elle, Vogue*) have featured overweight actresses or models on the cover recently. Other government and nonprofits have undertaken ad campaigns aimed at suggesting all body types are normal and acceptable (e.g., the "No body shame" campaign).

Generally the campaigns, policies, and images that set out to enhance women's body-esteem and protect consumers from exposure to unrealistic images have been widely applauded (Rappaport, 2011; Simmons, 2006). This is presumably because people believe such efforts (a) reduce the stigma and prejudice felt by consumers with larger bodies (Crandall, 1994), (b) discourage consumers from "chasing" a thin body for themselves that they likely can never attain, and/or (c) encourage consumers to be happy with their present body type, even if it is overweight. Interestingly, while public reaction toward normalizing overweight bodies seems to be positive (even though most recognize obesity as a public health concern), most people are abhorred by "thinspiration" (pro-ana [anorexia]) Web sites, often on the grounds that such Web sites normalize or glorify eating disorders (Heffernan, 2008). I should note, however, that such websites, beyond promoting extreme thinness, also promote other harmful eating behaviors that introduce their own health consequences.

Although there is scant research on the effects of "normalizing" obesity, a wealth of research from other domains suggests that the normalizing of a behavior or concept has consequences such as reducing the stigma or negativity associated with it. This can result in its increased pervasiveness. For example, when originally introduced by Louis Réard in 1946, the bikini bathing suit was deemed so inappropriate that the designers had to hire stigmatized individuals (e.g., showgirls) to model it ("The history of the bikini," 2013). Now, of course, the bikini is completely normalized; there is virtually no stigma to adults wearing it. In addition, social commentators and researchers have noted that carrying a large debt load has become more normalized and socially acceptable. This results in consumers justifying poor financial choices, and it may have contributed to the financial crisis (Peñaloza & Barnhart, 2011). One important property of social norms is that they need not be true in any objective sense to have an influence. For instance, people may make poorer financial decisions because they correctly know others do so as well (e.g., data show a consistent rise in US household debt; Federal Reserve Board, 2008) or because they simply feel that others are also taking out massive debt loads (e.g., a few salient friends mention doing so). Both of these social norms would likely increase people's willingness to take on additional debt.

One study (Lin & McFerran, 2014) examines normalizing explicitly and shows that exposure to models with body types that are more representative of the "average" weight (i.e., overweight) shifts perceptions of how normal and acceptable it is to be overweight. We also show that "normalizing" obesity can lower people's intentions to exercise and eat well, as well as increase their actual unhealthy eating behavior. This suggests that the incidence of obesity should also rise as it becomes more normal and socially acceptable, at least partly because the stigma associated with it dissipates.

The opposite of normalizing is, of course, stigmatizing. There are many strong social stigmas, such as powerful norms against polygamy and incest. While clearly not as stigmatized as incestuous relationships, people who are obese are still subject to considerable stigma and prejudice (e.g., Bacon, Scheltema, & Robinson, 2001; Crandall, 1994; Puhl & Heuer, 2009; Puhl & Latner, 2007). For example, obesity is associated with poorer job prospects and those who are obese earn less money (Organisation for Economic Cooperation and Development [OECD], 2012). Some organizations perpetuate this norm through their messaging. The rationale behind "fat shaming" campaigns is that the stigma may be leveraged to motivate overweight individuals to lose weight. For example, the "Strong4Life" campaign from Children's Healthcare of Atlanta, which featured photos of overweight children and taglines such as "Warning. . . . It's hard to be a little girl if you're not" (Johnson, 2012). Shaming also manifests itself more subtly: Abercrombie & Fitch does not carry XL and XXL size clothing and the company's CEO, Mike Jeffries, stated that his company's clothing should only be worn by attractive individuals (Lutz, 2013a). Similarly, the former chairperson of Lululemon, Chip Wilson, stated that their pants "don't work on some women's bodies" and the brand has placed larger size clothing items in the back of the store, which could be perceived as stigmatizing overweight customers (Lutz, 2013b). However, research tends to show that fat shaming is unlikely to be an effective strategy for most individuals. It is associated with social isolation and rejection. These feelings may enhance overeating and psychological stress, and decrease the pursuit of other healthy behaviors (Friedman & Puhl, 2012; Puhl & Brownell, 2001, 2003, 2006; Puhl & Heuer, 2010).

It is interesting and relevant to contrast obesity with smoking. In brief, smoking is now a stigmatized behavior in many places (see Bayer, 2008). Some have argued (e.g., Bell, Salmon, Bowers, Bell, & McCullough, 2010) that stigmatizing (or "denormalizing") has been used by public health officials in two ways: attacking the behavior (e.g., campaigns aimed at highlighting the risk of smoking to the self and others, restricting where tobacco can be sold or marketed, and through the banning of smoking in many public places) and attacking the industry (e.g., demonize the tobacco industry, expose industry marketing tactics). At least a few differences between smoking and obesity are notable. First, the food industry is much more fragmented and there are many likely "culprits." Second, smoking (the behavior) and tobacco (the industry) have been actively stigmatized more so than smokers (the people) in messaging. In many ways it is hard to draw a parallel to food here: Obesity is an outcome, while smoking is an activity; people clearly need to eat, but nobody needs to smoke. Third, there now exist many policies (such as clean indoor air laws, advertising bans, and tobacco taxes) that have helped individuals stop the behavior. Currently, there are few policies to support individuals in making healthy eating habits. Unlike smokers, obese consumers are subject to stigma in an environment that does a poor job of helping them change the behavior that is the basis of the stigma. Given that normalizing and stigmatizing obesity may both lead to potentially negative outcomes, at least for some, more research is clearly needed on the best media and public health messaging to promote health. It will be important to gain a greater understanding of how the interaction between society's changing body types and social norms influence health behaviors.

Beliefs About the Underlying Causes of Obesity

Obesity is a complex problem with many causes. These causes can generally be divided into three main sources that each play some role: factors that affect intake (diet), factors that affect energy expenditure (exercise), and genetic factors. However, there is growing scientific consensus that diet plays a more important causal role in obesity than physical activity or genes. The conclusion that overnutrition is the primary cause of obesity is based on many scientific studies across the globe (e.g., Pontzer et al., 2012). The *Journal of the American Medical Association* in a recent editorial concluded, "clearly, environmental causes of obesity are far more influential than genes ... Obesity results from overnutrition and the primary therapeutic target is preventing or reversing overeating. . . . Exercise is associated with weight loss but its duration or intensity has minor effects on weight loss relative to diet" (Livingston & Zylke, 2012; see also Hays et al., 2002; Jakicic, Marcus, Gallagher, Napolitano, & Lang, 2003; Swinburn, Caterson, Seidell, & James, 2004).

Why are exercise and genes thought to be less crucial than diet? First, it is simply impossible for the human genome to have morphed over

20 years to fully explain the rapid change in obesity rates (Comuzzie & Allison, 1998; Stunkard, Harris, Pedersen, & McClearn, 1990), and people's activity levels have remained stable over decades while obesity rates have increased (Young & Nestle, 2002). Immigrants also gain weight in proportion to the number of years they have been in the United States, suggesting the cause cannot be fully attributed to genes (Goel et al., 2004). Further, from 1980 to 2000 the number of people who self-report that they regularly exercise actually increased from 47% to 57%, and gym memberships in the United States nearly doubled from 1993 to 2009 (Cloud, 2009). Other empirical studies suggest that people are burning as many calories today as in the early 1980s (Westerterp & Speakman, 2008). Of course, regular exercise is beneficial in many ways, but when it comes to weight loss, it does not help to the same degree as dietary changes.

Even if it were possible to substantially increase the duration or intensity of one's exercise, for most people, it would simply be easier to shed those calories through intake rather than expenditure. It is much easier to simply skip the can of soda than to jog for an hour to burn it off. Almost no one has enough waking hours to burn off the 8,000 calories in the Quadruple Bypass burger at Heart Attack Grill restaurants (approximately 9 hours of swimming for someone weighing 150 lb, for example). Further, efforts to increase one's exercise are often accompanied by an increase in caloric intake as well. This can happen because the body is using more energy and thus people feel hungrier, or because people sometimes reward themselves for the exercise efforts with extra caloric intake (e.g., Church et al., 2009). This additional intake can result in a net caloric increase, rather than decrease, from exercise (Sonneville & Gortmaker, 2008). In sum, although exercise rates are relatively stable, Americans now eat at least 200 more calories a day on average than they did in 1980 (e.g., CDC, 2004). Unfortunately, the quality of food may have also declined over this time with an increase in eating away from home at places offering high-calorie food low in nutritional content. In summary, medical consensus shows that diet is a stronger predictor of obesity than either exercise or genetics, but has this knowledge passed down to laypeople? Do regular citizens know this to be the case? Such a question is important because word of mouth and folk wisdom are transmitted through an individual's social circle, shaping the lay beliefs of others, and the beliefs about the causes of obesity have a bearing on eating behaviors and weight gain.

Lay Beliefs

Lay theories are implicit assumptions that ordinary people hold about themselves and their world (Dweck, 1996). People have lay theories (sometimes called "naïve beliefs" or "common-sense" beliefs) about the causes and consequences of various phenomena. These beliefs may or may not dovetail with scientific or empirical facts. For example, some laypeople believe that larger objects fall more quickly or that higher priced products always have higher quality. Information and beliefs diffuse throughout cultures and individuals' smaller social networks get communicated through a variety of channels.

We tested the lay theories people have about the causes of obesity (McFerran & Mukhopadhyay, 2013, see also Brogan & Hevey, 2009; Dryer & Ware, 2014; Harvey, Summerbell, Kirk, & Hills, 2002; Ogden & Flanagan, 2008; Okonkwo & While, 2010), and as with many lay theories, there is considerable variance. We conducted six separate surveys in four different countries to determine the extent to which people indict diet, exercise, and/or genes as causes of obesity.

Across the studies, we used different question formats to assess people's lay theories. For example, sometimes we asked people to choose the primary cause in their minds, from a list of diet, exercise, or genetics. In others, we asked them to allocate 100 points among these factors according to how culpable they believed each to be. We also used a scale item as well as an open-ended measure to ensure that we were not simply suggesting "preferred" alternatives to respondents.

In one study, typical of the set, a nationally representative sample of South Koreans was asked to indicate what they believed to be the *primary* cause of obesity: eating too much, not exercising enough, or genetics. Diet theorists, that is, people who have a lay theory that poor diet is the primary cause of obesity, accounted for 50% of the respondents, exercise theorists for 41%, and gene theorists for 8%. The pattern across the studies suggests that only a little more than half the population holds beliefs in line with the scientific literature. This percentage was, perhaps not surprisingly, much higher among a sample of family physicians.

These results are similar to a 2004 US poll conducted by Harris Interactive. In their sample of 2,275 adults, a large majority (83%) blamed a lack of exercise for the obesity epidemic, while only 34% chose excessive calorie consumption. In sum, although medical research has come to a fairly decisive conclusion about the relative importance of a proper diet, many people believe (often erroneously) that they can exercise their way to a normal weight.

Why Do These Beliefs Matter?

Are there consequences of a misbelief about the cause of obesity? Other research on lay theories suggests there should be. Lay theories are guides to behavior. If I believe that I am doing poorly in school because I am not trying hard enough, under sufficient motivation I should be likely to try harder, since my belief suggests that this is the appropriate course of action. If, however, I believe I am doing poorly because I lack intelligence, then I view my effort as less consequential, and I am less likely to put in more time. Across several domains (including food), research has shown that lay theories significantly impact judgments and behaviors (Dweck, 1996).

In the domain of obesity, a belief that a lack of exercise is the cause of obesity should result in pursuit of weight loss by increasing the amount of physical exertion one puts forth. A diet belief should result in aiming to lose (or maintain) weight via reducing one's caloric intake. Given research that changing one's diet is likely to be more effective in weight-loss efforts, we expected that people's actual body mass should be predicted by their lay theory (among other factors). In other words, since lay theories should affect caloric intake (we also tested this), and other research shows intake is a strong predictor of body mass, one's mere beliefs about the cause of obesity should predict an individual's body mass. In several studies we found empirical support for the hypothesis that diet theorists should have lower body mass than exercise theorists. This relationship held even after controlling for numerous other variables known to be associated with body mass index. Further, supplementary studies showed that reverse causation was unlikely to contribute to our effect.

These results were also corroborated by at least one polling agency. In 2010, Harris Interactive/HealthDay found in a US-based adult sample of 2,418 people that "Most respondents who felt they were heavier than they should be blamed lack of exercise as the main cause, with 52% of overweight people, 75% of obese people and 75% of morbidly obese people saying they did not exercise enough. Food consumption was seen as the lesser of two culprits, with 36% of overweight respondents, 48% of obese respondents and 27% of morbidly obese feeling that they ate more than they should in general" (Harris Interactive, 2010, http://www.

harrisinteractive.com/NewsRoom/HarrisPolls/tabid/447/mid/1508/arti-cleId/558/ctl/ReadCustom%20Default/Default.aspx).   Another   study showed that stronger beliefs in genes as a cause of obesity was associated with lower exercise levels and lower consumption of fruits and vegetables (Wang & Coups, 2010). Others have shown that beliefs about the cause of obesity can have effects beyond influencing body mass. For example, Monterosso and colleagues (2005) showed that the stigma associated with overeating (and presumably obesity more generally) was attenuated if a genetic cause was given for an individual's obesity.

Where Do the Lay Beliefs Come From?

Lay theories are real, varied, and important, but where do they originate (or perpetuate, or propagate)? A variety of sources play a role, includ-ing people's social and cultural environments (Morris, Menon, & Ames, 2001). If your friends and family tell you how to lose weight, we often assume that they are credible sources of information. In addition, popular media and corporate communications play a role in influencing people's lay theories of why people are overweight (and/or how best to combat being overweight). Given the amount of public discussion about obesity, it is likely that most people, overweight or not, have arrived at some personal beliefs about the causes of obesity.

Indeed, a quick Internet search reveals outright contradictory views about obesity from popular media headlines:

"Exercise holds key to keeping weight off" (Colihan, 2008)

"An hour of daily exercise 'needed to stay slim'" ("An hour of . . ." 2010)

"Why exercise won't make you thin" (Cloud, 2009)

"Diet not exercise, plays role in weight loss" (LiveScience, 2009)

"Researchers identify 'fat gene' associated with obesity" (Jiang, 2014)

"Scientists debunk so-called fat gene" (Helm, 2007)

Although people's lay theories about the cause of obesity are likely shaped by many sources, there is a role for public health communications to more accurately shape these beliefs. At a simple level, we know from decades of human judgment and decision making that we place greater emphasis on salient exemplars we encounter. People will say, "She eats whatever she wants and does not gain weight," suggesting that diet may not play as much of a role as genes or exercise. Of course, such a statement makes wide judgments about the rest of the person's consumption throughout the week, which is almost certainly unobserved. When we see overweight (or thin) people and their parents, siblings, or children who also look similar, we may conclude that genes really matter, even though the similar body masses are likely also due to the fact that such individuals have similar dietary and exercise habits. Finally, we may observe someone who looks very fit and is frequently at the gym and conclude that his or her exercise is the key to keeping the weight off. Again, many fitness professionals do not simply exercise; they eat well, too, but because most eating is unobserved, it is easy to discount its importance.

We argue (Karnani, McFerran, & Mukhopadyay, 2014) that this (mis) information about the causes of obesity is spread and diffused into the public both unintentionally and intentionally. Because weight loss is an important goal, we share (and seek out) advice from others. Well-meaning people tout their (often short-term) success on the latest fad diet or exercise plan. Some of these suggest you can eat anything you want, so long as you follow a set exercise plan. Journalists often report stories and headlines that only loosely resemble the study they are reporting on, or they ignore other relevant papers in making sweeping generalities. Making errors or simplifying the science can play a role in shaping the discourse about the causes of obesity, a discussion that is shared and disseminated socially as we aim to quench our thirst for more information on the topic.

We (Karnani et al., 2014) argue as well for a more malignant source of misinformation about what is responsible for obesity. Specifically, we make the case that food and beverage industry corporations are motivated to deflect the spotlight away from their own products, some of which are the calorie-dense, nutrient-poor offerings that contribute to obesity in the first place. Although every food company in its corporate social responsibility statement proclaims its commitment to be a part of the solution to the obesity epidemic, at the same time, the food companies have a fiduciary responsibility to their shareholders to target growth and increase profits, the majority of which come from unhealthy offerings. This creates a dilemma for the food companies, and the profit motive most often dominates. Indeed, our research suggests corporate messaging is a prominent source of false messages regarding the probable causes of obesity. We contend the food industry's messaging—which emphasizes the importance of exercise in maintaining a healthy weight—is far from unbiased and is inconsistent with the scientific evidence.

Specifically, we argue that communication and promotional activities of the food companies reveal a concerted effort to deflect attention from bad diet and on to exercise (and other factors) as the causes of obesity. We call this effort, overlaid as it is with the theme of social responsibility, "leanwashing." We argue that leanwashing manifests itself in several ways. One is focused messaging and public statements about how exercise rather than diet causes obesity, or at the very least emphasize the importance of "energy balance." A second is to actively sponsor events that encourage exercise (playgrounds, sporting events, and athletes) and promote this as a solution to obesity. A third is to lobby aggressively against any effort on the part of government to reduce or ban the sale of unhealthy food, including by painting such efforts as infringing on personal choice and freedoms. The end result is misinformation about the causes of obesity, and an impaired understanding of what measures might be expected to have the highest efficacy in combatting it.

Conclusions

This chapter underscores the importance of understanding the influence of social norms and beliefs in the context of obesity, and it highlights some of the research that has been conducted in the area. Obesity is serious and costly in many terms. When items such as production losses (e.g., from missed work days) are added to healthcare costs, obesity accounts for over 1% of GDP in the United States, or over $150 billion (OECD, 2012). Beyond economic, there are also social and psychological costs that are considerable. It is unlikely that obesity for most people stems from a lack of motivation. Despite its normality, weight gain still seems to be some-thing most people want to avoid. It is frequently noted as the most common New Year's resolution. The dieting industry is growing, not shrinking, and is now worth over $40 billion annually in the United States alone (Reisner, 2008; Sherrid, 2003). Approximately one third of all women and a quar-ter of all men are on a diet (Crossen, 2003; Fetto, 2002) in the United States. If obesity frequently does not stem from a lack of motivation, there must be other causes. I suggest that social norms and misinformation are two important contributors to weight gain among a host of other factors. Although correcting false information might be easier than changing social norms, it might not be as efficacious, and indeed some of the misinforma-tion is shared socially as well.

There are a range of ways in which social norms influence eating. Understanding how social norms influence people opens up an opportu-nity for public health to leverage this information to combat obesity. First, although we are susceptible to normative influence, implied in that statement is that we also contribute to influence. When we serve a meal for others, we set the tone for the meal. When we choose to serve ourselves first, we set the anchor (or norm) for others to follow. An individual can put himself or herself in situations to not only eat smaller portions but also to influence others to do so as well. This works even better if we use smaller plates (see http://www.smallplatemovement.org). As mentioned earlier, seeking out groups to eat with that you know eat more modest portions might be helpful if you are concerned about overeating. However, by doing so you potentially remove yourself from eating with a different group, for whom you might serve as a positive influence as well.

Some of the norms discussed in this chapter are clearly widespread and cultural. A skeptic might argue that an individual is in little position to make changes that are large enough to affect others (indeed, perhaps not even himself or herself). Although there are clearly many important environmental factors to obesity, research suggests that local norms are more powerful than more global ones. In a seminal paper, Goldstein et al. (2008) show that norms set by a smaller set of individuals (guests staying in this hotel room) set a more powerful norm than those set by larger groups (guests of the hotel). Simply framing the norm more locally resulted in more prosocial behavior (i.e., towel reuse). Similarly, when eating, the norms set by those dining with us (particularly if we are similar to them or we wish to emulate them) are likely to be much more powerful than what "society" eats. The choices we make do matter in the world of those around us.

I also discuss some social norms associated with body weight. The fact that obesity may have reached a tipping point in terms of its normality is a large societal concern. This "normality" is interesting in that most social epidemics (e.g., fads) are popular and desirable when they spread widely. There seems to be little evidence suggesting that the normality of obesity has even led to reduced prejudice against the overweight, let alone widespread desire to gain weight. But what are some of the consequences of normalization, and where does it originate? Clearly more research is needed before these questions can be answered definitively.

Relatedly, what messaging is most useful to support public health? Current messaging takes many forms, as I note earlier. Some messages suggest being overweight is normal (in a descriptive sense) by using overweight models. Others suggest that being overweight is (or is not) acceptable in a more overt, injunctive sense. Research is clearly needed to understand if, when, and to whom each of the messages is effective.

For instance, the receiver can interpret a message like "real beauty" in several ways. It could promote body esteem, suggest that many people are obese, suggest it is OK to be overweight, or some combination thereof. Putting faces to bodies has been used in other disease campaigns, usually to reduce the stigma people hold against those who have the disease (e.g., HIV). Here lies a different scenario than HIV, however: There is little someone with HIV can do to reduce his or her HIV. And we would never dream of normalizing HIV if we thought it might increase the incidence rates of actual HIV. Of course, stigmatizing either the obese or those with HIV is likely to be problematic and ineffective for a whole host of reasons noted earlier. It is important to pretest messaging strategies and focus them on target audiences, as some messages that are effective for one group can be ineffective (or even counterproductive) for another.

I highlighted some concerns about normalizing obesity but also some known drawbacks of stigmatizing it. How can this be reconciled? One possibility is that more messaging about obesity is simply problematic in and of itself. In other words, steps taken to normalize or stigmatize may both be detrimental to public health. It could be that drawing attention to any body (large, small, or medium sized) and stating it is some normative standard is likely a poor idea. Ads like the Dove Real Beauty campaign draw attention to body types (even with noble intentions), increasing its psychological salience. We know from research in social psychology that the more attention that is devoted to something, the more of a focus and source of concern it can become (Wegner, Schneider, Carter, & White, 1987), and the more consumers find themselves struggling with self-regulation. It very well may be that efforts to normalize *or* stigmatize bodies are both increasing weight and body shape concerns, which can lead to either over- or undereating (Groesz, Levine, & Murnen, 2002; Polivy & Herman, 2002). From the perspective of norms, it might be more effective for public health to promote *behaviors* as normative, rather than promote a certain body type. Having generations chase a thin ideal has contributed to eating disorders, psychological challenges, and backfire effects (e.g., binge eating). Suggesting instead that it is normative to eat vegetables and smaller portions might be more effective messaging to reduce unhealthy eating. This merits further examination.

Finally, while I have I have focused on obesity in this chapter, the principles underlying social norms and beliefs likely apply across a range of health behaviors. Public health policies and interventions play a role in shaping what is normative. Using tools that shape social norms should play an important part in reducing obesity and other public health problems worldwide. However, when designing norm-based interventions, one must be mindful that they can lead to stigmatization and various unintended (and potentially harmful) consequences if not done carefully and evaluated rigorously.

References

American Medical Association (AMA). (2011). *Body image and advertising to youth.* Retrieved November 2013, from http://www.ama-assn.org/ama/pub/news/news/a11-new-policies.page

An hour of daily exercise needed to stay slim. (2010). *BBC News.* Retrieved February 2015, from http://news.bbc.co.uk/2/hi/health/8586767.stm

Asch, S. E. (1956). Studies of independence and conformity. A minority of one against a unanimous majority. *Psychological Monographs, 70*, 1–70.

Bacon, J. G., Scheltema, K. E., & Robinson, B. E. (2001). Fat phobia scale revisited: The short form. *International Journal of Obesity, 25*, 252–257.

Barthes, R. (1997). Toward a psychosociology of contemporary food consumption. In C. Counihan & P. Van Esterik (Eds.), *Food and culture: A reader* (pp. 20–27). New York, NY: Routledge.

Bayer, R. (2008). Stigma and the ethics of public health: Not can we but should we. *Social Science and Medicine, 67*, 463–472.

Bell, K., Salmon, A., Bowers, M., Bell, J., & McCullough, L. (2010). Smoking, stigma and tobacco 'denormalization': Further reflections on the use of stigma as a public health tool. A commentary on Social Science & Medicine's Stigma, Prejudice, Discrimination and Health Special Issue (67: 3). *Social Science and Medicine, 70*, 795–799.

Bell, R., & Pliner, P. L. (2003). Time to eat: The relationship between the number of people eating and meal duration in three lunch settings. *Appetite, 41*, 215–218.

Berger, J., & Rand, L. (2008). Shifting signals to help health: Using identity signaling to reduce risky health behaviors. *Journal of Consumer Research, 35*, 509–518.

Birch, L. L., & Fisher, J. O. (1998). Development of eating behaviors among children and adolescents. *Pediatrics, 101*, 539–549.

Brogan, A., & Hevey, D. (2009). The structure of the causal attribution belief network of patients with obesity. *British Journal of Health Psychology, 14*(1), 35–48.

Campbell, M. C., & Mohr, G. S. (2011). Seeing is eating: How and when activation of a negative stereotype increases stereotype-conducive behavior. *Journal of Consumer Research, 38*, 431–444.

Centers for Disease Control and Prevention. (2004). *National Health and Nutrition Examination Survey.* Retrieved February 2015, from http://www.cdc.gov/nchs/nhanes.htm

Christakis, N. A., & Fowler, J. H. (2007). The spread of obesity in a large social network over 32 years. *New England Journal of Medicine, 357*, 370–379.

Christakis, N. A., & Fowler, J. H. (2008). The collective dynamics of smoking in a large social network. *New England Journal of Medicine, 358*, 2249–2258.

Church, T. S., Martin, C. K., Thompson, A. M., Earnest, C. P., Mikus, C. R., & Blair, S. N. (2009). Changes in weight, waist circumference and compensatory responses with different doses of exercise among sedentary, overweight postmenopausal women. *PLoS One, 4*, e4515.

Cialdini, R. B. (2003). Crafting normative messages to protect the environment. *Current Directions in Psychological Science, 12*, 105–109.

Cialdini, R. B., Reno, R. R., & Kallgren, C. A. (1990). A focus theory of normative conduct: Recycling the concept of norms to reduce littering in public places. *Journal of Personality and Social Psychology, 58*, 1015–1026.

Cialdini, R. B., & Trost, M. R. (1998). Social influence: Social norm, conformity, and compliance. In D. T. Gilbert, S. T. Fiske, & G. Lindzey (Eds.), *Handbook of social psychology* (Vol. 2, pp. 151–192). New York, NY: McGraw-Hill.

Clay, D., Vignoles, V. L., & Dittmar, H. (2005). Body image and self esteem among adolescent girls: Testing the influence of sociocultural factors. *Journal of Research on Adolescence, 15*, 451–477.

Cloud, J. (2009). Why exercise won't make you thin. *Time.* Retrieved February 2015, from http://content.time.com/time/magazine/article/0,9171,1914974,00.html

Cohen-Cole, E., & Fletcher, J. M. (2008). Is obesity contagious? Social networks vs. environmental factors in the obesity epidemic. *Journal of Health Economics, 27*, 1382–1387.

Colihan, K. (2008). Exercise holds key to keeping weight off. *WebMD.* Retrieved February 2015, from http://www.webmd.com/diet/news/20080728/exercise-holds-key-to-keeping-weight-off

Comuzzie, A. G., & Allison, D. B. (1998). The search for human obesity genes. *Science, 280*(5368), 1374–1377.

Conger, J. C., Conger, A. J., Costanzo, P. R., Wright, L. K., & Matter, J. A. (1980). The effect of social cues on the eating behavior of obese and normal subjects. *Journal of Personality, 48*, 258–271.

Crandall, C. S. (1988). Social contagion of binge eating. *Journal of Personality and Social Psychology, 55*, 588–598.

Crandall, C. S. (1994). Prejudice against fat people: Ideology and self-interest. *Journal of Personality and Social Psychology, 66*, 882–894.

Crossen, C. (2003, July 16). Americans are gaining, but 'ideal' weight keeps shrinking. *Wall Street Journal,* Retrieved March 24, 2015, from http://www.wsj.com/articles/SB105830232931443000

de Castro, J. M. (1990). Social facilitation of duration and size but not rate of the spontaneous meal intake of humans. *Physiology and Behavior, 47*, 1129–1135.

de Castro, J. M. (1994). Family and friends produce greater social facilitation of food intake than other companions. *Physiology and Behavior, 56*, 445–455.

de Castro, J. M., & de Castro, E. S. (1989). Spontaneous meal patters of humans: Influence of the presence of other people. *American Journal of Clinical Nutrition, 50*, 237–247.

Dryer, R., & Ware, N. (2014). Beliefs about causes of weight gain, effective weight gain prevention strategies, and barriers to weight management in the Australian population. *Health Psychology and Behavioral Medicine, 2*, 66–81.

DuBois, D., Rucker, D. D., & Galinsky, A. (2012). Super size me: Product size as a signal of status. *Journal of Conusmer Research, 38*, 1047–1062.

Dumas, N. E., Sciacca, R. R., Decolongon, J., Rodriguez, J. K., & Giardina, E. V. (2011). *Obese and overweight women, children underestimate true weight.* Poster Session, American Heart Association's Nutrition, Physical Activity and Metabolism/ Cardiovascular Disease Epidemiology and Prevention Scientific Session, March 22–25, Atlanta, GA.

Dweck, C. S. (1996). Implicit theories as organizers of goals and behavior. In P. M. Gollwitzer & J. A. Bargh (Eds.), *The psychology of action: Linking cognition and motivation to behavior* (pp. 69–90). New York, NY: Guildford Press.

Federal Reserve Board. (2008). *Flow of funds accounts of the United States: Flows and outstandings 2005-2008.* http://www.federalreserve.gov/releases/z1/20091210/annuals/a2005-2008.pdf

Fetto, J. (2002). A moment on the lips. *American Demographics, 24,* 18.

Festinger, L., Schachter, S., & Back, K. (1950). *Social pressure in informal groups.* New York, NY: Harper & Row.

Friedman, R. R., & Puhl, R. M. (2012). *Weight bias. A social justice issue: A policy brief.* New Haven, CT: Rudd Center for Food Policy and Obesity, Yale University.

Goel, M. S., McCarthy, E. P., Phillips, R. S., & Wee, C. C. (2004). Obesity among US immigrant subgroups by duration of residence. *Journal of the American Medical Association, 292,* 2860–2867.

Goldman, S. J., Herman, P. C., & Polivy, J. (1991). Is the effect of social influence on eating attenuated by hunger? *Appetite, 17,* 129–140.

Goldstein, N. J., Cialdini, R. B., & Griskevicius, V. (2008). A room with a viewpoint: Using social norms to motivate environmental conservation in hotels. *Journal of Consumer Research, 35,* 472–482.

Graham, J. W., Marks, G., & Hansen, W. B. (1991). Social influence processes affecting adolescent substance abuse. *Journal of Applied Psychology, 76,* 291–298.

Groesz, L. M., Levine, M. P., & Murnen, S. K. (2002). The effect of experimental presentation of thin media images on body satisfaction: A meta-analytic review. *International Journal of Eating Disorders, 31,* 1–16.

Guendelman, M. D., Cheryan, S., & Monin, B. (2011). Fitting in but getting fat: Identity threat and dietary choices among US immigrant Groups. *Psychological Science, 22,* 959–967.

Halliwell, E., & Dittmar, H. (2005). The role of self-Improvement and self-evaluation motives in social comparisons with idealised female bodies in the media. *Body Image, 2,* 249–261.

Harris Interactive. 2010. *Overweight? Obese? Or normal weight? Americans have hard time gauging their weight.* Retrieved February 2015, from http://www.harrisinteractive.com/vault/HI-Harris-Healthday-Weight-2010-09-02.pdf

Harvey, E. L., Summerbell, C. D., Kirk, S. F. L., & Hills, A. J. (2002). Dieticians' views of overweight and obese people and reported management practices. *Journal Human Nutrition and Dietetics, 15,* 331–347.

Hays, N., Bathalon, G. P., McCrory, M. A., Roubenoff, R., Lipman, R., & Roberts, S. B. (2002). Eating behavior correlates of adult weight gain and obesity in healthy women aged 55–65. *American Journal of Clinical Nutrition, 75,* 476–483.

Heatherton, T. F., & Polivy, J. (1991). Development and validation of a scale for measuring state self- esteem. *Journal of Personality and Social Psychology, 60,* 895–910.

Heffernan, V. (2008). The girls of thinspo. *The New York Times*. Retrieved January 2014, from http://themedium.blogs.nytimes.com/2008/04/30/the-girls-of-thinspo/

Helm, J. (2007). Scientists debunk so-called "fat gene." *ABC News*. Retrieved February 2015, from http://abcnews.go.com/Health/Diet/story?id=2802503&page=1

Herman, C. P., & Polivy, J. (1980). Restrained eating. In A. J. Stunkard (Ed.), *Obesity* (pp. 208–225). Philadelphia, PA: Saunders.

Herman, C. P., Roth, D. A., & Polivy, J. (2003). Effects of the presence of others on food intake: A normative interpretation. *Psychological Bulletin, 129*, 873–886.

Jakicic, J. M., Marcus, B. H., Gallagher, K. I., Napolitano, M., & Lang, W. (2003). Effect of exercise duration and intensity on weight loss in overweight, sedentary women: A randomized trial. *Journal of American Medical Association, 290*, 1323–1330.

Jiang, K. (2014), Researchers identify fat gene associated with obesity. *UChicago News*. Retrieved February 2015, from http://news.uchicago.edu/article/2014/03/14/researchers-identify-fat-gene-associated-obesity

John, L., & Norton, M. I. (2013). Converging to the lowest common denominator in physical health. *Health Psychology, 32*, 1023–1028.

Johnson, C. (2012). Are health ads targeting "fat kids" too much? *HLN*. Retrieved February 2015, from http://www.hlntv.com/article/2012/01/04/are-georgia-anti-obesity-ads-too-harsh

Johnston, L. (2002). Behavioral mimicry and stigmatization. *Social Cognition, 20*, 18–35.

Karnani, A., McFerran, B., & Mukhopadhyay, A. (2014). Leanwashing: A hidden factor in the obesity crisis. *California Management Review, 56*, 5–30.

Khan, U., & Dhar, R. (2006). Licensing effect in consumer choice. *Journal of Marketing Research, 43*, 259–266.

Latané, B. (1981) The psychology of social impact. *American Psychologist, 36*, 343–356.

Leary, M. R., & Kowalski, R. M. (1990). Impression management: A literature review and two-component model. *Physiology and Behavior, 107*, 34–47.

Lin, L., & McFerran, B. (2014). The (ironic) Dove effect: Normalizing obesity leads to increased consumption of unhealthy food and lowers desire to engage in healthy behaviors. Working paper.

LiveScience Staff. (2009). Diet, not exercise, plays key role in weight loss. *NBC News*. Retrieved February 2015, from http://www.msnbc.msn.com/id/28524942/

Livingston, E., & Zylke, J. W. (2012). JAMA obesity theme issue. Call for papers. *Journal of American Medical Association, 307*, 970–971.

Lutz, A. (2013a). Abercrombie & Fitch refuses to make clothes for large women. *Business Insider*. Retrieved February 2015, from http://www.businessinsider.com/abercrombie-wants-thin-customers-2013-5

Lutz, A. (2013b). Lululemon workers say larger sizes are relegated to the back of the store. *Business Insider*. Retrieved February 2015, from http://www.businessinsider.com/lululemon-keeps-larger-sizes-hidden-2013-7

Martin, M. C., & Kennedy, P. F. (1993). Advertising and social comparison: Consequences for female preadolescents and adolescents. *Psychology and Marketing, 10*, 513–530.

Mazar, N., & Zhong, C. B. (2010). Do green products make us better people? Psychological Science, 21, 494–498.

McFerran, B., Dahl, D. W., Fitzsimons, G. J., & Morales, A. C. (2010a). I'll have what she's having: Effects of social influence and body type on the food choices of others. *Journal of Consumer Research, 36,* 915–929.

McFerran, B., Dahl, D. W., Fitzsimons, G. J., & Morales, A. C. (2010b). Might an overweight waitress make you eat more? How the body type of others is sufficient to alter our food consumption. *Journal of Consumer Psychology, 20,* 146–151.

McFerran, B., Dahl, D. W., Fitzsimons, G. J., & Morales, A. C. (2011). How the body type of others impacts our food consumption. In R. Batra, P. A. Keller, & V. Strecher (Eds.), *Leveraging consumer psychology for effective health communications: The obesity challenge* (pp. 151–167). Armonk, NY: M.E. Sharpe.

McFerran, B., & Mukhopadhyay, A. (2013). Lay theories of obesity predict actual body mass. *Psychological Science, 24,* 1428–1436.

Monin, B., & Miller, D. T. (2001). Moral credentials and the expression of prejudice. *Journal of Personality and Social Psychology, 81,* 33–43.

Monterosso, J., Royzman, E. B., & Schwartz, B. (2005). Explaining away responsibility: Effects of scientific explanation on perceived culpability. *Ethics and Behavior, 15,* 139–158.

Morris, M. W., Menon, T., & Ames, D. R. (2001). Culturally conferred conception of agency: A key to social perception of persona, groups, and other actors. *Personality and Social Psychology Review, 5,* 169–182.

Myers, P. N., & Biocca, F. A. (1992). The elastic body image: The effect of television advertising and programming on body image distortions in young women. *Journal of Communication, 42,* 108–133.

Ng, M., Fleming, T., Robinson, M., Thomson, B., Graetz, N., Margono, C., … Gakidou, E. (2014). Global, regional, and national prevalence of overweight and obesity in children and adults during 1980—2013: A systematic analysis for the Global Burden of Disease Study 2013. *Lancet, 384,* 766–781.

Nolan, J., Schultz, P. W., Cialdini, R. B., Goldstein, N., & Griskevicius, V. (2008). Normative social influence is undetected. *Personality and Social Psychology Bulletin, 34,* 913–923.

Ogden, J., & Flanagan, Z. (2008). Beliefs about the causes and solutions to obesity: A comparison of GPs and lay people. *Patient Education and Counselling, 71,* 72–78.

Okonkwo, O., & While, A. (2010). University students' views of obesity and weight management strategies. *Health Education Journal, 69,* 192–199.

Organisation for Economic Cooperation and Development (OECD). (2012). *Obesity update* 2012. Retrieved February 2015, from http://www.oecd.org/health/49716427.pdf

Oyserman, D., Fryberg, S. A., & Yoder, N. (2007). Identity-based motivation and health. *Journal of Personality and Social Psychology, 93,* 1011–1027.

Peñaloza, L., & Barnhart, M. (2011). Living U.S. capitalism: The normalization of credit/debt. *Journal of Consumer Research, 38,* 743–762.

Polivy, J., & Herman, C. P. (2002). Causes of eating disorders. *Annual Review of Psychology, 53,* 187–213.

Pontzer, H., Raichlen, D. A., Wood, B. M., Mabulla, A. Z. P., Racette, S. B., & Marlowe, F. W. (2012). Hunter-gatherer energetics and human obesity. *PLoS One, 7,* e40503.

Prentice, D. A., & Miller, D. T. (1993). Pluralistic ignorance and alcohol use on campus: Some consequences of misperceiving the social norm. *Journal of Personality and Social Psychology, 64*, 243–256.

Puhl, R. M., & Brownell, K. D. (2001). Bias, discrimination, and obesity. *Obesity Research, 9*, 788–805.

Puhl, R. M., & Brownell, K. D. (2003). Psychosocial origins of obesity stigma: Toward changing a powerful and pervasive bias. *Obesity Review, 4*, 213–227.

Puhl, R. M., & Brownell, K. D. (2006). Confronting and coping with weight stigma: An investigation of overweight and obese adults. *Obesity, 14*, 1802–1815.

Puhl, R. M., & Heuer, C. A. (2010). Obesity stigma: Important considerations for public health. *American Journal of Public Health, 100*, 1019–1028.

Puhl, R. M., & Heuer, C. A. (2009). The stigma of obesity: A review and update. *Obesity, 17*, 941–964.

Puhl, R. M., & Latner, J. D. (2007). Stigma, obesity, and the health of the nation's children. *Psychological Bulletin, 133*, 557–580.

Rappaport, S. D. (2011). *Listen first! Turning social media conversations into business advantage*. Hoboken, NJ: Wiley.

Reisner, R. (2008). The diet industry: A big fat lie. *Business Week*. Retrieved February 2015, from http://www.businessweek.com/debateroom/archives/2008/01/the_diet_indust.html

Rosenthal, B., & Marx, R. D. (1979). Modeling influences in the eating behavior of successful and unsuccessful dieters and treated normal weight individuals. *Addictive Behaviors, 4*, 215–221.

Roth, D. A., Herman, C. P., Polivy, J., & Pliner, P. (2001). Self-presentational conflict in social eating situations: A normative perspective. *Appetite, 36*, 165–171.

Schroeder, C. M., & Prentice, D. A. (1998). Exposing pluralistic ignorance to reduce alcohol use among college students. *Journal of Applied Social Psychology, 28*, 2150–2180.

Schultz, P. W., Nolan, J. M., Cialdini, R. B., Goldstein, N. J., & Griskevicius, V. (2007). The constructive, destructive, and reconstructive power of social norms. *Psychological Science, 18*, 429–434.

Sherif, M. (1936). *The psychology of social norms*. New York, NY: Harper.

Sherrid, P. (2003, March 16). Piling on the profit: There's no slimming down for companies selling diet products. *U.S. News and World Report*, pp. 41–43.

Simmons, T. (2006). Real women, real results: A look at dove's best of silver anvil-winning campaign. *Public Relations Society of America*. Retrieved February 2015, from http://www.prsa.org/SearchResults/view/471/105/Real_women_real_results_A_look_at_Dove_s_best_of_S#.UuxyRrQ9v2Q

Sonneville, K. R., & Gortmaker, S. L. (2008). Total energy intake, adolescent discretionary behaviors and the energy gap. *International Journal of Obesity, 32*, S19–S27.

Stice, E., & Shaw, H. E. (1994). Adverse effects of the media portrayed thin-ideal on women and linkages to bulimic symptomatology. *Journal of Social and Clinical Psychology, 13*, 288–308.

Stunkard, A. J., Harris, J. R., Pedersen, N. L., & McClearn, G. E. (1990). The body-mass index of twins who have been reared apart. *New England Journal of Medicine, 322*, 1483–1487.

Sunstein, C. (1996). Social norms and social roles. *Columbia Law Review*, *96*, 903–968.

Surowiecki, J. (2004) *The wisdom of crowds: Why the many are smarter than the few and how collective wisdom shapes business, economies, societies and nations*. New York, NY: Doubleday.

Swinburn, B., Caterson, I., Seidell, J., & James, W. P. T. (2004). Diet, nutrition and the prevention of excess weight gain and obesity. *Public Health Nutrition*, *7*, 123–146.

The history of the bikini. (2013). *Time*. Retrieved February 2015, from http://content.time.com/time/photogallery/0,29307,1908353_1905442,00.html

Upton, J. (2011). Is overweight the new normal weight? *The Huffington Post*. Retrieved February 2015, from http://www.huffingtonpost.com/2011/09/11/normalizing-obesity_n_956111.html

Wansink, B. (2006). *Mindless eating: Why we eat more than we think*. New York, NY: Bantam-Dell.

Wansink, B., Kent, R. J., & Hoch, S. J. (1998). An anchoring and adjustment model of purchase quantity decisions. *Journal of Marketing Research*, *35*, 71–81.

Wansink, B., Payne, C. R., & Chandon, P. (2007). Internal and external cues of meal cessation: The French paradox redux? Obesity, 15, 2920–2924.

Wang, C., & Coups, E. (2010). Causal beliefs about obesity and associated health behaviors: Results from a population-based survey. *International Journal of Behavioral Nutrition and Physical Activity*, *7*, 19.

Wegner, D. M., Schneider, D. J., Carter, S. R., 3rd, & White, T. L. (1987). Paradoxical effects of thought suppression. *Journal of Personality and Social Psychology*, *53*, 5–13.

Westerterp, K. R., & Speakman, J. R. (2008). Physical activity energy expenditure has not declined since the 1980s and matches energy expenditure of wild mammals. *International Journal of Obesity*, *32*, 1256–1263.

White, K., & Dahl, D. W. (2006). To be or not be: The influence of dissociative reference groups on consumer preferences. *Journal of Consumer Psychology*, *16*, 404–413.

White, K., & Dahl, D. W. (2007). Are all outgroups created equal? The influence of consumer identity and dissociative reference groups on consumer preferences. *Journal of Consumer Research*, *34*, 525–536.

White, K., & Simpson, B. (2013). When do (and don't) normative appeals influence sustainable consumer behaviors? Journal of Marketing, 77, 78–95.

World Health Organization (WHO). (2013). Global database on body mass index. Retrieved February 2015, from http://apps.who.int/bmi/

Young, L. R., & Nestle, M. (2002). The contribution of expanding portion sizes to the US obesity epidemic. *American Journal of Public Health*, *92*, 246–249.

6 | Communicating for Action

THE IMPORTANCE OF MEMORABILITY
AND ACTIONABILITY

JASON RIIS AND REBECCA K. RATNER

F OR MANY PUBLIC HEALTH PROBLEMS, individuals behave in ways that are inconsistent with their beliefs. People smoke, overeat, fail to exercise, and engage in unsafe sex even in cases where they believe the risks outweigh the hedonic benefits. This happens, at least in part, because humans have limited self-control. But another part of the problem is that the human mind has limited memory (Schacter, 2001) and attention (Kahneman, 2011). In light of these well-documented limitations, public health communicators need a toolkit that can work within these constraints to disseminate messages and encourage individuals to engage in healthy behaviors. This chapter describes principles that have proven effective for several different types of communication tools (health guidelines, behavioral prompts, and food labels), but the basic principles apply in many domains and for many other types of health communication as well. The intention of this chapter is to help health communicators develop tools that will lead to behavior change by targeted segments of the consumer population.

Memorable and Actionable Guidelines

One communication tool that directly addresses the limitations of memory and attention is what we have called the memorable and actionable guideline (Ratner & Riis, 2014). Memorable and actionable guidelines are suggestions or recommendations that ordinary people can use in their day-to-day lives. Checklists, although useful in some contexts (Gawande, 2009), are only a reference tool, and they are thus not memorable and actionable in the sense we mean. In a later section, we review some research showing that one of America's most famous guidelines, the USDA Food Pyramid (variations of which were used from 1992 to 2005), largely failed to be memorable and actionable, and thus failed as a guideline that could influence behavior on a day-to-day basis. The research on the Food Pyramid is useful in highlighting the limits of human cognition, and in highlighting just how challenging it can be for public health communicators to work within those limits.

Why Memorability and Actionability Are Key Criteria

Cognitive psychologists have been studying the limitations of the human memory system for over 100 years. Two of the most problematic limitations are that memory traces decay very quickly, and that relevant facts are not remembered when they are most needed. The psychologist Daniel Schacter (2009) refers to these as the "sins" of transience and absentmindedness. Health communicators thus need to develop guidelines that do not decay quickly, and that will come to mind at the time the desired behavior is needed. That is what we mean by memorable guidelines.

But even when they are memorable, guidelines can still fail to influence action if they do not account for the fact that much of human behavior and human thought is driven by automatic processes, or what the psychologist Daniel Kahneman (2011) calls System 1. These automatic processes are different from more deliberative attentional processes of System 2. This more deliberative system allows people to exhibit self-control and can make important corrections to automatic behavior. However, there are capacity constraints on System 2, and it cannot operate as a check on all the actions that people take. For this reason, a guideline should recommend behaviors that can be enacted easily, without much effort or attention.

Behaviors that require minimal attention and effort can be enacted more spontaneously within the tasks of daily life. It is also easier to rehearse actions that require minimal attention and effort, and this rehearsal facilitates these behaviors themselves becoming habitual and automatic (Duhigg, 2012; Rothman, Sheeran, & Wood, 2009). Finally, guidelines that require minimal effort and attention to follow will tend to be more amenable to planning. That is because it is easier to make simple plans than to make complicated plans. And plans are often important because some recommended actions will only be performed if thought goes in to considering how and when they will be enacted. This is particularly likely for behaviors that require coordination with other people or planning around other activities (e.g., scheduling a vaccination or planning a new exercise routine). Even for these types of more complex behaviors, some will be easier to plan than others, and those that are planned will be more likely to be enacted (Schweiger Gallo & Gollwitzer, 2007). Behavioral guidelines that require minimal attention and effort will thus be more actionable in virtue of being (1) easier to do spontaneously, (2) easier to rehearse, and/or (3) easier to plan and coordinate. Such guidelines will be more likely to lead to behavior change.

How Can Memorability and Actionability Be Achieved?

Several characteristics will tend to be features of guidelines (and other communications) that are memorable and actionable. We highlight three (simple, easy to visualize, and embedded triggers), but there are several others.

Simple

One of the best known findings in cognitive psychology is that our ability to recall information falls sharply as the information becomes more complex (Heath & Heath, 2007; Miller, 1956). Early experiments showed that people could only hold a few pieces of information in mind at a time, before they would lose track and forget some of the information. You can demonstrate this yourself by listing just seven or eight words for a friend and seeing how many she can recall even just a few moments later. For items to make it into long-term memory, the need for simplicity is even greater (Schacter, 2001).

This basic result has clear implications for communications. Some information will need to be left out of an otherwise complex message if the audience is to remember it. Prioritizing will thus be necessary, and communicators will have to make sometimes difficult decisions about exactly what their core message ought to be (Heath & Heath, 2007).

Consider one well-known campaign: "Friends Don't Let Friends Drive Drunk." The message did not list all the things that one could do to reduce drunk driving. It focused on one simple idea: Intervene before a friend drinks and drives. Even 20 years after this tagline was introduced, over 90% of Americans are aware of it (Ad Council, 2014).

The simplicity of this message allowed it to become a powerful and memorable phrase.

In terms of actionability, simplicity helps to prevent people from stalling in the face of complexity (Greenleaf & Lehmann, 1995). A series of simple, clear steps gives the direction that people need to take the required actions (Iyengar & Lepper, 2000; Lusardi, Keller, & Keller, 2008). Although a streamlined recommendation loses some of the detail of a more comprehensive recommendation, this process of streamlining is essential when communicating with the general public.

Easy to Visualize

The well-known saying that "a picture is worth a thousand words" captures a fundamental truth about the human cognitive system. Even just imagining pictures (without seeing them) can help recall, and psychologists believe that this is the case because two different memory processes can encode the same information. When both perceptual (visual) and semantic processes are involved, recall improves (Paivio, Walsh, & Bons, 1994). Indeed, recall is generally better for words that are concrete and hence easy to visualize (e.g., bird) than for words that are abstract and hence hard to visualize (e.g., justice). Relatedly, to recall several pieces of information, it is more effective to create a single mental image than to create different mental images for each piece of information (Morris & Stevens, 1974).

Visualization helps actionability, too. In a classic demonstration of this, people were asked to either imagine putting a golf ball successfully into a hole or to imagine putting the ball but missing the hole. Those in the successful visualization did 30% better than they did in previsualization attempts, while those in the failure visualization condition did 20% worse (Woolfolk, Parrish, & Murphy, 1985). Visualization is thus associated with action. But easy-to-visualize recommendations are helpful in another way, too—a person can more readily see if he or she has failed to comply. Imagine being advised to drive one mile and then turn left versus being advised to drive one mile and turn left at the yellow house. The latter, where feedback is easily obtained, is more likely to result in the desired action (Ratner et al., 2008).

Embedded Triggers

Embedding triggers into a message helps people recall it at just the right time. This basic approach was demonstrated in a dining hall study where students were randomly assigned to see one of two messages. The first message did not embed a trigger: "Live the healthy way, eat five fruits and veggies a day." The alternate message did embed a trigger: "Each and every dining-hall tray needs five fruits and veggies a day." The tray reference was intended to remind people of the message whenever they saw a tray. In this study, the tray message was associated with a 25% increase in fruit and vegetable consumption (Berger & Fitzsimons, 2008).

Embedding triggers can help with actionability, too (Berger, 2013; Berger & Fitzsimons, 2008; Heath & Heath, 2007). A trigger can activate automatic processes that make action more likely even in environments where an individual might be distracted. The "Friends Don't Let Friends Drive Drunk" message actually embeds a trigger (a friend who is about to drive drunk) that might prompt this kind of automatic reaction. Triggers will be most effective if they are typically present when individuals need to engage in the desired behavior (Berger & Fitzsimons, 2008).

Example—MyPyramid and MyPlate

The USDA regularly updates its *Dietary Guidelines for Americans* and develops a related communications graphic to encourage healthful eating. The Food Pyramid graphic was launched in 1992 and was redesigned in 2005 as the MyPyramid food guidance system (see Figure 6.1). Both guidelines featured five food groups (grains, vegetables, fruits, milk, and meat/beans) and gave recommended quantities to be consumed each day. The MyPyramid system featured a Web site that would produce recommended quantities that were customized for a person's age, gender, and amount of weekly exercise.

Although the original Food Pyramid was a highly recognized, iconic image, the guideline program faced criticism because consumers were often confused about various aspects of the specific recommendations (Britten, Haven, & Davis, 2006), and because the American diet remained far from meeting the recommended quantities, especially in the categories of fruits and vegetables (Cerully, Klein, & McCaul, 2006). The original graphic was designed by the public relations firm Porter-Novelli, but interestingly, that same firm, in response to criticism of the Food Pyramid, also designed a much simpler guideline called the Half Plate guideline ("Fill half of your plate with fruits and vegetables at every meal"). This simpler guideline captures a key nutritional component of the more complex pyramid guideline (i.e., roughly half of one's diet consisting of fruits and vegetables).

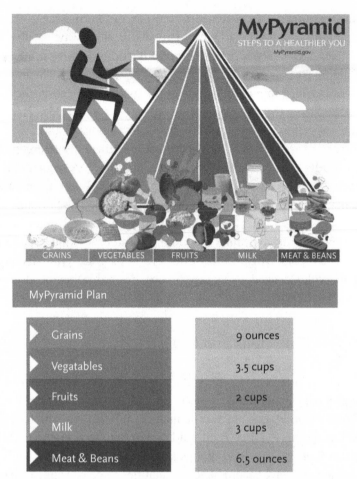

FIGURE 6.1 MyPyramid graphics and customized daily nutrition guideline (2005).

Quantitative Tests of MyPyramid Versus Half Plate

It would not be surprising to learn that people found the Half Plate guideline easier to remember than the MyPyramid guideline. But we sought to examine just how large this discrepancy was and to see if that discrepancy had consequences for behavior.

In one study, participants were randomly assigned to see either the MyPyramid guideline or the Half Plate guideline (Riis & Ratner, 2010). In the *MyPyramid* condition participants entered their age, sex, and exercise rates as they would on the USDA Web site and were then shown their customized food guidelines (e.g., 6 oz of grains, 1½ cups of fruit, etc.). In the *Half Plate* condition participants just saw the following guideline, identified as a nutrition tip: "Fill half of your plate with fruits and vegetables at every meal." In both conditions, participants were instructed to take as much time as they needed to study their guideline so that they would be able to describe that guideline to someone else.

The recall differences were very large. A large majority of the respondents (85%) who studied the Half Plate guideline described it correctly right after seeing it; however, only a minority (19%) who studied the MyPyramid guideline described it correctly (i.e., recalled the quantities and units in all five food categories). Recall for MyPyramid was much weaker than the Half Plate guideline, even though participants spent about three times as long studying the MyPyramid guideline (on average 30.3 seconds) compared to the Half Plate guideline (10.5 seconds). Participants' perceptions of the guidelines also reflected a benefit for Half Plate: Participants who saw the Half Plate (vs. MyPyramid) guideline reported that it was more motivating and beneficial and less complex (Riis & Ratner, 2010).

In another study, we examined actionability by asking people how easy the guidelines would be to follow. We compared Half Plate to MyPyramid and also to an even simpler guideline ("Eat a piece of fruit every day"). On a 1–7 scale (1 = not very easy, 7 = very easy), the Half Plate rating (M = 6.2) was significantly higher than the MyPyramid rating (M = 4.4) and not different from the piece-of-fruit guideline (M = 6.4). These lower ease-of-use ratings for MyPyramid suggest that MyPyramid is not being perceived by consumers as meeting the actionability criterion.

We examined people's food choices in a third study. Participants first studied either the MyPyramid or Half Plate guideline and then were asked approximately 1 month later which foods they would choose if selecting from a hypothetical cafeteria menu. Separately, they were also asked to recall the guideline. After the delay of 1 month, less than 1% of participants in the MyPyramid conditions could correctly report the numbers from all five categories, whereas over half (62%) of participants in the Half Plate condition recalled the guideline correctly. This memory difference translated into choice differences, as participants in the Half Plate condition selected more fruits and vegetables (M = 2.6 out 6 items) than did participants in the MyPyramid condition (M = 2.3 out of 6 items). This is a modest increase, but even small dietary changes can impact health (Lutes et al., 2008). The intervention itself was very modest, as participants saw the guidelines only one time, a month before the choice task. With exposure more on the scale of what one would see in a public service campaign, we expect that the effects would be larger.

The Half Plate guideline is more memorable and actionable than the MyPyramid guideline, and we see preliminary evidence that it may improve choice behavior as a result. The gains in memorability and action-ability were achieved in virtue of the guideline being simple (it is a short phrase), easy to visualize (with its plate imagery), and embedding a trigger for action (the image of the plate can remind people of the guideline when they see a real plate at mealtime). MyPyramid, on the other hand, has none of these properties: It is not simple (five categories and five quantities), is not easy to visualize (e.g., people can't easily visualize an ounce), and did not contain any embedded triggers to remind people to act (indeed, it does not even provide a moment of action since it gives daily totals that do not guide individual moments of decision—i.e., choices at mealtime).

MyPlate

In 2011, the USDA introduced a plate-based graphic in the new MyPlate guideline (Figure 6.2). Some of the key features of the Half Plate guideline are used in the MyPlate guideline. MyPlate is simple (at least simpler than MyPyramid), can be easily visualized, and it incorporates a trigger (a plate) that will be commonly present at mealtimes when food decisions are made.

The simpler MyPlate loses some information that was contained in MyPyramid. For example, it does not specify exact quantities to consume over a day. But since that information would have been hard to use anyway, we think that this represents a good prioritization. Ultimately, however, metrics will be needed to determine how the MyPlate messaging

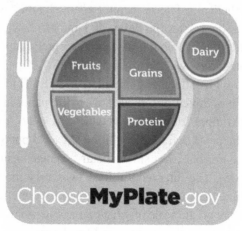

FIGURE 6.2 USDA MyPlate Nutrition Guideline (2011).

affects the American diet. Given our results, we believe it stands a much better chance of positively influencing consumer food choices than MyPyramid did.

Barriers to Memorable and Actionable Messages

Developing memorable and actionable messages is difficult and time consuming, and there can be a temptation to focus too much on the information that needs to be conveyed and not enough on how to convey it. This temptation is a challenge to the public health agenda. The development of effective messages is a craft, and professional involvement will help the cause.

Domain experts themselves are not always the best communicators, because it is easy for them to overestimate the information capacity of laypeople. This has been observed in the field of product development, where engineers and designers can focus too much on adding features, but not enough on usability (Gourville, 2006; Thompson, Hamilton, & Rust, 2005). Even if experts do appreciate the need for usability and simplified messages, the act of simplification requires prioritization and tradeoffs, and that can be a difficult process. Communication professionals can help, but domain experts need to be involved to ensure that the appropriate priorities are chosen.

Especially because these barriers are prevalent, memorability and actionability of guidelines should be measured explicitly during the message development process. Ratner and Riis (2014) give some specific suggestions as to how this can be done, in a preliminary fashion, in laboratory and survey studies. Full-blown field tests of effectiveness would be desirable, but they are extremely difficult to do since it is hard to limit exposure to randomly assigned groups through mass media. In the absence of random assignment, exposure would have to be measured, and that too is difficult to do with any accuracy.

Beyond Memorable and Actionable—Persuasion

Memorability and actionability are particularly useful when an audience finds a message generally acceptable but are falling short on action. There will be many other cases, however, when an audience is skeptical and needs to be convinced. In these cases different features may matter, and while not the focus of this chapter, we provide some examples here.

When persuasion is needed, one can look to findings from a large literature on attitude change. For example, message sources are more effective at changing attitudes when they are perceived as expert (Hovland & Weiss, 1951) and the message wording does not lead to a backfiring or "boomerang" effect (Quick & Stephenson, 2008). Messages that are repeated are more likely to be accepted as true (Skurnik, Yoon, Park, & Schwarz, 2005). Messages are more likely to be embraced when the audience first is prompted to engage in a small, token behavior that suggests their support for it (Stone & Focella, 2011). Moreover, what is persuasive to one individual may not be persuasive to another, and different message content and media channels may need to be used to meet the needs and motives of different audiences (Maibach et al., 2008).

Beyond Guidelines: Other Types of Health Communications

In this section we look at some other categories of health communications and see how they can be used effectively to address the limitations of the human mind. Many of these fall in the category of "nudges," a term introduced by the economist Richard Thaler and the legal scholar Cass Sunstein (2009). The most famous nudge is probably the use of default options that passively direct consumers to a wiser or healthier choice (discussed elsewhere in this volume). Defaults can be very effective, but they cannot be used in all settings. Sometimes more directive approaches are necessary. We discuss two types of directive nudges that have been shown to be effective, largely because they address the memory and attention limitations that we discussed at the beginning of this chapter.

Prompts and Reminders

One of the "sins" of memory discussed earlier was the tendency to forget to do things at key times. This limitation has been implicated in many health problems, including the failure to adhere to drug prescriptions (Cutler & Everett, 2010; Osterberg & Blaschke, 2005). Although lack of adherence has many causes, patients themselves consider forgetfulness to be the biggest contributor. Providing timely reminders through text messages or other prompts has been effective in improving drug adherence (Lester et al., 2010). But simple, timely reminders have also been effective in traditional public health contexts. Armstrong et al. (2009) randomly assigned adults to receive (or not receive) daily text message reminders to use sunscreen over a 6-week period. Sunscreen compliance in the control group (who received no texts) was 30%, but it was almost doubled, to 56% in the intervention group.

Prompts can do more than just remind you to do something like take a pill or apply sunscreen. Prompts can even remind you of your existing goals, at moments of weakness. Schwartz et al. (2012) invited customers at a fast-food restaurant to downsize their meal portions either with no discount or at a very nominal discount. In one study, 35% of customers agreed to downsize, and the nominal discount had no effect. This led to a savings reduction of roughly 200 calories per downsized meal. In subsequent studies, they measured food waste and found that getting less food on one's plate led to less food consumed. Plate waste was modest and it did not differ between groups who received downsize offers and those who did not (nor did it differ between those who accepted downsized offers and those who did not).

What is interesting about this study is that the prompt was helping people do something that they already believed was a good idea. The researchers report additional studies showing that (1) a majority of consumers believe that they often overeat at restaurants and that (2) while almost no consumers believed that restaurant portions were "usually too small," over a third believed that they were "usually too large." But consumers almost never spontaneously asked for smaller portions. This was seen both in survey studies and in field studies at the fast-food restaurant. Only when specifically asked if they would like a smaller portion would people get a smaller portion. A simple, well-timed prompt can help people remember that they do often overeat and that they could prevent overeating by getting less food on their plate. This prompt would not work if it was not consistent with existing goals.

The key thing about these prompts and reminders is that they are nudges that come right at a key moment of action. Their proximity to an action opportunity is what makes them so powerful as a behavioral influence.

Food Labels

Calorie labels have been mandated for fast-food restaurant chains in many jurisdictions, and the Affordable Care Act contains a provision to have them implemented nationwide. While these labels may be having supply side effects whereby restaurants are reformulating their meals to be lower in calories (Saelens et al., 2012), there is little evidence that they are having a large effect on consumers (Bollinger et al., 2011; Elbel, Kersh, Brescoll, & Dixon, 2009).

Calorie labels are limited in several ways in their ability to influence point-of-sale decisions. First, they are numeric so they require calculations and comparisons at a moment when an individual is distracted by her own cravings, by other customers, and by clerks eager to take their orders. Second, they are not visual, in the sense that people cannot visualize what 250 calories looks like. Third, they are not associated with action triggers—they do not directly prompt a particular action; they just provide information.

Traffic light labels, on the other hand, are much simpler, much more visual, and they do prompt or trigger specific action. These labels use red, yellow, or green traffic lights to indicate the healthfulness of foods; red is the least healthy, green the most. Although they have been in use in some forms on some packaged foods on a voluntary basis in the United Kingdom (Triggle, 2013), their use in food service has been very limited. Some workplace cafeterias have adopted the approach, and a series of studies have been conducted at a large hospital cafeteria in Boston. In a 2-year intervention, traffic light labels were associated with substantial changes in food and beverage choices. Selection of unhealthy red items declined by 15% (relative to baseline) and was entirely made up for by increases in healthier yellow and green items (Thorndike, Riis, Sonnenberg, & Levy, 2014).

The exact mechanism of the effect is not easily determined. But at least in some cases, the labeling is not simply informative; that is, it is not just giving people information that they did not have. Most people know that sugared soda is not healthy, and yet the presence of the red label greatly decreased consumption. An explicit reminder of the unhealthiness at the moment of decision may contribute, or perhaps the red label is seen as an implicit social norm that sugared soda is not something that people consume on a regular basis (Goldstein, Cialdini, & Griskevicius, 2008).

In addition to the efforts in food service, there are various programs to make packaged food labels simpler. Some grocery stores have licensed the NUVAL shelf labeling system, which assigns all foods and beverages scores of 0–100 (with higher scores indicating a better nutrition profile). The food industry (under a joint effort by the Grocery Manufacturers Association and Food Marketing Institute) has launched its own front-of-package label program (Facts Up Front), partly in response to concerns about the difficulty that most consumers have in using the mandated back-of-package nutrition facts panel. Although somewhat simplified from the back-of-package label, the Facts Up Front labels still display more information than most consumers can use at a glance, and the quantities mentioned are not particularly "easy to visualize," nor do they seem particularly likely to trigger action. Transparency is generally a good thing, so if people are looking for specific information (such as sodium amounts), it is good that they can find it more easily. But if people are not exactly sure about what to look for, or if they are too distracted or too busy to look closely, the impact on behavior will be minimal.

Conclusion

Communications that are aimed to influence people's actions as they navigate their daily lives need to be very sensitive to the way that the human cognitive system works. Major limitations of memory and attention have been documented by cognitive psychologists for decades (Kahneman, 2011; Schacter, 2001). We argue that to make their communications usable, and to make them likely to affect behavior, communicators need to pay careful attention to memorability and actionability. To achieve this, they can design communications that are simple, easy to visualize, and that embed triggers so that they are likely to be thought of at key moments of decision. These considerations are important for communications to all audiences, but they are even more important when targeting the millions of American with limited literacy skills (Panzer, Kindig, & Nielsen-Bohlman, 2004).

We have discussed the importance of these dimensions for some specific kinds of health communications, but the principles apply widely in regulatory efforts (Sunstein, 2013), product design (Siegel & Etzkorn, 2013), financial education (Fernandes, Lynch, & Netemeyer, 2014), and in the expanding field of health incentives (Volpp et al., 2008).

Designing memorable and actionable communications is not easy to do. The USDA's MyPlate does a better job than MyPyramid, but experts will always face the barrier of their own "privileged knowledge." It can be very easy for experts to underestimate the limitations of nonexperts, and providing less information will often seem counterintuitive. But the design efforts must be attempted, tradeoffs must be made, and memorability and actionability must be measured directly. Standard intervention research should be conducted as well, but the challenges of those kinds of studies are great. Direct tests of memorability and actionability are faster and easier, and they are an important first step that is too often ignored.

References

Ad Council. (2011). *Buzzed driving prevention*. Retrieved March 2014, from http://www. adcouncil.org/Impact/Case-Studies-Best-Practices/Drunk-Driving-Prevention.

Armstrong, A. W., Watson, A. J., Makredes, M., Frangos, J. E., Kimball, A. B., & Kvedar, M. (2009). Text-message reminders to improve sunscreen use. *Archives of Dermatology, 145*(11), 1230–1236.

Berger, J. (2013). Contagious: Why things catch on. New York, NY: Simon & Schuster.

Berger, J., & Fitzsimons, G. M. (2008). Dogs on the street, Pumas on your feet: How cues in the environment influence product evaluation and choice. *Journal of Marketing Research, 45*(1), 1–14.

Bollinger, B., Leslie, P., & Sorensen, A. T. (2011). Calorie posting in chain restaurants. *American Economic Journal: Economic Policy, 3*(1), 91–128.

Britten, P., Haven, J., & Davis, C. (2006). Consumer research for development of educational messages for the MyPyramid food guidance system. *Journal of Nutrition Education and Behavior, 38*, S108–S123.

Cerully, J. L., Klein, W. M. P., & McCaul, K. D. (2006). Lack of acknowledgement of fruit and vegetable recommendations among nonadherent individuals: Associations with information processing and cancer cognitions. *Journal of Health Communications, 11*, 103–115.

Cutler, D. M., & Everett, W. (2010). Thinking outside the pillbox—medication adherence as a priority for health care reform. *New England Journal of Medicine, 362*, 1553–1555.

Duhigg, C. (2012). *The power of habit: Why we do what we do in life and business.* New York, NY: Random House.

Elbel, B., Kersh, R., Brescoll, V., & Dixon, L. B. (2009). Calorie labeling and food choices: A first look at the effects on low-income people in New York City. *Health Affairs (Millwood), 28*(6), 1110–1121.

Fernandes, D., Lynch, J. G., & Netemeyer, R. G. (2014). Financial literacy, financial education, and downstream financial behaviors. *Management Science, 60*(8), 1861–1883. doi:10.1287/mnsc.2013.1849

Gawande, A. (2009). *The checklist manifesto.* New York, NY: Metropolitan Books.

Heath, C., & Heath, D. (2007). *Made to stick: Why some ideas survive and others die.* New York, NY: Random House.

Hovland, C. I., & Weiss, W. (1951). The influence of source credibility on communication effectiveness. *Public Opinion Quarterly, 15*(4), 635–650.

Goldstein, N. J., Cialdini, R. B., & Griskevicius, V. (2008). A room with a viewpoint: Using social norms to motivate environmental conservation in hotels. *Journal of Consumer Research, 35*(3), 472–482. doi:10.1086/586910

Gourville, J. T. (2006). Eager sellers and stony buyers: Understanding the psychology of new product adoption. *Harvard Business Review, 84*(6), 98–+.

Greenleaf, E. A., & Lehmann, D. R. (1995). Reasons for substantial delay in consumer decision making. *Journal of Consumer Research, 22*, 186–199.

Iyengar, S. S., & Lepper, M. (2000). When choice is demotivating: Can one desire too much of a good thing? *Journal of Personality and Social Psychology, 79*, 995–1006.

Kahneman, D. (2011). *Thinking, fast and slow*. New York, NY: Farrar, Straus and Giroux.

Lester, R. T., Ritvo, P., Mills, E. J., Kariri, A., Karanja, S., Chung, M. H., . . . Plummer, F. A. (2010). Effects of a mobile phone short message service on antiretroviral treatment adherence in Kenya (WelTel Kenya1): A randomised trial. *Lancet, 376*(9755), 1838–1845. doi:10.1016/S0140-6736(10)61997-6

Lusardi, A., Keller, P. A., & Keller, A. (2008). New ways to make people save: A social marketing approach. In A. Lusardi (Ed.), *Overcoming the saving slump: How to increase the effectiveness of financial education and savings programs* (pp. 209–236). Chicago, IL: University of Chicago Press.

Lutes, L. D., Winett, R. A., Barger, S. D., Wojcik, J. R., Herbert, W. G., Nickols-Richardson, S. M., & Anderson, E. S. (2008). Small changes in nutrition and physical activity promote weight loss and maintenance: 3-month evidence from the ASPIRE randomized trial. *Annals of Behavioral Medicine, 35*(3), 351–357. doi:10.1007/s12160-008-9033-z

Maibach, E. W., Roser-Renouf, C., & Leiserowitz, A. (2008). Communication and marketing as climate-change intervention assets. *American Journal of Preventive Medicine, 35*(5), 488–500.

Miller, G. (1956). The magical number seven, plus or minus two: Some limits on our capacity for processing information. *Psychological Review, 63*, 81–97.

Morris, P. E., & Stevens, R. (1974). Linking images and free recall. *Journal of Verbal Learning and Verbal Behaviour, 13*, 310–315

Osterberg, L., & Blaschke, T. (2005). Adherence to medication. *New England Journal of Medicine, 353*(5), 487–497. doi:10.1056/NEJMra050100

Paivio, A., Walsh, M., & Bons, T. (1994). Concreteness and memory: When and why? *Journal of Experimental Psychology: Learning, Memory, and Cognition, 20*(5), 1196–1204.

Panzer, L., Kindig, A. M., & Nielsen-Bohlman, D. A. (2004). *Health literacy: A prescription to end confusion*. Washington, DC: Institute of Medicine of the National Academies of Science.

Quick, B. L., & Stephenson, M. T. (2008). Examining the role of trait reactance and sensation seeking on perceived threat, state reactance, and reactance restoration. *Human Communication Research, 34*, 448–476.

Ratner, R. K., & Riis, J. (2014). Communicating science-based recommendations with memorable and actionable guidelines. *Proceedings of the National Academy of Sciences USA, 111*(Suppl. 4), 13634–13641.

Ratner, R. K., Soman, D., Zauberman, G., Ariely, D., Carmon, Z., Keller, P. A., . . . Wertenbroch, K. (2008). How behavioral decision research can enhance consumer welfare: From freedom of choice to paternalistic intervention. *Marketing Letters, 19*, 383–397.

Riis, J., & Ratner, R. (2010). Simplified nutrition guidelines to fight obesity. In R. Batra, P. A. Keller, & V. J. Strecher (Eds.), *Leveraging consumer psychology for effective health communications* (pp. 333–345). New York, NY: ME Sharpe.

Rothman, A. J., Sheeran, P., & Wood, W. (2009). Reflective and automatic processes in the initiation and maintenance of diet change. *Annals of Behavioral Medicine, 28*(Suppl.), 4–17.

Saelens, B. E., Chan, N. L., Krieger, J., Nelson, Y., Boles, M., Colburn, T. A., ... Bruemmer, B. (2012). Nutrition-Labeling Regulation Impacts on Restaurant Environments. *American Journal of Preventive Medicine. 4*(35), 505–511. doi:10.1016/j.amepre.2012.07.025

Schacter, D. (2001). *The seven sins of memory: How the mind forgets and remembers.* New York, NY: Houghton Mifflin.

Schwartz, J., Riis, J., Elbel, B., &Ariely, D. (2012). Inviting consumers to downsize fast-food portions significantly reduces calorie consumption. *Health Affairs, 31*(2), 399–407. doi:10.1377/hlthaff.2011.0224

Schweiger Gallo, I., & Gollwitzer, P. M. (2007). Implementation intentions: A look back at fifteen years of progress. *Psicothema, 19*, 37–42.

Siegel, A., & Etzkorn, I. (2013). *Conquering the Crisis of Complexity.* Grand Central Publishing.

Skurnik, I., Yoon, C., Park, D. C., & Schwarz, N. (2005). How warnings about false claims become recommendations. *Journal of Consumer Research, 31*, 713–724.

Stone, J., & Focella, E. (2011). Hypocrisy, dissonance and the self-regulation processes that improve health. *Self and Identity, 10*, 295–303.

Sunstein, C. R. (2013). *Simple(r), the Future of Government.* New York, NY: Simon & Schuster.

Thaler, R. H., & Sunstein, C. R. (2009). *Nudge: Improving decisions about health, wealth, and happiness.* New York: Penguin Books.

Thompson, D. V., Hamilton, R. W., & Rust, R. T. (2005). Feature fatigue: When product capabilities become too much of a good thing. *Journal of Marketing Research, 42*(4), 431–442.

Thorndike, A. N., Riis, J., Sonnenberg, L. M., & Levy, D. E. (2014). Traffic-light labels and choice architecture promoting healthy food choices. *American Journal of Preventive Medicine, 46*(2), 143–149. doi:10.1016/j.amepre.2013.10.002

Triggle, N. (2013). Food labelling: Consistent system to be rolled out. *BBC News.* Retrieved August 2014, http://www.bbc.com/news/health-22959239.

Volpp, K. G., Troxel, A. B., Pauly, M. V., Glick, H. A., Puig, A., Asch, D. A., ... DeGuzman, J. (2009). A randomized, controlled trial of financial incentives for smoking cessation. *New England Journal of Medicine, 360*(7), 699–709. doi:10.1056/NEJMsa0806819

Woolfolk, R. L., Parrish, W., & Murphy, S. M. (1985). The effects of positive and negative imagery on motor skill performance. *Cognitive Therapy and Research, 9*, 335–341.

7 | Nudging Individuals Toward Healthier Food Choices with the 4 P's Framework for Behavior Change

ZOË CHANCE, RAVI DHAR, MICHELLE HATZIS, AND KIM HUSKEY

D ESPITE MILLIONS OF DOLLARS BEING spent on nutritional and wellness education, people eat more and eat more fattening foods than they did 20 years ago, with rates of obesity skyrocketing as a result. In contrast to entreating people to marshal their limited energy toward self-control by providing them with more information, we present a framework that leverages principles of behavioral economics, psychology, and marketing to restructure the environment in ways that (1) maximize the benefits arising from sporadic efforts to achieve health goals and (2) minimize the willpower needed to make healthy choices. We propose the 4 P's Framework for Behavior Change, a comprehensive framework that integrates research findings to suggest ways of making desired behaviors like healthy eating less taxing. The framework can be applied by planners in any organizational context.

This chapter is structured as follows. First, we discuss five psychological barriers to making healthy choices. Next, we present the 4 P's Framework for Behavior Change: possibilities, process, persuasion, and person. Finally, we apply the framework in an organizational case study at Google.

Barriers to Change: How the Brain Short-Circuits Healthy Intentions

Although most people are familiar with the adverse health effects of smoking, weight gain, lack of exercise, and poor diet, people continue to engage in these behaviors at alarming rates. Most people are fully aware of what actions they need to take to improve their health, and many want to live healthier lives. Yet, despite good intentions, change is hard to achieve—most intentions to change behavior end in failure (Sheeran, Webb, & Gollwitzer, 2005).

When identifying the personal barriers to healthy change, many people point to insufficient time, financial resources, or motivation. Undoubtedly, these are among the reasons for the failure of our best-laid plans. However, there are additional processes operating outside our awareness that account for many of the difficulties we face in making optimal health decisions.

There are five major factors that often determine whether or not a desire to change actually leads to action.

We Are Wired to Favor Impulsive Choices

Behavioral economists describe decision making as a dual process, with two systems working together. The intuitive system, or "System 1," is emotional, automatic, and rapid. The deliberate system, "System 2," on the other hand, is conscious and takes effort to engage (Kahneman & Frederick, 2002; Stanovich & West, 2000). When you see a doughnut, the automatic urge to grab it is generated by the intuitive system, whereas considering the amount of fat and calories vis-à-vis the predicted enjoyment of the doughnut requires engaging the deliberate system. Choices emerge as an interplay of the two systems. The intuitive system has the first say because it comes online rapidly, responding to salient emotional stimuli. And unfortunately, healthy choices such as broccoli and jogging are less intuitively appealing than alternatives such as doughnuts and video games. So System 1 tends to favor unhealthy choices. System 2 tends to favor healthy choices that benefit us in the long run; however, since engaging a System 2 override is effortful, we often fail to engage System 2—particularly in small, everyday decisions such as food choices. Thus, System 1 has the advantage, and it leads us into temptation.

We're Too Busy to Make Clear-Headed Choices

Engaging System 2 requires both ability and motivation. However, when people are multitasking or otherwise distracted, extraneous thoughts compete for attention and siphon away the brain's limited conscious processing power, inducing "cognitive load." Cognitive load hampers System 2, reducing the ability to resist temptation. In a classic study involving food choices, people were asked to choose between fruit salad and cake. Those in the "cognitive load" condition were challenged to remember a seven-digit number while making the food selection, and they were 50% more likely to choose cake than those in the control group (Shiv & Fedorikhin, 1999). When individuals are busy or stressed, they have fewer cognitive resources for System 2 processing, leaving them especially likely to make indulgent System 1 choices without considering the long-term consequences.

We Have Limited Willpower

In a modern society with abundant opportunities to consume, willpower is tested all day, every day. And studies find resisting one impulse diminishes our ability to resist the next; that is, self-control is a limited resource (Baumeister, Bratslavsky, Muraven, & Tice, 1998; reviewed in Baumeister & Tierney, 2011). After a series of choices resulting in pain or self-denial, willpower reserves become depleted. In a field study of desire in which participants wore beepers for 1 week and were periodically asked whether they were experiencing a desire at that moment (System 1) and also whether they were resisting it (System 2), people reported spending a quarter of their waking hours using willpower to resist desires (Hofmann, Baumeister, Förster, & Vohs, 2012). Because people make so many food choices when already depleted by hunger, this is an area in which desire easily overwhelms attempts at self-control. Resistance is, too often, futile.

We Live for Today

Our thinking is biased toward the present: We heavily discount the future and privilege the here and now. Behavioral economists call this tendency "hyperbolic discounting" (see Chapter 2 by White and Dow). Awareness of hyperbolic discounting is important because so many of the potential benefits of our health decisions accrue in the distant future, while the costs tend to be borne in the present. And the ties between the costs and benefits are indirect. For example, spending a few moments to floss is costly now, and the potential benefit (avoiding a painful dentist visit) lies months or years in the future. The pleasure of smoking is immediate (at least for the smoker), while the potential cost (developing a tobacco-related disease) is in the future. Furthermore, we expect that in the future, we will make better decisions ... but when the future comes, it is once again our present-biased self making the decision. In one study, employees who had just eaten lunch were asked to choose which snack they wanted to receive the following week—either junk food or fruit. Most chose the fruit. However, when the snacks were delivered, the record of the planned choices was "lost," and the employees were asked to choose again the snack they wanted right then. The result: Only 20% stuck with fruit. The vast majority opted for the tempting treats (Read & van Leeuwen, 1998). The delayed impact of many short-term decisions can fool us into making the same bad choices again and again.

We Often Act Without Thinking

Contextual influences can stimulate automatic responses even without conscious attention. For example, when food is consumed from larger dishes, or in the company of others, people tend to eat more of it (Wansink, 2006). Over time, repeated cues can trigger consistent behaviors that solidify into habits that can be hard to break. In one study, moviegoers who habitually eat popcorn at the theater ate just as much popcorn when it was stale, despite complaining about it (Wansink & Kim, 2005). In much the same way we can drive home from work on autopilot, without making many conscious decisions at all, we mindlessly repeat other behaviors like finishing the food on our plate, buying popcorn at a movie theater, or reaching for a snack during a commercial break. Mindless eating is a particular risk when a person is under cognitive load from another activity, like watching television, driving, or working (see Chapter 9 by Wansink).

In the quest to improve health behaviors and choices, education, knowledge, and willpower are not enough. We have described five reasons the best intentions of System 2 are so often short-circuited by the automatic impulses of System 1. Because System 2 requires conscious attention and resources (cognitive capacity and willpower) that are in short supply, any interventions relying on System 2 for success will face tremendous challenges. We must search for ways to influence health choices that rely less on willpower and conscious determination. Fortunately, behavioral economics provides many inspirations. Research in behavioral economics has revealed a multitude of situations in which human behavior is seemingly irrational or counter to the individual's long-term self-interest—but is nonetheless predictable. The promise of behavioral economics is that these anomalies can be exploited opportunistically to nudge people in the direction of making healthier choices.

The 4 P's Framework for Behavior Change

To help practitioners apply some of the disparate insights from research in behavioral economics, psychology, and marketing, we have developed a framework called the 4 P's Framework for Behavior Change. The framework is consistent with Richard Thaler and Cass Sunstein's ideal of "libertarian paternalism"—nudging people in directions that align their behaviors with their long-term self-interest, without curtailing their ultimate freedom to choose (Thaler & Sunstein, 2003). Focusing on actionable, high-impact levers of change, it combines common sense with novel ways to make desirable behavior the path of least resistance. Although we focus on health and food choices here, the framework can be applied to any domain. The 4 P's are: possibilities (what choices are offered), process (how choices are made), persuasion (how choices are communicated), and person (how intentions are reinforced). (See Box 7.1 for a summary of the framework.) These four levers of change provide different paths to reduce resistance and nudge individuals toward healthy choices. Each component of the framework offers ways to make System 1 intuitive choices *healthier* or System 2 rational choices *easier.* Together, the 4 P's framework provides comprehensive suggestions for engineering the environment to make the healthy choice the easy choice. Any aspects of the 4 P's framework can be used together; it is not necessary to use all of them.

BOX 7.1 4 P'S FRAMEWORK FOR BEHAVIOR CHANGE

Possibilities
What choices are offered?
- Assortment
- Amount

Persuasion
How are choices communicated?
- Vividness
- Comparisons
- Moments of truth

Process
How are choices made?
- Accessibility
- Order
- Defaults

Person
How are intensions reinforced?
- Goals
- Habits
- Precommitment

In the following section of the paper, we describe the framework. Subsequently, we present a case study in which Google used many elements of the 4 P's framework, to provide ideas for how other planners might apply it in their own organizations.

Possibilities: What Choices Are Offered?

The first tool in the box is the simplest: Before strategizing how to steer people's choices, improve the options. While it may in rare cases be effective to ban undesirable behavior (such as smoking in restaurants) or to legislate desirable behavior (such as wearing seatbelts), the negative reactions against paternalism can often outweigh its benefits. Therefore, we advocate a gentler approach, maintaining freedom of choice while improving the options. When designing a choice set to facilitate healthy choices, the goals should be to make options healthier and to make healthy options more attractive (or make unhealthy options less attractive). The planning decisions around possibilities regard the assortment and the amount.

Assortment

The first decision a planner must make is what choices to offer: What will the assortment be? Availability has a strong impact on consumption: People tend to eat whatever is in front of them. Sometimes the existing options can be made healthier, either by modifying components (e.g., white to whole-grain pasta) or by switching the mode of delivery (e.g., salt shakers that dispense less salt per shake). Some manufacturers are engineering health creatively. PepsiCo has engineered "designer salt" with greater surface area, yielding more flavor per crystal and decreasing the amount of sodium required for a salty taste (McKay, 2010). Pharmaceutical companies promote safety through product design, with child safety caps on medicine bottles preventing fatal mistakes. In organizations, the addition of healthy choices will rarely face opposition if other options are retained. One study found people were more likely to choose a healthy option (fruit over a cookie) from a larger assortment than a smaller one (Sela, Berger, & Liu, 2009). Healthy menu options can be added to the list, and fun fitness activities and games can be made available. Vending machines might be upgraded to refrigerated machines, and fruit bowls might be stocked in conference rooms.

Relative appeal can be manipulated either by making healthy options more appealing or by making unhealthy items less so. In the Healthy Lunchrooms

Initiative, Wansink found that placing fruit in a nice bowl or under a light increased fruit sales by more than 100% ("Nutrition advice ...," 2014). Stairwells, too, could be made more aesthetically appealing to encourage their use, perhaps being decorated with art, carpeted, and well-lit.

Less-healthy options can be made less attractive, relative to the healthier alternatives. For example, elevator speed could be decreased to make the option of taking the stairs more appealing than taking a slow elevator, or an outdoor smoking area might be left unprotected from rain and snow. The city of London decided not to synchronize traffic lights, making driving there a slow and unpleasant experience, in order to encourage the use of public transportation.

Variety is a powerful stimulant of consumption. Generally, when consuming more than one thing is possible, more options means more consumption. This is true even when variation is more perceived than real. For example, people ate more M&Ms from a bowl containing more colors of M&Ms, even though the total quantity and flavors were identical to a bowl with fewer colors (Kahn & Wansink, 2004). Planners should consider the proportion of healthy to unhealthy options and decide whether to shift the balance in favor of healthy ones. This shift could be accomplished either by reducing the tempting options (risking backlash) or increasing the number of desirable options (risking an increase in overall consumption, if food is free).

Mindful attention to variety rotation cycles can nudge behavior as well. While we acknowledge that individuals often react strongly against the restriction of choice, we expect reactance to be tempered when choice is restricted only at certain times. Healthy or desirable options could be switched more frequently, to encourage sampling or consumption, while unhealthy or undesirable options could be switched less frequently, to encourage satiation. An advantage of selective restriction is that it helps to bolster self-control, while minimizing potential backlash from individuals who want to indulge periodically. Additionally, healthy options might be made available more often than they are currently. In fact, in a study of children's eating habits, availability was the number-one driver of consumption of fresh fruits and vegetables (Cullen et al., 2003). In an organization, this might translate to keeping the salad bar open all day. In other situations, making healthy options scarce could spur healthy purchase decisions—perhaps discounted gym memberships could be made available for only a short time.

Additionally, healthy options might be strategically bundled with other healthy options, or with less healthy options, For example, popular entrées might be paired with a side of salad or fruit. Or "lesser evils" might be paired with "greater goods" to increase the appeal of the desirable option. In a clever field experiment, Milkman, Minson, and Volpp (2014) paired addictive audiobooks with gym workouts to encourage exercise.

Amount

After the menu of options has been decided, the next question to answer about each item is, how much? What quantity and what price? Price changes have been found to be more effective than nutritional labeling in stimulating healthy behaviors (Horgen & Brownell, 2002), and one study found a 10% increase in fast-food prices led to a 0.7% decrease in obesity rate (Chou, Grossman, & Saffer, 2004). When prices of goods are set by an organization, for example, for cafeteria items and insurance plans, low prices or "sin taxes" can move behavior toward desired outcomes. Quantity discounts (supersized pricing) on healthy foods can increase the amount consumed (Haws & Winterich, 2013), due to a "unit bias" (Geier, Rozin, & Doros, 2006): People tend to believe the appropriate amount to eat is an entire portion (e.g., plate, bowl, or package). As a result, they serve themselves more and eat more when dishes or utensils are large. In one experiment, nutrition academics at an ice cream social served themselves 31% more ice cream when given larger bowls and 57% more when given both larger bowls and larger serving spoons (Wansink, van Ittersum, & Painter, 2006). People also pour and drink more from short, wide glasses than tall, thin ones: Children poured 70% more juice, and experienced bartenders poured 37% more alcohol into a short, wide glass of the same volume as a tall, thin one (Wansink & van Ittersum, 2003). Ice cream in a small cone is perceived to be more ice cream, and more satisfying, than the same amount in a large cone (Hsee, 1998). A small, full container conveys abundance, which leads to satisfaction.

Upgrading the possibilities through strategic influence on the assortment and the amount can improve the menu options either by making the options healthier or by making the healthy options more desirable. Next, we consider how the process can nudge individuals toward these healthy options.

Process: How Are Choices Made?

One of the major contributions of behavioral economics to behavior change lies in the application of small nudges in the "choice architecture" of the decision process that do not affect the number or type of options provided.

Small changes can be applied to the configuration of the different options or to the way that relevant information is presented. Firms can influence the architecture of the decision-making process through modifying either logistics (here, process) or information (here, persuasion).

One means of privileging healthy options is by modifying the structure or context of a choice. This can be accomplished through accessibility, order, and defaults.

Accessibility

Accessibility, actual or perceived, has a powerful effect on choices. Often, undesirable options are too accessible; for example, when fast-food restaurants offer free refills on sodas, they encourage consumption of empty calories not merely through the price discount but also by eliminating the need to wait in line again and pay at the counter.

Indeed, proximity of fast-food and full-service restaurants is the number-one predictor of local obesity trends (Chou et al., 2004). The goal of "choice architecture" interventions is to make a healthy choice the easy choice. Organizations might make healthy options more accessible by, for example, opening a health express line in the cafeteria to decrease waiting and provide a meaningful incentive to eat healthfully, at no cost. Many employers provide refrigerators and microwaves; food preparation (and cleanup) supplies could be increased, further encouraging employees to bring their lunch to work, saving them both money and calories. Unhealthy options might be made less accessible, for example, by moving junk foods and desserts to places harder to see and reach. Unhealthy vending machines might be relegated to the basement.

Just as subjective perceptions determine how quantity affects behavior, subjective perceptions also determine how accessibility affects behavior. For example, moving healthy foods to eye level increases their consumption (Thorndike, Sonnenberg, Riis, Barraclough, & Levy, 2012), even though they were already visible before. Visual cues might also make healthy options easier to identify; for example, healthy foods could be served on green plates.

Order

Order has a strong impact on preferences and choices between options. In a classic study, researchers found that when people touched and evaluated four pairs of stockings, they were four times as likely to choose the pair on the right as the one on the left—yet they had no awareness of the effect of order on their judgments (Nisbett & Wilson, 1977). More meaningfully, a political candidate whose name is listed first gains 3.5 percentage points in an election (Koppell & Steen, 2004). And sometimes the middle option can have an advantage, too—"extremeness aversion" leads many consumers to avoid, for example, the largest or smallest drink sizes (Sharpe, Staelin, & Huber, 2008). There are some conflicting findings in the research on order effects, but in general:

- In a pair, the first item has an advantage.
- In a set of three, the middle item has an advantage.
- In a larger group, both the first and last items have an advantage, with the last taking precedence if the items are experienced sequentially before the choice is made (touched, heard, tasted, etc., rather than seen all at one time).

These biases can serve health goals, if healthy options are offered in the advantaged positions in comparative choices.

Defaults

Much of the behavioral economics research on health has explored the effects of defaults and incentives. In many situations, multiple options are available, but one option has the privilege of being the default choice. Due to the power of the status quo bias, defaults have proven extremely effective in guiding choices, even in domains as weighty as organ donations (Johnson & Goldstein, 2003) and retirement savings (Thaler & Benartzi, 2004). Often people—including planners—are not even aware of any alternative to the default. For example, in one study at a Chinese takeout restaurant, patrons were asked if they would prefer a half-serving of rice (without any price discount). Many of them chose this option, which had always been available but had not occurred to them when the full-sized entrée was offered as the default (Schwartz, Riis, Elbel, & Ariely, 2012). Food planners could increase choices of healthy options by offering as the default: water as the beverage, vegetables or fruit as the side dish, small portion sizes, and low-fat and low-salt condiments as the default. Less healthy substitutes could be available upon request.

Strategic planning of the possibilities and process can gently shift behavior toward healthy choices without restricting the freedom to choose unhealthy alternatives; however, these levers can sometimes be costly, requiring major changes. Therefore, it is also advisable to implement nearly costless interventions to complement them or to substitute, when necessary, by focusing on persuasion.

Persuasion: How Are Choices Communicated?

To succeed in persuasive communication, planners should try to seize the moment and communicate the right message, the right way, at the time when the individual will be most receptive to it. Persuasion depends on vividness, comparisons, and moments of truth.

Vividness

Most communication by organizations is informative, addressing thoughtful, deliberate System 2. Planners can achieve better results by making sure their messages address intuitive, emotional System 1 as well. One way of tapping into the emotional response is to make the message more vivid. Vividness can be achieved with words or with a visual or tactile experience.

Names play an important role in expectations and evaluations. Understanding this, marketers have recently been changing the names of some popular products. To avoid the vivid and negative images of oiliness, Kentucky Fried Chicken has been officially shortened to KFC®, and Oil of Olay has been shortened to Olay®. To escape the vivid and visceral connection with constipation, prunes have become "dried plums." Healthy choices can be assisted by vivid names as well. Researchers found that adding adjectives like "succulent" or "homemade" made food not only more appealing but also tastier and more filling (Wansink, van Ittersum, & Painter, 2005). The Healthy Lunchroom initiative found that the simple intervention of naming fruit with vivid descriptors like "fresh Florida oranges" increased fruit consumption by up to 26% (Wansink, 2006). However, food descriptions can drive overconsumption too: Dieters thought a "salad special" was healthier and thus ate more of it than an identical "pasta special" (Irmak, Vallen, & Robinson, 2011). And people eat more when portions are called "small" or "medium," while believing they have eaten less (Aydinoglu, Krishna, & Wansink, 2009).

Using pictures or objects is another vivid way to engage the emotions, which can encourage persistence in healthy behaviors. For example, looking at bacteria cultured from their own hands led doctors to wash more often. And seeing a vial of fat from a gallon of whole milk caused many milk drinkers to switch to skim (Heath & Heath, 2010). Visuals can also simplify the decision process. In one cafeteria intervention, implementing a simple green/yellow/red color-coding system improved sales of healthy items (green) and reduced sales of unhealthy items (red).

Comparisons

The right message depends on relevant trade-offs and comparisons. For example, when a person is in a future-oriented mindset, thinking about an activity in the distant future, the more abstract properties of the activity, such as its purpose, take precedence. However, when the activity is in the near future, its more concrete properties, such as its process, gain importance (Trope & Lieberman, 2003, 2010). When considering going for a run today, individuals tend to focus on concrete details such as the momentary pleasure or pain they expect, what they will wear, and where and for how long they will run. However, when considering a run next month, they are more likely to focus on abstract aspects such as what it means to be runner, what the long-term effects of exercise may be, and why they have decided to run. This variation in mindset brings substantial variation in preferences and in willingness to attend to certain types of information. Trade-offs between momentary pleasure and long-term health will be made very differently when in a concrete mindset, with momentary pleasure being heavily weighted, than when in an abstract mindset, with long-term health receiving more attention. Like timing, the content of the message should match the goals.

Messages can also quantify the effects of a behavior, apply standards, or frame the outcome as a loss or gain. A quantifying message might say, "Taking the stairs for 5 minutes a day 5 days a week burns off 2.5 lb of fat in a year" or "1 Snickers bar = 20-minute run." Standards can increase goal compliance by making progress measurable. Using a pedometer with a stated goal (e.g., 10,000 steps) increases physical activity (Bravata et al., 2007); and 8 glasses of water or 5 fruits and vegetables per day provide helpful benchmarks for measuring desired health behaviors. Sometimes the comparison is implied, framed as loss or a gain. Although there are subtle qualifications, people are generally more sensitive to losses than gains, and more motivated by fear than pleasure (Baumeister, Bratskavsky, Finkenauer, & Vohs, 2001; Kahneman & Tversky, 1979). Perneger and Agoritsas (2011) surveyed more than 1,000 physicians to find that their beliefs about the effectiveness of a new drug depended on whether its outcomes were framed as a loss (the mortality rate) or a gain (the survival rate). Clearly, this has worrisome implications for public health. The planner, however, can leverage the strength of message framing and test multiple messages to find the one most effective in that situation.

Moments of Truth

An individual's evaluation of her choice alternatives depends on her underlying goals. While she pursues many goals, only a small number are active in any particular moment. One result is that decision processes are quite sensitive to timing—and for some marketing campaigns, timing is everything. People will be most receptive to persuasion when they are already thinking about the goal. Two creative campaigns illustrate the power of seizing the "moment of truth." In Beirut, Procter & Gamble's laundry detergent marketing team wanted to reach consumers when the goal of having clean clothes was already activated. This particular goal is rarely top-of-mind for most people, but the marketing team discovered the perfect opportunity. Because most Beirut residents live in tall apartment buildings and hang their laundry on balconies to dry, they see the street traffic below while thinking about clean clothes. Seizing the moment, Procter & Gamble bought advertising space on the tops of buses. Another creative marketing team was tasked with encouraging Americans to buy Campbell's soup. However, American families already had many cans of soup in their pantries. So Campbell's needed to first encourage people to eat soup, so that they would then consider buying more. Given that soup satisfies the goal of eating comfort food, Campbell's purchased local "storm spot" television advertising. They produced special commercials that would air only during a storm, when Americans would be most likely to desire to eat something warm and comforting.

Planners of behavioral change can take a page from the marketing playbook by asking themselves when the goal relevant to the desired behavior will be most salient. For example, in an office building, signs reminding employees to take the stairs can be placed next to or on the elevators, when people are thinking about their goal of getting upstairs. In the right locations, stair prompts with messages such as "Burn calories, not electricity" have been found to be highly effective, increasing stair use by as much as 40%, even 9 months later (Lee et al., 2012). Similarly, information or a hotline number for quitting smoking could be placed in the physical location where people go to smoke. And messages encouraging water consumption could be placed on tables where food is eaten, or at the top of the stairs, where thirsty stair climbers will see them. Sometimes the goals planners need to keep in mind are the goals that go *against* the desired behavior. For example, knowing that by lunchtime, the goal of getting full on a tasty meal may trump the goal of long-term health, planners can offer choosers the opportunity to decide their meals ahead of time, before the goal of assuaging hunger kicks in.

To leverage the power of persuasion, the right message needs to be delivered in the right place at the right time. Identifying moments of truth in which the relevant goal is most salient, communicating vividly, and choosing the right standards of comparison are three powerful ways to influence behavior. And persuasion is the least invasive and lowest cost way to nudge people toward better choices. Despite these strengths, even the best communication at the moment of truth will have only a limited influence on behavior in other situations. A planner's only hope of changing behavior across contexts is to focus on influencing the person.

Person: How Are Intentions Reinforced?

Most behavior change initiatives already focus on the individual person, attempting to influence his or her choices in general. Planners hope that exposure to the truth will improve behavior in every situation—at work, at home, on vacation, and so on. However, because of the barriers to change described in the opening section (impulsivity, cognitive load, bounded willpower, hyperbolic discounting, and automaticity), behavior change does not always follow a change in attitudes. Unfortunately, influencing the person can be much more challenging than influencing through possibilities, process, and persuasion. We can, however, provide some suggestions for influencing a person through goal setting and skill building in order to reinforce healthy intentions. The object of these interventions is to maintain healthy behaviors over time, eventually making them habitual and automatic.

Goals

An important component of self-improvement strategies is setting and tracking goals. To improve performance, a goal should be both motivational and measurable; therefore, it must be challenging, specific, and concrete (Locke & Latham, 1990). A goal to "lose weight" is merely a wish, whereas a goal to "run 3 miles 3 times a week until the wedding" entails both a reasonable challenge and a means of measuring success—and is therefore more likely to yield the desired outcome (Strecher et al., 1995).

Goals also become more manageable when broken into smaller steps. Like paying for a new car in monthly payments, a goal of losing 4 lbs or pounds per month becomes easier than losing 50 lbs or pounds in a year. And another important benefit of setting intermediate goals is building momentum by tracking small wins along the way—perception of progress toward a goal can itself be motivating (Kivetz, Urmisky, & Zheng, 2006). Planners might offer advice about goals, such as cutting them into "bite-size" pieces (skipping dessert for a week, rather than permanently cutting out sugar), or celebrating the small wins. Self-reinforcement gives people something to look forward to (a pedicure, a bubble bath, a new magazine) and creates a sense of progress along the way. The key to the long-term success of goal setting and measurement of health behaviors lies in making those new behaviors habitual.

Habits

Although people experience their own behavior as conscious and intentional, the majority of all actions are automatic, bypassing the conscious decision-making process entirely (Bargh & Chartrand, 1999). Because habits are enacted automatically, without requiring willpower or conscious effort, turning healthy behaviors into habits is the ideal way to sustain them. Habits should be shaped one at a time, and any positive reinforcement should take place during or immediately following the behavior (Pryor, 2002). To further reinforce the behavior, individuals can leverage contextual cues (Sutherland, 2008). Implementation intentions use cues to serve as reminders for triggering a desired behavior, and they can help to develop the behavior into a habit. Research has shown implementation intentions to be effective in developing healthy habits such as performing breast self-exams (Prestwich et al., 2005), exercising (Luszczynska, Sobczyk, & Abraham, 2007), and eating vegetables (Chapman, Armitage, & Norman, 2009)—simply by asking study participants to decide where, when, and how they plan to take action. Habits are more easily formed and broken in new environments, because they lack the contextual cues that triggered old habits (Wood, Tam, & Guerrero Witt, 2005). Therefore, behavior change efforts launched in coincidence with other changes such as moves, promotions, reorganizations, new relationships, new jobs, or even seasonal changes have a greater chance of success (Verplanken & Wood, 2006). Even in familiar environments, contextual cues can facilitate habit formation—laying out exercise clothes the night before can prompt a morning jog, or setting twice-a-day medications next to the toothbrush can improve medication compliance.

Precommitment

Even with the right goals, the right management, and the right reinforcement of habits, there will be times in which the desired behavior is particularly difficult or temptation is particularly strong. It has recently and repeatedly been confirmed that willpower is a depletable mental resource, and that when people are tired, hungry, stressed, or focused on something else, or have just expended willpower in another situation, they are less likely to perform actions requiring willpower (Baumeister & Tierney, 2011). And this effect is more than psychological—in fact, willpower seems to be impaired by low blood sugar (Gailliot et al., 2007). The good news is that willpower, like a muscle, can be developed over time (Mischel, 1996); and it can also be temporarily improved by eating or drinking—yet another reason that eating more small, healthy meals throughout the day may be beneficial (Katz & Gonzáles, 2004). Knowing that their willpower may falter, individuals can preplan when possible or create their own "commitment devices."

Preplanning allows System 2 to make a reasoned decision ahead of time, thus preventing the impulses of System 1 from resulting in rash and regrettable actions. Researchers have found that when people make decisions for the distant future, they save more money (Thaler & Benartzi, 2004) and choose healthier food (Milkman, Rogers, & Bazerman, 2010; Read & van Leeuwen, 1998).

Commitment devices increase the cost or difficulty of engaging in undesirable behaviors, thus reducing reliance on willpower. Many field experiments have asked participants to put their own money at risk as an incentive for following through on their intended behaviors, for example losing weight (John et al., 2011) and quitting smoking (Giné, Karlan, & Zinman, 2010). Observing the power of such interventions, behavioral economists Dean Karlan and Ian Ayres founded a Web site, http://www. Stickk.com, that helps users create their own commitment devices, staking their money or reputation on following through on their good intentions.

We have described many possible ways in which the well-meaning planner can support the healthy intentions of others, and we have provided some suggestions for reinforcing one's own healthy intentions as well. Given the many forces at work in every context, the only way to predict the precise impact of an intervention or "tweak" is to try it out in a small-scale experiment. And when possible, this is what the authors do.

Next, we shall describe how one team of people at one firm—the food team at Google—has put the 4 P's framework into action, testing many of these recommendations along the way.

Case Study: Google

In 2007 and the next 7 years, Google was rated by its employees ("Googlers") as one of the top five US companies to work for ("100 best companies ...", 2014). And in all those years, Googlers mentioned the free, homemade food as one of the keys to their satisfaction. The biggest challenge for the food team was figuring out how to help Googlers stay simultaneously healthy and satisfied: failing on either dimension would mean loss of productivity and morale, which could hurt business outcomes and employee retention. And inducing satisfaction meant not just providing a variety of foods (including some less healthy ones), but treating employees as adults capable of making their own decisions about their bodies and their health. Therefore, gentle nudges that did not restrict choices were appealing to the food team.

When the Google food team engaged Yale University to help them apply the 4 P's framework, they had already been using many "tweaks" inspired by behavioral economists that were consistent with the framework. In fact, they were on the vanguard of applying behavioral economics to the food environment. Here, we describe how the framework is being applied at Google, with results of some pilot studies and a few suggestions for possible future interventions. We do not include the person section of the framework in the case study; our joint endeavor has focused thus far on the low-hanging fruit of the first three areas, possibilities, process, and persuasion. Our hope is that describing how the framework can be applied to one challenge (serve food that keeps people healthy and satisfied) in one type of location (Google offices) will inspire ideas for applying the framework to other challenges and locations.

Possibilities: What Choices Are Offered?

Assortment

In the quest to help Googlers make healthy food choices that would satisfy them, the obvious first step was to try to serve an assortment of foods that were both delicious and nutritious. While each chef had considerable leeway for creativity, all served a variety of healthy foods on the menu each day. Kale quinoa salad, butternut squash soup, and fresh seasonal fruits were typical of the rotating healthy fare. Some food team members organized special programs at their locations; for example, one office held a 30-day juice challenge, offering fresh-pressed vegetable juices as an afternoon snack. Another office offered do-it-yourself dinners assembled at work and brought home, to help employees eat better outside the office. And in most locations, fresh fruits and vegetables were offered throughout the day in the many break areas known as "microkitchens."

As the food team shifted menus to accommodate more healthy foods, they also shifted recipes to make foods healthier. Chefs decreased salt, sugar, and cream in their dishes, and they modified their recipes to offer daily specials such as a rotating specialty sandwich with 500 calories or fewer. In some cases, healthy items were simply made more appealing; for example, tap water was upgraded to "spa water," with fruit-, herb-, or cucumber-infused water served from a water bar. Also, chefs bundled healthy items together in another daily special, the 600-calorie plate.

Since Google's cafes and microkitchens offered hundreds of delicious options daily, variety was a blessing and a curse. While the food team could have cut back on variety, taking back anything employees have come to count on is a risky proposition. Therefore, they would probably be better off focusing on the cycles of variety over time and on perceived variety. Rather than limiting unhealthy options, they could increase the perceived variety of healthy options through redundancy in multiple locations. For example, healthy dishes served in other parts of the café could be repeated in a colorful "eating well" or "super charge" station. The food team could lower the perceived variety of less healthy dishes by serving foods of the same color on the same day, side by side. When planning variety within each station, healthier items could be displayed in the privileged first position, where they would be more likely to be chosen, leaving less room on the plate for unhealthy alternatives.

Restricting choice is a sensitive matter, and its success depends on how the restriction is framed. An example of a success is one café's Pizza Wednesday. With this positive framing, many Googlers saw Wednesday as a day to look forward to, with pizza as an indulgent special treat. While actually restricting pizza during every day but one, Pizza Wednesday was successful because it framed the indulgence as gain rather than a loss. (We expect "Pizza-less Wednesday" would have been poorly received, despite entailing more frequent availability of pizza.)

In the future, Google chefs could further support health without taking choices away through careful planning of variety over time. Thus, healthier menu options could be rotated more frequently while indulgent items could be rotated less frequently, without shifting the balance of healthy versus indulgent items on any particular day. For example, prepared salads could change daily, with desserts changing weekly. The longer cycles for indulgent items would leverage satiation to decrease consumption, and the shorter cycles for healthy items would leverage variety seeking.

Amount

The Google food team was committed to not charging Googlers for meals or snacks, so the question of "how much" was limited to quantity in this case. Although Googlers were permitted to serve themselves unlimited helpings, in practice, seconds and thirds were rare. Therefore, serving size provided a strong anchor for the quantity of each food consumed. To reduce consumption of caloric beverages, the food team switched 22-oz cups to 16-oz cups. And in some locations, they offered smaller to-go boxes to help Googlers control their own food portions when bringing food back to their desks. Desserts in all cafés were plated or cut in small quantities. In microkitchens where bulk snacks were served, serving scoops were intentionally small.

While consumption frequency is affected by where and when a food is served, serving size is more affected by what the food is served in. For example, numerous studies (reviewed in Wansink, 2006; Wansink, van Ittersum, & Painter, 2006) have shown smaller plates and bowls to be effective in reducing consumption. When the food team surveyed Googlers about the idea of offering smaller plates, they found most Googlers (65%) supported the introduction of small plates, but most (75%) were also against the removal of large ones. Googlers did not want their choices restricted. When small plates were experimentally introduced, 30% of Googlers chose them over the large plates (Kang 2013).

Additionally, we conducted a field study to test the effect of switching out bulk candies for small packages. Most Google microkitchen snacks were served from bulk containers with 4-oz cups provided for convenience, and we had noticed that most snackers seemed to be filling the 4-oz cups. After taking baseline measures of individual consumption in two microkitchens, in one of those microkitchens, we replaced loose M&Ms (the most popular snack) with small individually wrapped packages. During the baseline period, the average serving size was identical between the two microkitchens, but the small packages treatment reduced the average serving size by 58%—from 308 calories to 130 calories.

Process

Accessibility

Whenever possible, healthy items were made easier to reach, and unhealthy items were made more difficult to reach. Accessibility stimulates mindless consumption—and sometimes this can be beneficial. For example, in a pilot study at Google, stocking water bottles in coolers at eye level behind glass, while moving sugary beverages to the bottom shelves behind frosted glass, increased water consumption 47%, while decreasing calories consumed in sugary beverages 6% (Kang, 2013). This manipulation impacted real accessibility, and also perceived accessibility. In many cafés, salad bars were set up near the café entrances, where everyone walked by, and desserts were relegated to a corner, where they were visible but not immediately accessible. The intent was to make a salad a mindless choice, and a dessert a conscious one. Accessibility can be harmful as well, of course, when it makes unhealthy foods mindless choices or leads to overconsumption. We conducted an observational field study to test the effect of accessibility on snacking.

This study was run at a large and busy microkitchen containing two beverage stations: a close one 6½ feet from the snack bar and a far one 17½ feet from the snack bar. Both beverage stations had a refrigerator containing bottled beverages and a brewing station for hot drinks. The snack bar contained a variety of nonperishable snacks such as nuts, crackers, candies, dried fruit, and cookies. For every Googler who took a drink during a 7-day observation period, we recorded which beverage station they used and whether they also took a snack. The results were dramatic: Drinkers at the close beverage station were 50% more likely to take a snack than those at the far beverage station. We found that for men, who showed a greater difference than women, the estimated "penalty" for using the close beverage station was equivalent to approximately 1 lbs or pounds of fat per year for each daily cup of coffee.[1]

Persuasion

Vividness

Visual labels had been used in Google cafés and microkitchens with varying success. Like Thorndike et al.'s (2012) hospital cafeteria field study, Google used stoplight labels, with green for the healthiest items, red for the least healthy items, and yellow for those in between. Many Googlers reported that the colored labels helped them make healthy choices. They also reported relying on the visual icons for vegetarian, gluten-free, and so on, to help them easily avoid foods conflicting with their dietary restrictions.

We experimented with showing visual serving sizes for snacks in a microkitchen, for example, showing how far to fill the snack cup for a proper serving; however, this intervention had no impact on consumption. Any kind of serving size suggestion requires multistage processing: seeing the suggestion, attending to it, deciding to what degree to follow the suggestion, and then acting on that decision. While serving size suggestions are undoubtedly useful in some situations for some people, we recommend portioning (as in the fun packs study) or relying on nudges such as the size of the dish or serving utensil whenever possible.

Comparisons

An additional persuasive and informative tool Google could make more use of in the future would be café menus, whether publicly displayed in high-traffic areas like microkitchens, or digital and customizable online. Even the simplest menu impacts choices through the order in which items are listed (privileging items at the top of the list) and by how the foods are named and described. There are many ways a menu can nudge people toward healthy choices.

First, healthy choices can be featured menu items, like chefs' specials at restaurants. Google chefs could star their recommendations, or recommendations might be treated like a featured online classified ad, for example, moved to the top of the list, boxed, bolded, shaded, accompanied by an attractive photograph, and so on. Second, menus would not need to be comprehensive; they could provide a subset of the day's dishes, highlighting healthy options and avoiding some of the unhealthy ones. Third, employees could be empowered to create their own menu filters. At Google, and in any work environment in which most employees work on computers, there would be an opportunity to allow employees to customize menus according to their own preferences. Besides allowing employees to easily view foods they would be likely to enjoy and to make a decision about where to eat lunch, individually customizable menus provide the benefit of allowing employees to take action when their willpower is strong that would provide benefits when their willpower is weak. For example, one could make the decision to permanently hide all desserts from the menu list, thereby avoiding that temptation in the future. A final benefit that a digital menu might provide would be links to healthy recipes, so that Googlers could reproduce some of their favorites at home.

Moments of Truth

When we ran a field study to test whether promotions could increase uptake of some widely disliked vegetables, we promoted the vegetables at the "moment of truth," right at the point of choice.

Five target vegetables were selected, based on being commonly disliked and seasonally available: brussels sprouts, parsnips, beets, cauliflower, and squash. For each of the target vegetables, Google chefs selected a recipe for a hot dish and a recipe for a cold salad containing that vegetable as the dominant ingredient. During a baseline period of five Mondays, chefs made a hot dish and a salad with the same main vegetable each week in both of two high-traffic cafés. During the following five Mondays, the same dishes were served again in both cafés and were advertised in only the treatment café with large colorful "Vegetable of the Day!" posters displaying an elegant picture of the raw vegetable and an uninformative bit of trivia, as well as flyers next to each dish. The moment-of-truth vegetable promotions increased the number of employees trying the hot dishes at the treatment café by 74%, even as the proportion decreased in the control café. Promotions also increased the average serving size of the hot dish at the treatment cafe by 64%. Although the effect was smaller for the salad, which had lower uptake and was served in a lower-traffic location, overall consumption of the promoted vegetables increased at the treatment café by 48%.

We have described many ways in which the 4 P's framework has nudged Googlers toward healthy choices and we have suggested other ways in which it might do so; however, we must emphasize that each intervention should be tested for efficacy in the relevant context. For example, persuasive signs at Google have shown mixed results. After fast-food consumption at many New York City fast-food restaurants decreased following mandated calorie labeling in 2008 (Dumanovsky et al., 2011), signs with warnings about calories in Coke were tested in a Seattle microkitchen. In that case, consumption of Coke and other sugary beverages did not change. On the other hand, the Vegetable of the Day experiment showed promising results. We have tried to provide as much guidance as possible to suggest types of interventions likely to succeed in nudging people toward healthy behaviors, but each situation and population is unique enough that the only way for planners to ensure success is to run small experiments, as the Google food team does.

Conclusion

We have suggested many potential ways a planner might help other people improve their health choices with as little effort as possible—reducing the burden of System 2—through the application of research findings from behavioral economics and psychology. These findings offer a toolbox of interventions leveraging a contextual approach aimed at influencing specific decisions via (1) the combination of choices people are exposed to, (2) the choice environment, and (3) the communication about the choices. Additionally, we have offered advice on supporting the individual in the development of healthy habits, to make healthier choices in any time or place. There is great potential in the contextual spheres of influence outlined here that will enable planners to make healthy choices easy choices.

Note

1. Assuming 150-calorie snacks.

References

100 best companies to work for (2007-2014). (2014). *Fortune*. Retrieved February 2015, from http://archive.fortune.com/magazines/fortune/best-companies/

Aydinoglu, N. Z., Krishna, A., & Wansink, B. (2009). Do size labels have a common meaning among consumers? In A. Krishna (Ed.), *Sensory marketing: Research on the sensuality of products* (pp. 343–360). New York, NY: Routledge.

Bargh, J. A., & Chartrand, T. L. (1999). The unbearable automaticity of being. *American Psychologist, 54*, 462–479.

Baumeister, R. F., Bratslavsky, E., Finkenauer, C., & Vohs, K. D. (2001). Bad is stronger than good. *Review of General Psychology, 5*(4), 323–370.

Baumeister, R. F., Bratslavsky, E., Muraven, M., & Tice, D. M. (1998). Ego depletion: Is the active self a limited resource? *Journal of Personality and Social Psychology, 74*(5), 1252–1265.

Baumeister, R. F., & Tierney, J. (2011). *Willpower: Rediscovering the greatest human strength*. New York, NY: Penguin Press.

Bravata, D. M., Smith-Spangler, C., Sundaram, V., Gienger, A. L., Lin, N., Lewis, R., ... Sirard, J. R. (2007). Using pedometers to increase physical activity and improve health: A systematic review. *Journal of the American Medical Association, 298*, 2296–2304.

Chapman, J., Armitage, C. J., & Norman, P. (2009). Comparing implementation intention interventions in relation to young adults intake of fruit and vegetables. *Psychology and Health, 24*(3), 317–332.

Chou, S., Grossman, M., & Saffer, H. (2004). An economic analysis of adult obesity: Results from the behavioral risk factor surveillance system. *Journal of Health Economics*, *23*, 565–587.

Cullen, K. W., Baranowski, T., Owens, E., Marsh, T., Rittenberry, L., & de Moor, C. (2003). Availability, accessibility, and preferences for fruit, 100% fruit juice, and vegetables influence children's dietary behavior. *Health Education and Behavior*, *30*, 615–626.

Dumanovsky, T., Huang, C. Y., Nonas, C. A., Matte, T. D., Bassett, M. T., & Silver, L. D. (2011). Changes in energy content of lunchtime purchases from fast food restaurants after introduction of calorie labelling: Cross sectional customer surveys. *British Medical Journal*, *343*, 1–11.

Gailliot, M. T., Baumeister, R. F., DeWall, C. N., Maner, J. K., Plant, E. A., Tice, D. M., ... Schmeichel, B. J. (2007). Self-control relies on glucose as a limited energy source: Willpower is more than a metaphor. *Journal of Personality and Social Psychology*, *92*, 325–336.

Geier, A. B., Rozin, P., & Doros, G. (2006). Unit bias a new heuristic that helps explain the effect of portion size on food intake. *Psychological Science*, *17*(6), 521–525.

Giné, X., Karlan, D., & Zinman, J. (2010). Put your money where your butt is: A commitment contract for smoking cessation. *American Economic Journal: Applied Economics*, *2*(4) 213–235.

Haws, K. L., & Winterich, K. P. (2013). When value trumps health in a supersized world. *Journal of Marketing*, *77*(3), 48–64.

Heath, C., & Heath, D. (2010). *Switch: How to change things when change is hard.* New York, NY: Crown Business.

Hofmann, W., Baumeister, R. F., Förster, G., & Vohs, K. D. (2012). Everyday temptations: An experience sampling study on desire, conflict, and self-control. *Journal of Personality and Social Psychology*, *102*, 1318–1335.

Horgen, K. B., & Brownell, K. D. (2002). Comparison of price change and health message interventions in promoting healthy food choices. *Health Psychology*, *21*(5), 505–512.

Hsee, C. K. (1998). Less is better: When low-value options are valued more highly than high-value options. *Journal of Behavioral Decision Making*, *11*, 107–121.

Irmak, C., Vallen, B., & Robinson, S. R. (2011). The impact of product name on dieters' and nondieters' food evaluations and consumption. *Journal of Consumer Research*, *38*(2), 390–405.

John, L. K., Loewenstein, G., Troxel, A. B., Norton, L., Fassbender, J. E., & Volpp, K. G. (2011). Financial incentives for extended weight loss: A randomized, controlled trial. *Journal of General Internal Medicine*, *26*(6), 621–626.

Johnson, E. J., & Goldstein, D. (2003). Do defaults save lives? *Science*, *302*, 1338–1339.

Kahn, B. E., & Wansink, B. (2004). The influence of assortment structure on perceived variety and consumption quantities. *Journal of Consumer Research*, *30*(4), 519–533.

Kahneman, D., & Frederick, S. (2002). Representativeness revisited: Attribute substitution in intuitive judgment. In T. Gilovich, D. Griffin, & D. Kahneman (Eds.), *Heuristics of intuitive judgment: Extensions and applications* (pp. 49–81). New York, NY: Cambridge University Press.

Kahneman, D., & Tversky, A. (1979). Prospect theory: An analysis of decision under risk. *Econometrica*, *47*, 263–291.

Kang, C. (2013, September 1). Google crunches data on munching in office. *The Washington Post*. Retrieved February 2015, from http://www.washingtonpost.com/business/technology/google-crunches-data-on-munching-in-office/2013/09/01/3902b444-0e83-11e3-85b6-d27422650fd5_story.html

Katz, D. L., & Gonzáles, M. H. (2004). *The way to eat*. Naperville, IL: Sourcebooks.

Kivetz, R., Urminsky, O., & Zheng, Y. (2006). The goal-gradient hypothesis resurrected: Purchase acceleration, illusionary goal progress and customer retention. *Journal of Marketing Research*, *43*, 39–58.

Koppell, J., & Steen, J. A. (2004). The effects of ballot position on election outcomes. *Journal of Politics*, *66*(1), 267–281.

Lee, K. K., Perry, A. S., Wolf, S. A., Agarwal, R., Rosenblum, R., Fischer, S., ... Silver, L. D. (2012). Promoting routine stair use: Evaluating the impact of a stair prompt across buildings. *American Journal of Preventive Medicine*, *42*(2), 136–141.

Locke, E. A., & Latham, G. P. (1990). *A theory of goal setting and task performance*. Englewood Cliffs, NJ: Prentice-Hall.

Luszczynska, A., Sobczyk, A., & Abraham, C. (2007). Planning to lose weight: Randomized controlled trial of an implementation intention prompt to enhance weight reduction among overweight and obese women. *Health Psychology*, *26*(4), 507–512.

McKay, B. (2010, March 22). PepsiCo develops 'designer salt' to chip away at sodium intake. *Wall Street Journal*. Retrieved May 2014, from http://www.wsj.com/articles/SB10001424052748704534904575131602283791566

Milkman, K., Minson, J. A., & Volpp, K. G. (2014). Holding the Hunger Games hostage at the gym: An evaluation of temptation bundling. *Management Science*, *60*(2), 283–299.

Milkman, K. L., Rogers, T., & Bazerman, M. H. (2010). I'll have the ice cream soon and the vegetables later: A study of online grocery purchases and order lead time. *Marketing Letters*, *21*(1), 17–35.

Mischel, W. (1996). From good intentions to willpower. In P. Gollwitzer & J. Bargh (Eds.), *The psychology of action* (pp. 197–218). New York, NY: Guilford Press.

Nisbett, R. E., & Wilson, T. D. (1977). Telling more than we can know: Verbal reports on mental processes. *Psychological Review*, *84*, 231–259.

Nutrition advice from nutrition expert Brian Wansink. (2014). *Smarter Lunchrooms Movement*. Retrieved May 2014, from http://smarterlunchrooms.org/news/nutrition-advice-nutrition-expert-brian-wansink

Perneger, T. V., & Agoritsas, T. (2011). Doctors and patients susceptibility to framing bias: A randomized trial. *Journal of General Internal Medicine*, *26*(12), 1411–1417.

Prestwich, A., Conner, M., Lawton, R., Bailey, W., Litman, J., & Molyneaux, V. (2005). Individual and collaborative implementation intentions and the promotion of breast self-examination. *Psychology and Health*, *20*, 743–760.

Pryor, K. (2002). *Don't shoot the dog*. Gloucestershire, UK: Ring Press.

Read, D., & van Leeuwen, B. (1998). Predicting hunger: The effects of appetite and delay on choice. *Organizational Behavior and Human Decision Processes*, *76*(2), 189–205.

Schwartz, J., Riis, J., Elbel, B., & Ariely, D. (2012). Inviting consumers to downsize fast-food portions significantly reduces calorie consumption. *Health Affairs*, *31*(2), 399–407.

Sela, A., Berger, J., & Liu, W. (2009). Variety, vice, and virtue: How assortment size influences option choice. *Journal of Consumer Research, 35*(6), 941–951.

Sharpe, K., Staelin, R., & Huber, J. (2008). Using extremeness aversion to fight obesity: Policy implications of context dependent demand. *Journal of Consumer Research, 35*, 406–422.

Sheeran, P., Webb, T. L., & Gollwitzer, P. M. (2005). The interplay between goal intentions and implementation intentions. *Personality and Social Psychology Bulletin, 31*, 87–98.

Shiv, B., & Fedorikhin, A. (1999). Heart and mind in conflict: The interplay of affect and cognition in consumer decision making. *Journal of Consumer Research, 26*, 278–292.

Stanovich, K. E., & West, R. F. (2000). Individual differences in reasoning: Implications for the rationality debate? *Behavioral and Brain Sciences, 23*, 645–726.

Strecher, V. J., Seijts, G. H., Kok, G. J., Latham, G. P., Glasgow, R., DeVellis, B., ... Bulger, D. W. (1995). Goal setting as a strategy for health behavior change. *Health Education Quarterly, 22*, 190–200.

Sutherland, A. (2008). *What Shamu taught me about life, love, and marriage: Lessons for people from animals and their trainers.* New York, NY: Random House.

Thaler, R. H., & Benartzi, S. (2004). Save More Tomorrow™: Using behavioral economics to increase employee saving. *Journal of Political Economy, 112*(S1), S164–S187.

Thaler, R. H., & Sunstein, C. R. (2003). Libertarian paternalism. *American Economc Review Papers and Proceedings, 93*, 175–179.

Thorndike, A. N., Sonnenberg, L., Riis, J., Barraclough, S., & Levy, D. E. (2012). A 2-phase labeling and choice architecture intervention to improve healthy food and beverage choices. *American Journal of Public Health, 102*(3), 527–533.

Trope, Y., & Liberman, N. (2003). Temporal construal. *Psychological Review, 110*, 403–421.

Trope, Y., & Liberman, N. (2010). Construal level theory of psychological distance. *Psychological Review, 117*, 440–463.

Verplanken, B., & Wood, W. (2006). Interventions to break and create consumer habits. *Journal of Public Policy and Marketing, 25*(1), 90–103.

Wansink, B. (2006). *Mindless eating: Why we eat more than we think.* New York, NY: Bantam.

Wansink, B., & Kim, J. (2005). Bad popcorn in big buckets: Portion size can influence intake as much as taste. *Journal of Nutrition, Education, and Behavior, 37*(5), 242–245.

Wansink, B., & van Ittersum, K. (2003). Bottoms up! Peripheral cues and consumption volume. *Journal of Consumer Research, 30*, 455–463.

Wansink, B., Van Ittersum, K., & Painter, J. E. (2005). How descriptive food names bias sensory perceptions in restaurants. *Food Quality and Preference, 16*(5), 393–400.

Wansink, B., Van Ittersum, K., & Painter, J. E. (2006). Ice cream illusions: bowls, spoons, and self-served portion sizes. *American Journal of Preventive Medicine, 31*(3), 240–243.

Wood, W., Tam, L., & Guerrero Witt, M. (2005). Changing circumstances, disrupting habits. *Journal of Personality and Social Psychology, 88*, 918–933.

8 | Incentivizing Health Behaviors

KRISTINA LEWIS AND JASON BLOCK

SMOKING, POOR NUTRITION, lack of physical activity, excess alcohol consumption, and noncompliance with medications explain much of the excess mortality in the United States and increasingly across the world (Danaei et al., 2009; Mokdad, Marks, Stroup, & Gerberding, 2004). Finding strategies to decrease these behaviors, and to sustain these changes, is the holy grail of medicine and public health. However, as anyone who has tried to change a behavior can attest, behaviors are often entrenched and intractable to change. A major impediment to change is the natural human tendency to discount the future and value the present (Laibson, 1997). Future discounting often prevents people from making decisions that have an abstract future benefit, such as a lower risk for a heart attack, while causing inconveniences in the present, such as forgoing the most palatable foods and taking medications with unpleasant side effects. Addictions and physiologic factors further confound behavior change. For example, patients who abuse substances must not only recognize the present and future benefits of quitting but also must overcome their addictions to the chemicals they abuse. Weight loss also requires overcoming physiologic barriers such as a lower metabolic rate and altered hormonal levels, leading to frequent weight regain (Ammerman et al., 2002; Leibel & Hirsch, 1984; Leibel, Rosenbaum, & Hirsch, 1995).

One oft-explored strategy to overcome the barriers of future discounting and addiction is paying people to change their behaviors. Studies extending back to the 1970s have examined financial incentives for behavior change (Cahill & Perera, 2011; Jeffery, 2012; Ryan et al., 2011). When used to encourage behavior change, most incentives include straightforward payments to patients or enrollment in lotteries for cash or prizes. In this chapter, many of the studies we present utilize these traditional approaches. However, several studies use principles arising from behavioral economics, including loss aversion, regret, and defaults (Choi, Laibson, Madrian, & Metrick, 2004; Connolly & Butler, 2006; Kahneman & Tversky, 1979; Thaler & Sunstein, 2009). These approaches, discussed in detail in Chapters 1 and 2, incorporate components that might help people overcome future discounting. In this way, behavioral economics might "supercharge" financial incentives.

Commitment contracts are an example of the type of incentives heavily influenced by behavioral economics (Halpern, Asch, & Volpp, 2012; Loewenstein, Brennan, & Volpp, 2007). Commitment contracts have a long legacy, extending back through the mists of time to Homer's *Odyssey*. To avoid temptation from the Sirens, Odysseus instructed his men to plug their ears with wax and tie him to his ship's mast. In so doing, he planned in advance to avoid a known temptation and successfully avoided an unfortunate consequence. When applied to behavior change, commitment contracts often take the form of a deposit contract in which individuals bet on their own success. If they achieve a predetermined outcome, they receive their money back in return, often with additional incentives. If they fail, they lose their money. In the language of the *Odyssey*, the bet is the wax and ropes, and the Sirens' song is the temptation that leads people toward unhealthy choices—cigarettes, food, inactivity, alcohol, drugs, and avoidance of medication. Several studies have found success with deposit contracts; however, success is typically for a finite period, during the active phase of the contracts (Gine, Karlan, & Zinman, 2010; Halpern et al., 2012; John et al., 2011; Kullgren et al., 2013; Volpp, John, et al., 2008; White, Dow, & Rungruanghiranya, 2013).

In this chapter, we discuss the array of studies on traditional financial incentives and those influenced by behavioral economics. We focus on studies of weight loss, smoking cessation, and medication compliance. We further present some literature on other health behaviors and then close the chapter by commenting on changes in the 2010 Affordable Care Act that might ignite the use of incentives and the ethics of using incentives.

Incentives for Obesity Treatment/Weight Loss

Over 30% of US adults are now classified as obese (Flegal, Carroll, Kit, & Ogden, 2012). Promotion of effective methods for helping these individuals lose weight is among the highest priorities in medicine and public health. As is all too familiar for many, achieving weight loss and keeping the weight off can be very difficult, requiring sustained decreases in caloric intake coupled with increases in caloric expenditure. Individuals must do this while overcoming the metabolic and hormonal processes that are working against their success. Scores of randomized trials and observational cohort studies provide clear evidence that diets are difficult for patients to comply with and that people often revert to old eating habits relatively quickly.

Behavioral economics helps explain why weight loss is so difficult, even though it is such a desirable outcome for most individuals who are overweight or obese. First, dieting and exercise may not be particularly pleasurable, especially for those who currently eat a fairly unhealthy diet and live a sedentary lifestyle. Swapping a juicy bacon cheeseburger, a sugar-laden soda, and fries for a salad with balsamic vinegar and water, or hitting the gym instead of the TV remote control button are some of the many tough choices that must be made regularly in order for people to lose weight. Secondly, not only are the requisite behavior changes somewhat unpleasant, but the end goal of weight loss is typically far in the future, after months or sometimes years of slogging through diet and activity changes. Lastly, unhealthful foods and inducements for a sedentary lifestyle are ubiquitous in today's environment; the default is set up for people to continue gaining weight. For the average future-discounting, default-loving human being, this makes the path to sustained weight loss fraught with difficulty.

In light of the rising prevalence of obesity, researchers and policy makers have rekindled interest in the use of financial incentives to help individuals lose weight. By shifting rewards into real time, with tangible dollars, people are offered a universally desirable outcome, earning money, to offset the often unpleasant feelings associated with decreased caloric intake and increased caloric expenditures. In studies, these incentives have taken various forms, from fixed payments to those influenced by behavioral economics. The research to date has been promising but also has a number of important limitations, which are reviewed here.

Size of Incentive

One of the first questions that comes to mind when considering the use of financial incentives to change behavior is "How much do you need to pay people for this to work?" For the outcome of weight loss, an intuitive answer is "more is better" (Jeffery, 2012). Beyond that, there is no agreed-upon amount that seems to be optimal (and, indeed, too large an incentive can backfire). Prior trials examining this issue have employed a wide range of dollar amounts. While those who paid people more found greater weight loss, clinically significant weight loss (at or above 5% of baseline body weight) was also observed in studies with relatively small financial incentives (Jeffery, 2012). For example, Finkelstein and colleagues (Finkelstein, Linnan, Tate, & Birken, 2007) conducted a workplace-based trial where 207 individuals were randomized to usual care or were paid $7 or $14 per percent of body weight lost. Among those receiving financial incentives, two thirds of participants lost weight. To these successful participants, the average payout was just $49.

As it turns out, paying people too much may also backfire. Tsai et al. tested the importance of size of financial incentive in a pilot randomized trial (Tsai, Felton, Hill, & Atherly, 2012). Within a 4-month clinical weight-loss program, they allocated 50 adult participants to one of two arms: a group that received a 40% subsidy to participate in the program and a group that received a complete subsidy. The expense of the program, without a subsidy, was costly because it included meal replacements and medical visits. Mean weight loss at the end of the trial was equal between the groups (5.3% in full subsidy arm and 5.1% in the 40% subsidy arm, $p = .71$). Interestingly, more participants dropped out in the full subsidy group than in the partial subsidy group. These results may imply that people need some "skin in the game" to contribute to their motivation to attend such programs. This study did not include a comparison group with 0% subsidy.

Finally, while the existing literature on this topic suggests that higher incentive amounts can lead to greater weight loss, Jeffery published a 2012 review of financial incentives for weight loss and noted that very high levels of financial reward have not yet been tested (Jeffery, 2012). Perhaps there is some threshold level beyond which employers or other users of financial incentives would see diminishing returns of increasing investment. There is a clear need for further research to inform this issue.

Structure of Incentives

The simplest way of providing financial incentives for weight loss is to directly reward all people who achieve a predetermined weight-loss goal. The simplicity enhances the feasibility of implementation for employers and health systems that might employ these incentives. Without sacrificing simplicity, however, guaranteed earnings could be structured to capitalize on the problem of future discounting, by rewarding people along the way to a weight-loss goal, rather than waiting to deliver a lump sum of money at the end of a weight-loss period. The pilot randomized trial by Finkelstein et al. discussed earlier used either "front-loaded" (provided at 3 months) or "back-loaded" (provided at 6 months) incentives (Finkelstein et al., 2007). As predicted by concepts in behavioral economics, participants in the front-loaded group lost the most weight. Perhaps even more effective than a front-loaded incentive is the notion of providing immediate financial rewards for incremental progress toward a goal. In the setting of weight-loss trials, this immediate feedback mechanism was most closely employed by Volpp and colleagues when they rewarded participants daily for weigh-ins (Volpp, John, et al., 2008).

Some researchers have tested deposit contracts, which, by their structure, are "supercharged" by loss aversion, as a means of improving weight loss. Deposit contracts often couple risk with the possibility of reward; those who succeed at meeting their weight-loss goals not only recoup their at-risk money but also receive some additional financial reward, such as a matched amount from an employer. Cawley and Price reported observational data pooled from several worksite wellness programs where overweight or obese employees participated in one of four possible programs: (1) a complex continuous repayment program where individuals were paid monthly on a variable scale per percent weight lost ($n = 1,580$), (2) a deposit contract (participants put forward \$9.95/month as a "bet" on their own ability to achieve a weight loss goal) with lump sum repayment by their employer upon meeting goals ($n = 765$), (3) a deposit contract with continuous repayment ($n = 161$), or (4) a more traditional nonincentivized "control" program ($n = 129$) (Cawley & Price, 2013). Employers selected which program they wanted to implement in their workplace. All participating employees had access to daily informational e-mails about habits to support weight loss, call center support, and quarterly weigh-ins at worksite kiosks. The investigators observed no significant difference in year-end weight loss between the control participants and those in the continuous repayment group (only 0.1 lb more weight loss), part of which they attributed to the complexity of the reward scheme. On the other hand, participants in both of the deposit arms lost significantly more weight—2 lbs on average more than those in the control group—when accounting for attrition by carrying the baseline weight forward. For the group enrolled in the deposit contract with continuous repayment, weight loss was consistently lower than in the control group, no matter how attrition was addressed. Overall, attrition rates were very high despite the incentives; 68% of all who initially signed up for one of the four programs had dropped out by year's end (and those who were less successful were more likely to drop out).

In another twist on the delivery mechanism for financial incentives for weight loss, some have tested the use of lotteries. Typically, in these studies, participants qualify for entry into a lottery based on whether they meet a predesignated weight target. In some cases, only those who meet their goal are entered into the lottery; in other cases, all are entered, but participants can only collect on their winnings if they have met their goal. The latter approach brings concepts of regret aversion into a lottery (i.e., being told "how much money they would have won if they had stuck to their goals"). At their most basic level, lotteries seem to work because people tend to overestimate their chances of winning, even if probabilities of winning are low, such as might be the case with aggressive weight-loss goals. A study by Volpp and colleagues is perhaps the best-known study using lotteries to promote weight loss (Volpp, John, et al., 2008). They randomized 57 participants to one of three groups—no incentive, a lottery arm, or a deposit contract arm—for a 4-month period. Lottery arm participants did not have to put any of their own money at risk but were only eligible for winnings if they met a daily weight goal. Deposit contract participants deposited $0.01 to $3.00 daily, with the amount at their discretion. If they met or exceeded their weight-loss goals, their deposit was refunded at the end of each month, plus a fixed incentive matched 1:1 by the investigators. At the end of 16 weeks, both incentive arms lost significantly more weight than the control group on average (deposit 14 lb, lottery 13 lb, control 4 lb); there was no significant difference in weight loss between lottery and deposit contract arm participants. When participants were reweighed 3 months after the trial ended (after removal of incentives), there was weight regain in both incentive groups (mean final weight losses: deposit 6.2 lb, lottery 9.2 lb, control 4.4 lb). While there was no longer a statistically significant difference in weight loss between the three groups at the 7-month mark, there was a significant pre-to-post decrease in weight among incentive participants that was not evident among control participants.

Lotteries may work better for some individuals and/or demographic groups than for others. John et al. pooled the results from two trials and explored whether certain demographic characteristics might predict the optimal delivery method for incentives (John, Loewenstein, & Volpp, 2012). They found that lotteries might be most effective for people with lower income. Additionally, fighting attrition is important. A variable lottery, with the amount increasing over time, may be needed to keep people interested and willing to participate.

Attrition is an ongoing concern of these programs, especially deposit contracts. While risk aversion may lead to more success with weight loss, attrition could thwart long-term success, especially if participants are asked to deposit a large amount (Jeffery, 2012). John et al. evaluated how the structure of deposit contracts might impact uptake (John et al., 2012). They postulated that deposit contracts relying on frequent small deposits could work better than large lump-sum deposits. John described this as the "peanuts effect," an effect driven by the perception that small losses spread over time are easier to tolerate than a one-time loss of a lump sum of equal size. The downside to small frequent deposits is the weakening of the loss aversion effect; that is, participants do not feel that the daily amount is worth much to them and do not mind losing it. A further challenge to small, frequent deposits is potential habituation to the process, referred to as the "status quo" effect. People get used to putting the same amount of money in the pot every day, and regardless of their weight outcome, they are unlikely to increase or decrease the amount deposited. If deposit contract programs are to be sustainable, they must strike a balance between the size and timing of deposits to maximize effect and tolerability.

A final, but very important, point pertaining to the structure and timing of financial incentives is the notion of "mental accounting" (Thaler, 1990). That is, people tend to categorize identical sums of money differently depending on whether the sum is paid out as a cash benefit or as a discount on an existing cost (e.g., $400 off of their annual health insurance premium). The discount is not going to change someone's ability to make a short-term decision like going out to dinner; on the other hand, receiving a check for cash in the same dollar amount could ("I'm definitely going to try out that new restaurant this weekend!"). The two incentives would leave a person with the same net value, but people are likely to respond more enthusiastically to a check in their mailbox than to a smaller sum deducted from their paychecks each pay period. Although some employer groups and health plans have engaged in incentives such as premium discounts to help promote weight management among employees (Kaiser Family Foundation and Health Research & Educational Trust, 2013), program designers might see better results with equal-value incentives provided as cash rather than savings on existing costs.

In What Programmatic Context Do Incentives Work Best for Weight Loss?

Recently, employers have increasingly turned to financial incentives to promote wellness program participation or explicitly reward (or penalize) behaviors, such as smoking cessation or weight loss. Often these incentives are embedded in robust wellness programs that offer health coaching, educational programs, and disease management (Kaiser Family Foundation and Health Research & Educational Trust, 2013). Interestingly, financial incentives for weight loss may still work in the absence of a comprehensive program (Jeffery, 2012). In the Pounds for Pounds program, Relton and colleagues evaluated a financial incentive for weight loss among 402 National Health Service staff members in the United Kingdom (Relton, Strong, & Li, 2011). This study utilized a simple pre-post evaluation of a real-world program without a control group. The program consisted primarily of the incentive (ranging from £70 to £425 per year depending on a person's weight-loss plan); there was no accompanying behavioral instruction or education, other than a small booklet of weight-loss tips. The incentive was based solely on achievement of weight loss, without any deposit contract component. At the end their participation, almost half of the participants achieved weight loss of at least 5% of baseline body weight. The study had several limitations, however. Participation lengths varied, both due to attrition (>50% dropped out without completing a weight-loss plan) and variable time goals (some people set a goal for weight loss at 6 months, for example). By the end of a year, approximately 25% of initial participants remained in the program.

Who Gets the Money? Applying Incentives to the Individual Versus a Group

Incentives for weight loss can be given at the individual level or applied to groups of people who are asked to work as a team to lose weight. Applying incentives to a group is hypothesized to increase motivation among all group members, capitalizing on the notion that people would be motivated not just out of a desire for personal success but also out of a fear of failing teammates. In a comprehensive review of the literature, this norm-based approach for promoting weight loss seems to hold, at least for those who have more difficultly losing weight. In contrast, the "biggest losers" (people who lose the most weight) do so regardless of whether they work alone or in a group (Jeffery, 2012). In one recent trial that specifically tested this issue of individual- versus group-based incentives, Kullgren et al. randomized 105 obese employees (89% were female) to one of three arms: control versus individual incentive ($100/month) or group incentives ($500/group/month) for 6 months, followed by 12 weeks without incentives (Kullgren et al., 2013). At 6 months, group incentive participants lost more weight (4.4 kg more than the control group) than those receiving individual incentives (3.2 kg relative to control). Although all three groups regained weight after the cessation of incentives, group participants still had significantly greater weight loss than the other two arms at the 36-week mark. Mean earnings for group participants were highest at $514 versus just $128 for the individual participants. In another 3-month weight-loss trial, Morgan et al. randomized 110 overweight or obese male shift workers to a group-based financial incentive or a control group, in which participants received access to a standard wellness program. In the incentive arm, the group with highest mean weight loss at both 1 and 3 months into the program could earn $AU50 gift vouchers for each member (Morgan et al., 2011). Although the trial was brief, those in the incentive arm lost 4.0 kg at 3 months, compared to those in the usual wellness program arm who gained an average of 0.3 kg.

Financial Incentives for Weight-Loss Maintenance

Little research has been done on using incentives to promote weight-loss maintenance. Weight loss in most of the existing studies peaks at 6 months into the intervention, followed by a period of regain, often accelerated if financial incentives are removed (Jeffery, 2012). In fact, this pattern of weight loss is consistent even with purely behavioral diet studies without incentives (Sacks et al., 2009). In his review article focusing on incentives for weight loss, Jeffery suggested that escalating rewards may be required to promote either weight-loss maintenance or continued weight loss after about 6 months, a strategy that could be costly for employers or other groups with wellness programs. One trial by John et al. evaluated incentives for both weight loss and a brief weight-loss maintenance period following the main intervention (John et al., 2011). The intervention lasted 32 weeks, with 6 months for weight loss and 2 months for weight-loss maintenance. Participants were randomized to one of three arms (22 people in each arm): a control group, a deposit contract for weight loss, or a deposit contract for both weight loss and maintenance. At the 8-month mark, there was no difference in weight loss between the two incentive arms (but both incentive arms lost more than the control group). Weight regain after the removal of financial incentives was significant in both incentivized groups—about 1 year after the trial ended, the participants (regardless of whether they received a weight maintenance incentive during the first year) had essentially returned to their pretrial weight.

Summary of Incentives for Weight Loss

Although financial incentives can be effective for promoting weight loss, little is known about the durability of that weight loss, the optimal incentive size or structure, or the reproducibility of research results in real-world programs. Some experts have speculated that, as is often the case with translating trials into practice, pragmatic weight-loss programs using incentives might achieve more modest success than what has been observed in trials to date (Jeffery, 2012). Incentive-based weight-loss interventions supercharged by behavioral economics have tremendous promise as well. However, there is a need for more evidence to judge whether lotteries or deposit contracts work better than traditional incentives.

In the general population, the uptake of traditional incentives might be greater than the uptake of commitment contracts. Few people are at the behavioral stage of change (preparation) that would compel them to agree to what may be onerous conditions presented by deposit contracts. Fixed incentives might help nudge people to advance along to the next stage of behavior change (i.e., transition from a contemplation stage to a preparation stage). More research should therefore be done to determine whether the complexity introduced by behavioral economics is worth the effort.

Incentives for Smoking Cessation

Smoking is another key, relatively intractable public health problem that is one of the leading causes of death, if not the leading cause. This intractability lends itself, perhaps, to financial incentives that might further motivate someone to quit. Several prior studies have used financial incentives to induce smoking cessation. The largest of these was a landmark randomized controlled trial conducted at General Electric by Volpp and coauthors (Volpp et al., 2009). Approximately 65% of participants were male, nearly 90% were White, and the mean age was about 45 years. Mean daily cigarette use was about one pack per day with prior cessation attempts ranging from 6 to 7. For the intervention arm, the study provided fixed monetary incentives to compel cessation: $100 for completing a community smoking-cessation program; $250 for quitting within

6 months of enrollment, verified by salivary cotinine measurement; and $400 for sustained abstinence from smoking for 6 months after quitting. Control and intervention participants received information about community resources for cessation. By 6 months into the study, 21% quit smoking in the incentive arm compared to 12% in the control group. Incentivized participants maintained a higher quit rate than nonincentivized participants; 15% remained abstinent 6 months after quitting compared to just 5% of the nonincentivized group.

Interestingly, most demographic and behavioral factors were not associated with quitting except that participants who had frequent prior attempts to quit or were in the preparation stage of behavior change were more likely to have success. Participants received their last incentive payment if they were abstinent for 6 months after initially quitting. Yet differences in quit rates remained persistently higher for an additional 6 months after incentives stopped (9% vs. 4%, $p < .001$). Despite this measureable difference in long-term quit rates, this study reinforced the challenging nature of quitting smoking. Quit rates were low regardless of study arm.

In an accompanying process evaluation, participants, in hindsight, did not endorse incentives as a major factor in their efforts to quit. Only 30% of quitters in the incentive arm identified the incentive as very or extremely important in encouraging cessation (Kim, Kamyab, Zhu, & Volpp, 2011). Nearly all of the quitters were confident they would have quit even without an incentive. Most of the nonquitters were not motivated by an incentive regardless of size; only 26% indicated that they would have quit with a larger incentive (median desired incentive was $1,500 among all nonquitters). Willingness to quit upon study entry (precontemplation, contemplation, or preparation) was an important predictor of how much monetary "nudge" nonquitters felt would have helped them quit. Nearly 50% in the precontemplation stage felt that only an incentive of ≥$3,400 could have led them to quit compared to 20% of those in the preparation stage.

This General Electric study stands out in many ways. It was one of the larger studies to examine incentives and smoking cessation, and it is the only US incentive study to find persistence after incentives ceased. Furthermore, participants were paid much more than in most prior studies. In a systematic review of 19 studies covering 1980 to 2009, Cahill and colleagues examined studies with varied incentives, from fixed payments and/or lotteries to deposit contracts inspired by the principle of loss aversion. Only 2 of 11 studies showed a significant benefit of incentives on cessation at 6 months (Cahill & Perera, 2011; Jason, Salina, McMahon, Hedeker, & Stockton, 1997; Volpp et al., 2009). The Volpp study, of eight studies measuring persistence of cessation, was the only one demonstrating success of incentives through 12 months and beyond. But, ultimately, most studies reviewed did not pay participants much, or had small sample sizes (Troxel & Volpp, 2012). Given the highly addictive nature of nicotine, smokers are likely to have highly inelastic demand for smoking. They are willing to continue to smoke despite high monetary cost of cigarettes, thereby foregoing a built-in financial incentive to quit. To overcome the barrier of addiction, incentive payments may need to be quite high.

The other study demonstrating a benefit from incentives at 6 months was a cluster randomized controlled trial of 63 worksites (58 completed the study) and 844 participants (Jason et al., 1997). Clusters included a control arm that received only self-help information, an incentive arm that added on a $1 per day incentive for every day of abstinence over 6 months (max of $175), and a group plus incentive arm that further added on 20 group counseling sessions. Across clusters, those participating were 58% to 72% female, 63% to 78% White, and had a mean age of nearly 38 years. Quit rates at 6 months were 8%, 20%, and 39%, in the control, incentive, and incentive plus group arms with significant differences across all groups. At 12 months, the only significant differences remaining were between the group plus incentive arm and the other two arms (quit rates 16%, 18%, and 33%). Based on this study, perhaps small monetary contributions distributed frequently can have the same impact as a large lump sum.

A notable, well-conducted negative study was among 181 participants with severe mental illness (Gallagher, Penn, Schindler, & Layne, 2007). Over a 36-week period, all participants received intensive smoking-cessation counseling, and intervention groups received up to $480 in incentives for quitting and remaining abstinent, or this incentive plus nicotine replacement. Among all participants, nearly 40% to 60% were female, nearly three quarters were White, and mean age was around 43 years. Quit rates were similar across groups, with limited objectively documented cessation, assessed using salivary cotinine (2% in the control arm, 7% in the incentive, and 0% in the incentive plus nicotine replacement at 20 weeks with only slight differences at 36 weeks). There was some evidence of reduced smoking (but not cessation) in the intervention arms, measured via self-report, expired carbon monoxide levels, or salivary cotinine.

Behavioral economics has influenced incentive trials for smoking cessation as well. In the 1980s, Paxton completed several trials in the United Kingdom using deposit contracts for cessation. These studies had some limitations, including inadequate randomization and blinding processes.

But they were unique in their use of deposit contracts. The first of these examined deposit contracts of £20 (33 subjects) versus no deposit (27 subjects) for participants in a 4-month smoking-cessation program that consisted of approximately 13 group sessions (Paxton, 1980). Subjects randomized to deposit contracts provided the £20 as a lump sum and then received a £5 refund per week if abstinent (confirmed by urinary cotinine); they then made a second equivalent deposit during the fifth week with refunds of £10 every other week for the remaining 4-week period. At two months, abstinence was greater in the deposit contract group (approximately 75% vs. 55%; exact rates not provided), but by 6 months, rates were equivalent, around 40%. Paxton repeated this study without a control group but varied the structure of contracts: contracts for 2 months versus 4 months; contracts with an increasing interval between refunds ("thinning of reinforcement," refunds at 2, 4, 8, and 16 weeks instead of every 1 to 2 weeks in the standard contract); and contracts in which subjects deposited weekly for 4 weeks rather than as a lump sum at the beginning of the 4-week period (Paxton, 1983). Throughout this 1-year study, abstinence rates were similar across groups; however, quit rates at 1 year were higher for subjects receiving contracts with thinning (38% vs. 27%) versus no thinning. Similar to studies on the acceptability of different types of deposit contracts for weight loss, subjects providing weekly deposits were more likely to contribute the full requested deposits over the study period (68%) compared to those requested to provide lump sums every 4 weeks (37%).

While these studies do not analyze how much people are willing to deposit, interestingly, people may bet larger amounts of money to perform a more difficult commitment. For example, they may be willing to deposit (and risk forfeiting) a larger amount of money to quit for 12 months instead of quitting for 3 months. Intuitively, it makes more sense for people to be risk averse and thus risk less for more difficult tasks because of the higher risk of failure. The psychology of precommitment may be the opposite. If we want people to precommit to a more onerous action (e.g., getting their colonoscopy, quitting smoking), we should consider asking them to place more money at risk in their deposit contract. While there is evidence of this for weight loss, there is no clear evidence in smoking cessation.

In all, studies on financial incentives and smoking cessation are rather limited. The best conducted of them show modest success of large incentives for smoking cessation with persistence after incentives stopped. Studies using incentives influenced by behavioral economics are fairly dated with rare contemporary studies of deposit contracts only available from developing countries. One such example comes from Thailand (White et al., 2013). White and colleagues enrolled 201 smokers across 42 Thai villages in a study that compared a one-time smoking-cessation program (control) to an incentive group that had several components: a deposit contract of at least $1.67 over 10 weeks with $5 provided by study staff and an additional $5 provided if a participant's deposits were over $5, a group-based incentive in which participants received $40 if both the participant and their chosen or assigned team partner had quit smoking by 3 months, and frequent text messaging to encourage deposits. Participants only received the deposits back if they quit at 3 months, verified by urinary cotinine. Researchers continued to follow participants for 14 months. At the 3-month mark, 46% of participants in the intervention group versus 14% in the control had quit; these differences remained significant at 6 months (44% and 19%), even though the incentive had ceased after 3 months. Differences persisted over 14 months, with sustained quit rates of 42% and 25%; these results were marginally significant.

Another similar study in the Philippines found small but significant effects of commitment contracts on smoking cessation (Gine et al., 2010). The study randomized 2,000 participants to either 1) open an account that functioned as a commitment contract with an initial investment of 50 pesos (approximately $1), 2) receive cue cards that graphically depicted consequences of smoking, or 3) a control group. Only 11% of those randomized to the commitment contract actually opened an account, probably reflecting those smokers in the preparation stage for cessation. Participants that opened an account deposited additional money, on average, every 2 weeks, for a closing balance at 6 months of 553 pesos. If participants quit by 6 months, objectively determined by urine cotinine, they received their full deposit back, but if not, they forfeited it. In intent-to-treat analyses of all those randomized, the commitment contract was associated with a 3% to 6% higher quit rate at 6 months than the control group. Similar to the Volpp study, there was evidence for persistence, with a 4% to 6% higher quit rate at 12 months, even though the commitment contract only last for 6 months. Not surprisingly, because of such low uptake of the intervention, the rates of quitting among those using the accounts was substantially higher.

These studies provide further evidence that behavioral economics might supercharge incentives, with group-based support an important add-on as well. Further research should tell us which components of these incentives might be most effective.

Incentives for Medication Adherence

Adhering to prescribed medication regimens is a challenge for a variety of reasons: acceptance of being diagnosed with a medical condition, the cost of medications, side effects, and the logistics of remembering to take a pill daily, among others. Adherence in developed countries is quite low, estimated to be 50% by the World Health Organization (Sabaté, 2003). Because the health consequences of many chronic conditions, such as hypertension, diabetes, and asthma, directly relate to whether patients are compliant with their medication regimen, the costs of nonadherence, both monetarily and for population health are staggering (Osterberg & Blaschke, 2005; Sabaté, 2003).

Paying patients to comply with medical treatment has been a commonly investigated strategy. In a 2012 review of 18 studies, DeFulio and colleagues examined studies using incentives for compliance with antihypertensives, anticoagulation therapy, nicotine replacement, and regimens for HIV, tuberculosis, or substance abuse (DeFulio et al., 2012). Most of these 18 demonstrated some benefit of incentives on adherence, but the studies were small and short term. None of the five examining adherence after incentives stopped demonstrated persistent benefits. Further, few of the studies showed any effect on objectively measured health metrics, such as screening for illicit drugs or HIV viral load. For example, DeFulio et al. enrolled 38 heroin users (nearly all Black race, ages 42 to 45 years, 26% to 58% female across conditions), into an treatment program that involved using injectable naltrexone, an opioid receptor antagonist that blocks the effect of opiates such as heroin, and is associated with lower rates of use (DeFulio et al., 2012). They randomized participants into two groups: one that had free access to a therapeutic workplace in which they could receive payments for completing training programs ("prescription" arm) and a second group that could only access the program if they were compliant with naltrexone injections ("contingent" arm). Over the 6-month study period, 26% of participants in the prescription arm received all prescribed doses of naltrexone injections compared to 74% of those in the contingent group. Yet, despite much higher compliance with naltrexone, the study found no differences in urine samples positive for either opiates or cocaine.

A randomized controlled trial promoting adherence to antiretrovirals for HIV found similar results, this time using a lottery (Rosen et al., 2007). The trial enrolled 56 patients with HIV who had a history of substance abuse. Over 16 weeks, all subjects received weekly counseling sessions to promote adherence with the "contingent" group additionally earning lottery tickets when adherent. Participants were >50% Black with a mean age of 42 to 46 years. The lotteries occurred weekly, and participants could redeem winnings for goods such as clothes, bus tokens, and gift certificates to stores. After 16 weeks, those in the contingent group were more compliant (76% vs. 44%), but this difference abated after the lottery finished (61% vs. 46% at 32 weeks). HIV viral load, a measure of how well the medication suppresses HIV virus, improved more in the contingency group at 16 weeks than for controls, but no difference was evident at 32 weeks.

More recent studies have incorporated sophisticated comparisons and behavioral economics. At the Philadelphia Veteran Affairs Medical Center, a recent study of 118 Black veterans with uncontrolled diabetes compared usual care to either a peer mentorship program or a financial incentive (Long, Jahnle, Richardson, Loewenstein, & Volpp, 2012). Nearly all participants were male with mean age of 59 to 60 years. Usual care included providing patients with basic information about their hemoglobin A_{1c} (HbA_{1c}), a measure of glucose control, and the goals of treatment. The peer mentorship arm assigned a study participant to a mentor who previously had uncontrolled diabetes. The incentive arm offered $100 to participants who lowered their HbA_{1c} by 1% and $200 if lowered it by 2% or to ≤6.5%. Peer mentorship was the most effective intervention, leading to a significant reduction in HbA_{1c} of −1.08 (95% CI, −1.62, −0.54) compared to nonsignificant reductions for participants receiving the financial incentive (−0.46, 95% CI −1.02, 0.10) or usual care (−0.01, 95% CI −0.52, 0.51).

A study of 141 patients with psychosis (schizophrenia, schizoaffective, bipolar disorders) spread across 73 mental health teams in the United Kingdom was an important test of how incentives might work for patients in desperate need of adherence (Priebe et al., 2013). Patients were eligible for the study if they had ≤75% adherence with depot injections of prescribed antipsychotic medications (depot injections lead to medication slowly being released, requiring injections only every 1 to 4 weeks). Patients were randomized by mental health team, one half to usual care and one half to receive $22 for each monthly injection. Over 12 months, the incentive group increased their compliance from 69% to 85% (adjusted effect estimate of 11.5%, 95% CI 3.9%, 19%); control participants increased compliance from 71% to 75%. Physician reported assessments of symptoms were no different between groups, but patient-reported quality of life was improved in the incentive arm.

Compliance with anticoagulation treatment, specifically with warfarin, has been studied more thoroughly, including using lotteries.

Kimmel and colleagues tested a lottery-based compliance program among 100 patients enrolled in the University of Pennsylvania anticoagulation clinic (Kimmel et al., 2012). The outcome was the percentage of measurements in which patients were out of range (<2 or >3.5) for their measure of anticoagulation (the international normalized ratio, INR), meaning they were either underdosed or overdosed. Specifically, an electronic system monitored whether participants took their prescribed dose of warfarin (the system registered when a patient opened the pill container and prompted them to confirm whether he or she took the proper dose). The researchers conducted a daily drawing of all participants in the incentive arm, with each participant having a 1 in 5 chance of winning $10 and a 1 in 100 chance of winning $100. Yet the lottery was infused with loss aversion in that participants could not collect winnings if they had failed to take their daily medication. If participants were compliant and won the day's lottery, they received notification of their winnings via the electronic system, further incorporating rapid reinforcement of behaviors. If they missed their medication dose but still won the lottery, they received notification of the amount of money they forfeited because of their nonadherence. The primary outcome of the study, percentage of INR measures out of range, was no different for intervention and control participants. However, the lottery appeared to work for participants starting the study with an INR below range. These participants had 61% fewer out-of-range measures compared to the control arm and also had better overall compliance with warfarin. This study was an expanded version of a prior uncontrolled trial of 20 participants which showed substantial benefits of lotteries on adherence to warfarin and out-of-range INRs (Volpp, Loewenstein, et al., 2008).

In all, incentive-based interventions to improve medication compliance have demonstrated some success, especially with inducing better medication adherence during the active phase of incentives. This holds true both for fixed incentives and lotteries. Demonstrating that incentive both improve adherence and health outcomes has been more elusive. Few studies demonstrate any benefit of an incentive after it stops. Figuring out how to induce a persistent behavior change or how to incorporate incentives over long periods is a critical area for future research. Also, it remains unclear whether incentives are more effective than, or add value to, other established methods of encouraging compliance, such as pharmacist-based education programs and teaching self-management (Ryan et al., 2011).

Other and Emerging Individual and Public Health Uses of Financial Incentives

Substance Abuse

Perhaps more than any of the other topics covered in this chapter, substance abuse poses a huge problem for behavior change due to future discounting. Withdrawal from an addictive substance has dramatic physical and emotional manifestations and relapsing with the substance is often highly pleasurable. Compounding this is the fact that substance abusers tend to discount the future to a greater degree than do non–substance abusers (Jaroni, Wright, Lerman, & Epstein, 2004).

As is the case with weight loss, more may be better for inducing abstinence when it comes to financial incentives, and the combination of financial incentives with behavioral programs seems to have variable effects (Lussier, Heil, Mongeon, Badger, & Higgins, 2006). In a randomized trial among recovering cocaine users in a methadone-maintenance program (MMP), Rawson et al. explored the relative efficacy of financial incentives (referred to in this trial as contingency management [CM]) versus cognitive-behavioral therapy (CBT) sessions (Rawson et al., 2002). They randomized 120 participants to one of four arms: CM plus CBT, CM alone, CBT alone, and usual care. During the 16-week study period, the highest rates of cocaine-free urine were observed in the CM-only (financial incentives) group (30%). The next highest were in the CBT plus CM group (26%), with the CBT group exhibiting only 20% cocaine-free urine samples, and the controls at 11%. Interestingly, between the CBT and CBT/CM group, participant attendance at CBT sessions was significantly higher among CM recipients (25% vs. 18%).

Unfortunately, as is also the case for the application of incentives to promote weight loss, little is known about how much money should be paid to promote drug abstinence. Most work has focused on the use of monetary vouchers, provided only to individuals when drug abstinence is confirmed. A meta-analysis on this topic suggests that timing of the incentive is especially sensitive in this population—rewards should be given immediately rather than delayed in order to achieve maximum effect (Lussier et al., 2006).

Family Planning and Teen Pregnancy

Particularly in the developing world, financial incentives have been tested as a way to promote uptake of contraception, including sterilization, or have focused on the outcome of limiting family size, with the method of birth control left up to individuals (Heil, Gaalema, & Herrmann, 2012). As with other health-related financial incentives that have been reviewed, larger incentives appear to have larger effects on outcomes. Also, choosing a measure to incent that is truly outcome based (e.g., no pregnancy this year) compared to more process based (e.g., attend meetings to discuss safer sex options) appears to be more effective (Heil et al., 2012). Unfortunately, there are many limitations to the existing studies in this topic area. Many have been quasi-experimental studies and relied upon softer outcomes such as contraception by self-report.

One US-based randomized trial examined the use of financial incentives to promote support group attendance for teen moms, in an effort to reduce repeat pregnancies (Stevens-Simon, Dolgan, Kelly, & Singer, 1997). Stevens-Simon et al. randomized 286 primiparous girls ages 18 and under to one of four arms: peer support (weekly group meeting), peer support plus financial incentive ($7/weekly meeting), financial incentive alone ($7/week), and a control arm, and followed them for 24 months. While they found that those who received financial incentives were far more likely to participate in group sessions (58%) than those who did not (9%), there were no statistically significant differences between the arms with respect to repeat pregnancy rates (35% in the peer support/incentive arm, 56% in the peer support arm, 42% in the incentive only arm, and 34% in the control arm).

Physical Activity Promotion

Many incentives in worksite programs and other general wellness programs focus on promoting healthy behaviors, rather than requiring a health outcome of some kind. One example of this is the use of financial incentives to promote physical activity. As we outlined in the section on weight loss, for people who are sedentary at baseline, initiating routine physical activity can be difficult due to time demands and the fact that it often produces unpleasant feelings for those who are not very physically fit. In a 2009 review, Zimmerman (2009) outlined key concepts from behavioral economics and considered how they might apply to the promotion of physical activity. He noted that when applying financial incentives to an outcome such as physical activity, or other health behaviors, the framing of that incentive is critical. If the financial incentive makes it appear that the behavior is undesirable, then it may backfire and make people less likely to comply. However, if incentives are used as part of a generally positive informational campaign rather than in isolation, they may help to increase the attractiveness of an activity that is already being portrayed in a positive light.

Despite this theoretical framework supporting the use of incentives to promote physical activity, the experimental evidence for their effectiveness is scant. In a 2013 quasi-experimental study, Hunter et al. group-randomized 406 employees in Northern Ireland to one of two arms—a financial incentive arm where participants could collect points for physical activity (points could be used toward retail purchases) ($n = 199$), or an arm where participants self-monitored their activity but received no incentives ($n = 207$) (Hunter, Tully, Davis, Stevenson, & Kee, 2013). They found no significant difference in physical activity levels between the two groups, and recorded physical activity levels at the 6-month mark were quite low overall (26 min/week for the incentive arm, 24 min/week for the control arm). Objective measures of physical activity were not obtained.

A few other short-term studies have found some benefit to incentives among college students. Charness and Gneezy conducted two experiments using monetary incentives to encourage use of campus gyms on two university campuses (Charness & Gneezy, 2009). In the first experiment, they randomized 120 students to either a control group, a group that received $25 to visit the gym once during a designated week ("one visit"), or a group that received both the $25 for one visit and an additional $100 to visit the gym eight times over the subsequent 4-week period ("eight visits"). Before and after the intervention, they obtained records of gym use from magnetic swipe cards that students were required to use to gain entrance. Students in the control group maintained steady gym attendance before and after the intervention—0.59 visits/week in the 8 weeks prior to 0.56 during the 7 weeks after the study began, as did students receiving the "one-visit" incentive (0.7 to 0.76). Students receiving the higher incentive for "eight visits" increased their gym membership from 0.6 visits/week prior to 1.24 after, different than the other two groups ($p < .001$). The increase among the eight-visits group was persistent during the 7-week period after the incentive ceased, suggesting possible habit formation. When stratified by baseline gym attendance, the increases in the eight-visits group were only evident among students who were not regular gym attendees prior to the study (<1 visit/week).

The second experiment ($n = 168$) was similar but provided up to $175 in incentives to all participants, if they attended three meetings to have biometric tests measured (Charness & Gneezy, 2009). The control group had no further requirements to obtain the incentive, but the two intervention groups had additional gym attendance requirements—either attending the campus gym once over 4 weeks or eight times. Results were nearly identical to the first experiment except that all groups demonstrated increased gym membership during the study; gym membership attendance was significantly higher in the eight-visit group compared to the other two groups. This change, again, was only noted among students who were not regular attenders prior to the study, and the increase in attendance was persistent over a 15-week period after that study finished.

Two very similar studies examined additional features regarding incentives for gym attendance. Babcock and Hartman conducted a study among 222 students and found increases in gym attendance among students receiving $80 for eight visits (Babcock & Hartman, 2010). They captured friendship networks within their study sample and found greater gym attendance when incentivized study participants had friends who were also in this incentive treatment condition. Acland and Levy conducted a nearly identical study to Charness and Levy (Acland & Levy, 2013). However, they maintained measurement for a longer follow-up period, including over a semester break. They found that the short-term persistent increase in gym attendance among those incentivized for eight visits was no longer evident after a semester break, suggesting some limitations to persistence after a substantial schedule disruption.

Promotion of Public Health

In addition to incenting behaviors or outcomes that mainly impact individual health, financial incentives can be applied to individuals to promote their uptake of services that have a large impact on population health. For example, obtaining vaccines and getting communicable disease screenings are inherently unpleasant activities with perhaps greater benefits at the population level than the individual level. Additionally, because most vaccines are administered as one or a few doses, their health benefits can be conferred without the persistence required for meaningful physical activity and dietary changes. Screenings have similar characteristics but may require persistence if risky behavior, such as having multiple sexual partners, is ongoing. Thus, these types of activities are attractive targets for the application of financial incentives. In a 2014 systematic review and meta-analysis by Giles et al. (2014), authors examined five studies of cash incentives to increase vaccination rates and cancer screening. All studies evaluated the impact of the incentive relative to no intervention. The authors concluded that the provision of cash or cash-like incentives improved uptake of vaccines and screening relative to no intervention (pooled RR 1.92 [1.46–2.53]).

The Affordable Care Act: Fanning the Flames for Incentives to Change Behaviors?

One of the hallmark reforms of the 2010 Affordable Care Act (ACA) was to extend existing employer-based insurance market policies that prohibit the denial of health insurance based on preexisting conditions ("guaranteed issue") or charging more based on health status ("community rating"). The ACA established guaranteed issue and community rating for the individual insurance market as well. Yet the ACA also aggressively endorsed the use of financial incentives to promote wellness, doubling down on earlier provisions in the 1996 Health Insurance Portability and Accountability Act (HIPAA) (Internal Revenue Service, Employee Benefits Security Administration, Centers for Medicare and Medicaid Services, 2013; Madison, Schmidt, & Volpp, 2013). HIPAA allowed employers to alter employee health insurance premiums by 20% if employees (or their dependents) participated in wellness programs. Under the ACA, the premium reduction or increase allowed rose to 30% of the cost of the insurance policy, or up to 50% if the incentive included smoking-cessation programs. Certain restrictions apply to incentive programs that are "health contingent" (i.e., requiring an activity related to a specific health condition or changing a health outcome): The incentive must be available annually and to all employees with adequate alternative goals available when medical conditions might inhibit achievement of standard goals. Also, the incentive program must have a reasonable chance of success and be transparent to employees. For "participatory" programs (i.e., requiring an activity unrelated to a specific health condition, such as completing a health risk assessment or reimbursing the cost of a gym membership), most restrictions do not apply; these programs only need to be made available to all employees.

Employers are taking advantage of these provisions. In a 2013 survey of 1,865 employers that offered health benefits (public or private employers with three or more employees), nearly all of the large employers (99%) and a large majority of small companies (76%) offered some type of wellness program (Kaiser Family Foundation and Health Research & Educational Trust, 2013). Incentives were common, especially among large employers (≥200 employees), with 36% offering some type of incentive; only 8% of small employers (3 to 199 employees) provided a wellness incentive. Most of the incentives were to complete a health risk assessment, a standardized survey capturing health data. Other incentives were for biometric screening (i.e., measurement of cholesterol, blood sugar, body weight, and blood pressure) or to complete a program to address a specific health problem. Few employers imposed penalties on employees not participating in their wellness programs.

The present lack of penalties may change over time. Under the ACA, employers are equally free to incentivize wellness program participation or penalize nonparticipation. With the restrictions set forward, they can also incentive or penalize based on achievement or failure to achieve specified health goals. Volpp and Galvin describe how the $750 smoking-cessation incentive program at General Electric was later turned into a penalty, a $625 surcharge on health insurance (Volpp & Galvin, 2014). This charge resulted from logistical and financial challenges of administering an incentive program as well as concerns regarding fairness to nonsmokers. Even without using penalties, employers offering incentives may circumvent provisions that prevent them from charging different premiums based on health status (Schmidt, Voigt, & Wikler, 2010). For those employees with hard-to-manage obesity or diabetes or a long-time smoking addiction, the lack of an incentive could be a de facto penalty, especially if employers decide to increase background insurance premiums to cover the costs of their incentive programs.

Further evidence of the Affordable Care Act's endorsement of incentives came in the form of $100 million in funding for a 5-year, 10-state financial incentive demonstration project called the Medicaid Incentives for Prevention of Chronic Diseases (Section 4108) (Blumenthal et al., 2013; Center for Medicare and Medicaid Innovation, 2013). Starting in 2012, the Center for Medicare and Medicaid Innovation awarded grants to a diverse mix of states; most states implemented programs to address obesity, smoking, hyperlipidemia, diabetes, or hypertension. The programs all provide fixed incentives, ranging from $20 to $1,150 per year, paid in various ways: cash, gift cards, a wellness reimbursement account, or items to encourage wellness, such as food vouchers, exercise equipment, or childcare funds. Most states implemented the programs as randomized controlled trials with robust evaluation components. In the next several years, these evaluations should render important verdicts about the programs, and financial incentives generally. Prior Medicaid incentive programs in Florida, Idaho, and West Virginia provided relatively small incentives that only could be used for healthcare expenditures; these programs lacked rigorous evaluation and met with limited success (Blumenthal et al., 2013). The exception was Idaho's program to increase well-child visits by providing points to offset premium expenses. The percent of children in families participating in the program increased from 23% before the incentive program to 49% after (Greene, 2011).

Ethics of Financial Incentives: Are We Creating a Slippery Slope?

Can Incentives Backfire and Undermine an Individual's Intrinsic Motivation?

The growth of financial incentives to promote health behaviors or outcomes has engendered greater concerns about their use. One of the most common concerns, often expressed by behavioral scientists, is the notion that financial incentives may undermine an individual's inherent motivation to perform a behavior (or achieve an outcome) and, thus, once removed, leave the individual less motivated than he or she was at baseline. But is this phenomenon truly a threat with respect to most health behaviors or outcomes?

Self-determination theory argues that people can be more motivated to change by rewards intrinsic to the actual behavior (e.g., feeling great after going for a run, feeling happy after eating a healthy meal), rather than by an extrinsic reward (e.g., money) (Moller, McFadden, Hedeker, & Spring, 2012). Because of the close connection to the activity, this intrinsic reward should, therefore, be more predictive of long-term behavior change and thus long-term maintenance of health outcomes than the extrinsic rewards. Most of the literature on this concept comes from laboratory-based psychological experiments that involved teaching people a task that was somewhat enjoyable, then paying them to do it, followed by a removal of the payment (Promberger & Marteau, 2013). For a narrow range of behaviors, several real-world studies confirm these findings. In one real-world study, embedded within an existing program at the University of Zurich, temporary incentives permanently reduced motivation levels. In this field experiment, providing a charitable donation "match" increased student donations in the short run, but after the match was removed, donations decreased below prematch levels, suggesting a reduction in motivation to give (Gneezy, Meier, & Rey-Biel, 2011; Meier, 2007). In an earlier study also conducted by Gneezy, the initiation of a small fine (approximately $3, a negative financial incentive) for late pickup at daycare actually led to higher rates of late pickups than had existed prior to the fine (Gneezy et al., 2011). Even after lifting the fine, late pickups were more common than at baseline. These findings illustrate that assigning a relatively small penalty for an undesirable behavior can backfire by devaluing a preexisting social norm. In the daycare experiment, parents at baseline likely tried to be on time for picking up their children because they wanted to be courteous to staff. When a small dollar value was assigned to the behavior, parents recalibrated the intrinsic value they placed on the behavior. The fine simply monetized being late, and, at a measly value of $3 per late pickup, they became permanently more likely to engage in this negative behavior.

Health behaviors may be different, especially when there is a clear intrinsic benefit. In the case of physical activity, as was discussed earlier, people may become habituated to the behavior because they eventually discover the activity to be pleasurable, which in turn transforms the extrinsic motivator of cash to a more powerful intrinsic motivation (Acland & Levy, 2013; Charness & Gneezy, 2009). The extrinsic motivation may help people overcome the initial unpleasantness, with the intrinsic benefits later taking over. In a recent review, Promberger and Marteau expounded on this notion (Promberger & Marteau, 2013). They noted that there is little evidence that extrinsic motivation thwarts intrinsic motivation for persistence of health behavior change. Additionally, they note that for most people who are not currently engaging in healthy behaviors, they have a very low (or no) existing intrinsic motivation. You cannot undermine what did not exist. Furthermore, they argue that many healthy behaviors (e.g., eating vegetables, getting a vaccine) are by nature not very enjoyable in the moment. Thus, any impetus to change is likely to be an external factor similar to an incentive, such as a college reunion coming up or preventing a heart attack. If these factors are removed, the sustainability of behavior change depends entirely on whether that change stuck and engendered intrinsic motivation.

One example of incentives promoting health behavior change, as opposed to detracting from it, comes from a recently published study by Just and Price that compared paying school children to eat produce to requiring that they take a fruit or vegetable (or simply putting one on their tray automatically) (Just & Price, 2013). The researchers were concerned about whether monetizing the behavior ("eat your veggies") would eliminate a child's intrinsic motivation, particularly for kids who were high consumers of veggies at baseline. In fact, the study showed that the intervention did not cause this kind of "boomerang" effect. The preintervention norm was no vegetable consumption. After the incentive began, the norm shifted to eating one vegetable. Moreover, paying kids to eat their veggies resulted in less waste at the end of the meal compared to the "default" option (putting a fruit or vegetable on every child's tray).

Moller et al. examined intrinsic motivation by conducting a secondary analysis of participants in a randomized trial of financial incentives for weight loss (Moller et al., 2012). The goal of the analysis was to elicit participant motives for joining the trial and for changing their behavior. They found that people who were motivated by money were equally likely to *initiate* behavior changes for improving their health; those who were *less* motivated by money were more likely to *maintain* the behavior changes in the long run. They also noted that personal characteristics, such as gender, may modify the effect of financial incentives on motivation—men who were financially motivated were less able to maintain healthy lifestyle changes than women who were financially motivated.

In summary, there is limited evidence that incentives pose much risk of undermining behavior change initiation. But, there will need to be careful consideration and thought put toward how to promote long-term maintenance of health behavior changes in programs after being triggered by incentives. Whether behavioral economics–inspired incentives, such as deposit contracts and lotteries, affect long-term motivation differently than pure financial incentives is not yet known.

Can Incentives Be Coercive or Be Viewed as Penalties on Nonrecipients?

Another commonly cited ethical concern is that, as incentives are frequently imposed by an employer on an employee group, they may feel coercive. This concern is especially relevant in the case of the Affordable Care Act, when a critical need of employees—health insurance—is altered by penalties, or even incentives that might lower the price of health insurance.

A related question is whether or not incentives should target health outcomes (e.g., smoking cessation, reaching a target body mass index) instead of process measures along the way to permanent behavior change (e.g., signing up for a smoking-cessation class or eating more healthfully). Because some health outcomes are so difficult to achieve, it may be that setting too unrealistic a target can backfire, leading people to become demoralized. Tackling this question, Schmidt and colleagues discussed whether outcome-based measures (e.g., lose 20 lb, lower LDL by 20 points) are inherently less fair than process-based measures (e.g., sign up for gym membership, take statin medication) (Schmidt, Asch, & Halpern, 2012). They argued that instead of focusing on this process-outcome distinction when considering the fairness, we should consider personal control over whatever measure is being chosen. For example, if someone is a low-income worker living in a bad neighborhood, a process measure such as joining a gym or logging 10,000 steps a day on a pedometer might be very difficult to achieve due to personal circumstances. Such circumstances may call for a recalibration of chosen outcomes, providing flexibility so that individuals can tailor them based on their personal ability to accomplish goals. Allowing individuals to tailor their goals to their life circumstances and abilities could minimize the risk for coercion or inadvertent discrimination. Of course, there are limitations in that such flexibility could lead to outcomes being too watered down for meaningful change. Regulations for new Affordable Care Act provisions on incentives do require some of this flexibility, but how these provisions impact the implementation of incentives is not yet clear.

Should We Be Using Financial Penalties (Sticks) Instead of Financial Rewards (Carrots)?

Although financial incentives can be either positive (rewards or "carrots") or negative (fines/penalties or "sticks"), the carrots tend to be more popular than the sticks, especially among those who are being encouraged to change a behavior. On the other hand, if bystanders are asked about the best way to motivate other people's behavior (e.g., your coworkers who smoke or who need to lose weight), those who view themselves as already "at goal" with the behavior tend to prefer that sticks be used for the noncompliers. Some of these so-called bystanders may argue: "If I already stopped smoking by myself, why should my employer reward others for doing something that I already did without being paid? Shouldn't that money be spent on me instead?" (Loewenstein, Asch, Friedman, Melichar, & Volpp, 2012). Further, according to the theory of loss aversion, people ought to be more responsive to a stick than to a carrot; that is, they would find it twice as aversive to be penalized for failing to lose weight than to be rewarded some amount of cash to perform the same behavior. When constructing incentives, organizations must fully consider these trade-offs, balancing preferences, fairness, and effect, and be fully transparent about them.

Public Perception of Financial Incentives for Health

Despite a clear interest in financial incentives on the part of the research and health and wellness community, it is critical that we also gain a solid understanding for public perception of financial incentives. If most people are inherently turned off by financial incentives, then programs relying on them are unlikely to be widely effective or widely implemented. Promberger et al. recently surveyed 1,350 individuals from the United States and United Kingdom, asking them to rate the fairness and acceptability of using financial incentives to improve health outcomes (Promberger, Brown, Ashcroft, & Marteau, 2011). They found that people generally perceived incentives as less acceptable and less fair than equally priced, equally effective medical interventions for health conditions such as obesity, drug addiction, and smoking cessation. Additionally, people generally disliked the idea of applying a financial penalty to a health behavior. In a series of discrete choice experiments, the same investigator and her team looked at the acceptability of using financial incentives for two common areas—smoking cessation and weight loss (Promberger, Dolan, & Marteau, 2012). They found that the acceptability of incentives was highly dependent on the likely effect of the incentive. When incentives were framed as being effective at changing behaviors, participants were more likely to view them favorably. Yet a minority of participants ($n = 26$, 6%) remained opposed to the use of financial incentives in any context, even when they were told that the incentive was four times as effective as a hypothetical, similarly priced medical intervention for a given condition. Furthermore, participants found the idea of incentives delivered as direct cash payments less acceptable than giving vouchers for grocery store use, for example. Finally, these participants also felt that acceptability of using financial incentives varied based on the target condition. People were generally more comfortable with the use of financial incentives for weight loss than for smoking cessation, a phenomenon the authors attribute to differing levels of "moralization" between the two behavior types (Promberger et al., 2012). Based on these findings, it would seem that, if structured carefully, most people would be open to the idea of financial incentives to improve some health outcomes; however, there is likely to remain a small, but vocal, fraction who object to the concept regardless of evidence of its effectiveness.

Conclusion

Financial incentives can influence health behaviors. But results are mixed and still relatively early in their evolution. Future studies should compare a variety of incentives with time-honored methods of inducing behavior change, such as intensive lifestyle counseling, for a variety of conditions and use of medications, such as for smoking cessation. These comparisons should take into account efficacy and effectiveness as well as cost because even if incentives are noninferior to other programs they may be more cost-effective. Incentives also may add value to these programs, especially when structured with clever behavioral economics–inspired components. Most critically, the issue of persistence with behavior change must be explored. This holds true not only for incentives but really with any behavior change program. To date, very little data support persistent behavior change with incentives (Volpp et al., 2009; White et al., 2013) with rare data showing persistence with comprehensive behavior change programs (Knowler et al., 2009).

References

Acland, D., & Levy, M. R. (2013). Naivete, projection bias, and habit formation in gym attendance. *Social Science Research Network*. Retrieved February 2015, from http://ssrn.com/abstract=2233004

Ammerman, A., Pignone, M., Fernandez, L., Lohr, K., Jacobs, A., Nester, C., ... Whitener, L. (2002). Behavioral counseling in primary care to promote a healthy diet. In US Preventive Services Task Force (Ed.), *Guide to clinical preventive services* (3rd ed.). Rockville, MD: Agency for Healthcare Research and Quality.

Babcock, P., & Hartman, J. (2010). *Exercising in herds: Treatment size and status specific peer effects in a randomized exercise intervention*. Retrieved February 2015, from the University of California, Santa Barbara website, http://www.econ.ucsb.edu/~hartman/Research_papers_files/ExerciseHerd_2010_08.pdf

Blumenthal, K. J., Saulsgiver, K. A., Norton, L., Troxel, A. B., Anarella, J. P., Gesten, F. C., ... Volpp, K. G. (2013). Medicaid incentive programs to encourage healthy behavior show mixed results to date and should be studied and improved. *Health Affairs (Millwood)*, 32(3), 497–507. doi:32/3/497 [pii] 10.1377/hlthaff.2012.0431

Cahill, K., & Perera, R. (2011). Competitions and incentives for smoking cessation. *Cochrane Database of Systematic Reviews*, 4, CD004307. doi:10.1002/14651858. CD004307.pub4 [doi]

Cawley, J., & Price, J. A. (2013). A case study of a workplace wellness program that offers financial incentives for weight loss. *Journal of Health Economics*, 32(5), 794–803. doi:10.1016/j.jhealeco.2013.04.005

Center for Medicare and Medicaid Innovation. (2013). *Initial report to Congress: Medicaid incentives for prevention of chronic diseases evaluation.* Retrieved March 2014, from http://innovation.cms.gov/Files/reports/MIPCD_RTC.pdf

Charness, G., & Gneezy, U. (2009). Incentives to exercise. *Econometrica, 77*(3), 909–931.

Choi, J., Laibson, D., Madrian, B., & Metrick, A. (2004). For better or for worse: Default effects and 401(k) savings behavior. In D. A. Wise (Ed.), *Perspectives in the economics of aging* (pp. 81–121). Chicago, IL: University of Chicago Press.

Connolly, T., & Butler, D. (2006). Regret in economic and psychological theories of choice. *Journal of Behavior and Decision Making, 19,* 139–158.

Danaei, G., Ding, E. L., Mozaffarian, D., Taylor, B., Rehm, J., Murray, C. J., & Ezzati, M. (2009). The preventable causes of death in the United States: Comparative risk assessment of dietary, lifestyle, and metabolic risk factors. *PLoS Medicine, 6*(4), e1000058. doi:10.1371/journal.pmed.1000058

DeFulio, A., Everly, J. J., Leoutsakos, J. M., Umbricht, A., Fingerhood, M., Bigelow, G. E., & Silverman, K. (2012). Employment-based reinforcement of adherence to an FDA approved extended release formulation of naltrexone in opioid-dependent adults: a randomized controlled trial. *Drug Alcohol Depend, 120*(1–3), 48–54. doi:S0376-8716(11)00301-2 [pii] 10.1016/j.drugalcdep.2011.06.023

Finkelstein, E. A., Linnan, L. A., Tate, D. F., & Birken, B. E. (2007). A pilot study testing the effect of different levels of financial incentives on weight loss among overweight employees. *Journal of Occupational Environmental Medicine, 49*(9), 981–989. doi:10.1097/JOM.0b013e31813c6dcb

Flegal, K. M., Carroll, M. D., Kit, B. K., & Ogden, C. L. (2012). Prevalence of obesity and trends in the distribution of body mass index among US adults, 1999–2010. *Journal of the American Medical Association, 307*(5), 491–497. doi:10.1001/jama.2012.39

Gallagher, S. M., Penn, P. E., Schindler, E., & Layne, W. (2007). A comparison of smoking cessation treatments for persons with schizophrenia and other serious mental illnesses. *Journal of Psychoactive Drugs, 39*(4), 487–497.

Giles, E. L., Robalino, S., McColl, E., Sniehotta, F. F., & Adams, J. (2014). The effectiveness of financial incentives for health behavior change: systematic review and meta-analysis. *PLoS One, 9*(3), e90347. doi:10.1371/journal.pone.0090347

Gine, X., Karlan, D., & Zinman, J. (2010). Put your money where your butt is: A commitment contract for smoking cessation. *American Economics Journal: Applied Economics, 2*(4), 213–235.

Gneezy, U., Meier, S., & Rey-Biel, P. (2011). When and why incentives (don't) work to modify behavior. *Journal of Economic Perspectives, 25*(4), 191–210.

Greene, J. (2011). Using consumer incentives to increase well-child visits among low-income children. *Medical Care Research and Review, 68*(5), 579–593. doi:1077558711398878 [pii] 10.1177/1077558711398878

Halpern, S. D., Asch, D. A., & Volpp, K. G. (2012). Commitment contracts as a way to health. *British Medical Journal, 344,* e522.

Heil, S. H., Gaalema, D. E., & Herrmann, E. S. (2012). Incentives to promote family planning. *Preventive Medicine, 55*(Suppl.), S106–112. doi:10.1016/j.ypmed.2012.06.014

Hunter, R. F., Tully, M. A., Davis, M., Stevenson, M., & Kee, F. (2013). Physical activity loyalty cards for behavior change: a quasi-experimental study. *American Journal of Preventive Medicine, 45*(1), 56–63. doi:10.1016/j.amepre.2013.02.022

Internal Revenue Service, Department of the Treasury; Employee Benefits Security Administration, Department of Labor; Centers for Medicare and Medicaid Services, Department of Health and Human Services. (2013). Incentives for nondiscriminatory wellness programs in group health plans: Final rule. *Federal Register*, *78*(106), 33157–33192.

Jaroni, J. L., Wright, S. M., Lerman, C., & Epstein, L. H. (2004). Relationship between education and delay discounting in smokers. *Addictive Behaviors*, *29*(6), 1171–1175. doi:10.1016/j.addbeh.2004.03.014

Jason, L. A., Salina, D., McMahon, S. D., Hedeker, D., & Stockton, M. (1997). A work-site smoking intervention: A 2 year assessment of groups, incentives and self-help. *Health Education Research*, *12*(1), 129–138.

Jeffery, R. W. (2012). Financial incentives and weight control. *Preventive Medicine*, *55*(Suppl.), S61–67. doi:S0091-7435(11)00526-3 [pii]

John, L. K., Loewenstein, G., Troxel, A. B., Norton, L., Fassbender, J. E., & Volpp, K. G. (2011). Financial incentives for extended weight loss: A randomized, controlled trial. *Journal of General Internal Medicine*, *26*(6), 621–626. doi:10.1007/s11606-010-1628-y

John, L. K., Loewenstein, G., & Volpp, K. G. (2012). Empirical observations on longer-term use of incentives for weight loss. *Preventive Medicine*, *55*(Suppl.), S68–S74. doi:10.1016/j.ypmed.2012.01.022

Just, D., & Price, J. (2013). Default options, incentives and food choices: Evidence from elementary-school children. *Public Health and Nutrition*, *16*(12), 2281–2288. doi:10.1017/S1368980013001468

Kahneman, D., & Tversky, A. (1979). Prospect theory: An analysis of decision under risk. *Econometrica*, *47*, 263–291.

The Kaiser Family Foundation and Health Research & Educational Trust. (2013). *Employer health benefits: 2013 annual survey*. Retrieved April 2014, from http://kaiserfamilyfoundation.files.wordpress.com/2013/08/8465-employer-health-benefits-20132.pdf

Kim, A., Kamyab, K., Zhu, J., & Volpp, K. (2011). Why are financial incentives not effective at influencing some smokers to quit? Results of a process evaluation of a worksite trial assessing the efficacy of financial incentives for smoking cessation. *Journal of Occupational and Environmental Medicine*, *53*(1), 62–67. doi:10.1097/JOM.0b013e31820061d7

Kimmel, S. E., Troxel, A. B., Loewenstein, G., Brensinger, C. M., Jaskowiak, J., Doshi, J. A., ... Volpp, K. (2012). Randomized trial of lottery-based incentives to improve warfarin adherence. *American Heart Journal*, *164*(2), 268–274. doi:10.1016/j.ahj.2012.05.005

Knowler, W. C., Fowler, S. E., Hamman, R. F., Christophi, C. A., Hoffman, H. J., Brenneman, A. T., ... Nathan, D. M. (2009). 10-year follow-up of diabetes incidence and weight loss in the Diabetes Prevention Program Outcomes Study. *Lancet*, *374*(9702), 1677–1686. doi:10.1016/S0140-6736(09)61457-4

Kullgren, J. T., Troxel, A. B., Loewenstein, G., Asch, D. A., Norton, L. A., Wesby, L., ... Volpp, K. G. (2013). Individual- versus group-based financial incentives for weight loss: A randomized, controlled trial. *Annals of Internal Medicine*, *158*(7), 505–514. doi:10.7326/0003-4819-158-7-201304020-00002

Laibson, D. I. (1997). Golden eggs and hyperbolic discounting. *Quarterly Journal of Economics, 62*, 443–477.

Leibel, R. L., & Hirsch, J. (1984). Diminished energy requirements in reduced-obese patients. *Metabolism, 33*(2), 164–170. doi:0026-0495(84)90130-6 [pii]

Leibel, R. L., Rosenbaum, M., & Hirsch, J. (1995). Changes in energy expenditure resulting from altered body weight. *New England Journal of Medicine, 332*(10), 621–628. doi:10.1056/NEJM199503093321001 [doi]

Loewenstein, G., Asch, D. A., Friedman, J. Y., Melichar, L. A., & Volpp, K. G. (2012). Can behavioural economics make us healthier? *British Medical Journal, 344*, e3482. doi:10.1136/bmj.e3482

Loewenstein, G., Brennan, T., & Volpp, K. G. (2007). Asymmetric paternalism to improve health behaviors. *Journal of the American Medical Association, 298*(20), 2415–2417. doi:298/20/2415 [pii] 10.1001/jama.298.20.2415 [doi]

Long, J. A., Jahnle, E. C., Richardson, D. M., Loewenstein, G., & Volpp, K. G. (2012). Peer mentoring and financial incentives to improve glucose control in African American veterans: a randomized trial. *Annals of Internal Medicine, 156*(6), 416–424. doi:10.7326/0003-4819-156-6-201203200-00004

Lussier, J. P., Heil, S. H., Mongeon, J. A., Badger, G. J., & Higgins, S. T. (2006). A meta-analysis of voucher-based reinforcement therapy for substance use disorders. *Addiction, 101*(2), 192–203. doi:10.1111/j.1360-0443.2006.01311.x

Madison, K., Schmidt, H., & Volpp, K. G. (2013). Smoking, obesity, health insurance, and health incentives in the Affordable Care Act. *Journal of the American Medical Association, 310*(2), 143–144. doi:10.1001/jama.2013.7617

Meier, S. (2007). Do subsidies increase charitable giving in the long run? matching donations in a field experiment. *Journal of the European Economic Association, 5*(6), 1203–1222.

Mokdad, A. H., Marks, J. S., Stroup, D. F., & Gerberding, J. L. (2004). Actual causes of death in the United States, 2000. *Journal of the American Medical Association, 291*(10), 1238–1245. doi:10.1001/jama.291.10.1238 [doi]

Moller, A. C., McFadden, H. G., Hedeker, D., & Spring, B. (2012). Financial motivation undermines maintenance in an intensive diet and activity intervention. *Journal of Obesity, 2012*, 740519. doi:10.1155/2012/740519

Morgan, P. J., Collins, C. E., Plotnikoff, R. C., Cook, A. T., Berthon, B., Mitchell, S., & Callister, R. (2011). Efficacy of a workplace-based weight loss program for overweight male shift workers: The Workplace POWER (Preventing Obesity Without Eating like a Rabbit) randomized controlled trial. *Preventive Medicine, 52*(5), 317–325. doi:10.1016/j.ypmed.2011.01.031

Osterberg, L., & Blaschke, T. (2005). Adherence to medication. *N Engl J Med, 353*, 487–497.

Paxton, R. (1980). The effects of a deposit contract as a component in a behavioural programme for stopping smoking. *Behavior Research and Therapy, 18*(1), 45–50. doi:0005-7967(80)90068-6 [pii]

Paxton, R. (1983). Prolonging the effects of deposit contracts with smokers. *Behavior Research and Therapy, 21*(4), 425–433. doi:0005-7967(83)90012-8 [pii]

Priebe, S., Yeeles, K., Bremner, S., Lauber, C., Eldridge, S., Ashby, D., ... Burns, T. (2013). Effectiveness of financial incentives to improve adherence to maintenance treatment with antipsychotics: Cluster randomised controlled trial. *British Medical Journal, 347*, f5847.

Promberger, M., Brown, R. C., Ashcroft, R. E., & Marteau, T. M. (2011). Acceptability of financial incentives to improve health outcomes in UK and US samples. *Journal of Medical Ethics, 37*(11), 682–687. doi:10.1136/jme.2010.039347

Promberger, M., Dolan, P., & Marteau, T. M. (2012). "Pay them if it works": Discrete choice experiments on the acceptability of financial incentives to change health related behaviour. *Social Science and Medicine, 75*(12), 2509–2514. doi:10.1016/j.socscimed.2012.09.033

Promberger, M., & Marteau, T. M. (2013). When do financial incentives reduce intrinsic motivation? Comparing behaviors studied in psychological and economic literatures. *Health Psychology, 32*(9), 950–957. doi:10.1037/a0032727

Rawson, R. A., Huber, A., McCann, M., Shoptaw, S., Farabee, D., Reiber, C., & Ling, W. (2002). A comparison of contingency management and cognitive-behavioral approaches during methadone maintenance treatment for cocaine dependence. *Archives of General Psychiatry, 59*(9), 817–824.

Relton, C., Strong, M., & Li, J. (2011). The 'Pounds for Pounds' weight loss financial incentive scheme: An evaluation of a pilot in NHS Eastern and Coastal Kent. *Journal of Public Health (Oxford), 33*(4), 536–542. doi:10.1093/pubmed/fdr030

Rosen, M. I., Dieckhaus, K., McMahon, T. J., Valdes, B., Petry, N. M., Cramer, J., & Rounsaville, B. (2007). Improved adherence with contingency management. *AIDS Patient Care STDS, 21*(1), 30–40. doi:10.1089/apc.2006.0028

Ryan, R., Santesso, N., Hill, S., Lowe, D., Kaufman, C., & Grimshaw, J. (2011). Consumer-oriented interventions for evidence-based prescribing and medicines use: An overview of systematic reviews. *Cochrane Database Syst Rev, 5*, CD007768.

Sabaté, E. (2003). (Ed.). *Adherence to long-term therapies: Evidence for action.* Geneva, Switzerland: World Health Organization.

Sacks, F. M., Bray, G. A., Carey, V. J., Smith, S. R., Ryan, D. H., Anton, S. D., ... Williamson, D. A. (2009). Comparison of weight-loss diets with different compositions of fat, protein, and carbohydrates. *New England Journal of Medicine, 360*(9), 859–873. doi:10.1056/NEJMoa0804748 [doi]

Schmidt, H., Asch, D. A., & Halpern, S. D. (2012). Fairness and wellness incentives: What is the relevance of the process-outcome distinction? *Preventive Medicine, 55*(Suppl.), S118–S123. doi:10.1016/j.ypmed.2012.03.005

Schmidt, H., Voigt, K., & Wikler, D. (2010). Carrots, sticks, and health care reform—problems with wellness incentives. *New England Journal of Medicine, 362*(2), e3. doi:10.1056/NEJMp0911552 [doi]

Stevens-Simon, C., Dolgan, J. I., Kelly, L., & Singer, D. (1997). The effect of monetary incentives and peer support groups on repeat adolescent pregnancies. A randomized trial of the Dollar-a-Day Program. *Journal of the American Medical Association, 277*(12), 977–982.

Thaler, R. (1990). Anomalies: Saving, fungibility, and mental accounts. *Journal of Economic Perspectives, 4*(1), 193–205.

Thaler, R., & Sunstein, C. (2009.). *Nudge: Improving decisions about health, wealth, and happiness.* New York, NY: Penguin Books.

Troxel, A. B., & Volpp, K. G. (2012). Effectiveness of financial incentives for longer-term smoking cessation: Evidence of absence or absence of evidence? *American Journal of Health Promotion, 26*(4), 204–207. doi:10.4278/ajhp.101111-CIT-371

Tsai, A. G., Felton, S., Hill, J. O., & Atherly, A. J. (2012). A randomized pilot trial of a full subsidy vs. a partial subsidy for obesity treatment. *Obesity (Silver Spring), 20*(9), 1838–1843. doi:10.1038/oby.2011.193

Volpp, K. G., & Galvin, R. (2014). Reward-based incentives for smoking cessation: How a carrot became a stick. *Journal of the American Medical Association, 311*(9), 909–910. doi:10.1001/jama.2014.418

Volpp, K. G., John, L. K., Troxel, A. B., Norton, L., Fassbender, J., & Loewenstein, G. (2008). Financial incentive-based approaches for weight loss: A randomized trial. *Journal of the American Medical Association, 300*(22), 2631–2637. doi:10.1001/jama.2008.804

Volpp, K. G., Loewenstein, G., Troxel, A. B., Doshi, J., Price, M., Laskin, M., & Kimmel, S. E. (2008). A test of financial incentives to improve warfarin adherence. *BMC Health Services Research, 8*, 272. doi:10.1186/1472-6963-8-272

Volpp, K. G., Troxel, A. B., Pauly, M. V., Glick, H. A., Puig, A., Asch, D. A., . . . Audrain-McGovern, J. (2009). A randomized, controlled trial of financial incentives for smoking cessation. *New England Journal of Medicine, 360*(7), 699–709. doi:10.1056/NEJMsa0806819

White, J. S., Dow, W. H., & Rungruanghiranya, S. (2013). Commitment contracts and team incentives: A randomized controlled trial for smoking cessation in Thailand. *American Journal of Preventive Medicine, 45*(5), 533–542.

Zimmerman, F. J. (2009). Using behavioral economics to promote physical activity. *Preventive Medicine, 49*(4), 289–291.

9 | Slim by Design

MOVING FROM CAN'T TO CAN

BRIAN WANSINK

W HEN WE THINK OF "POLICY," we think of Congress and laws—that is, policy with a capital P. But every person and household has policies. They are the habits and daily patterns, like the policy to hang up your keys when you get home or to take off your shoes. It might be a policy to eat breakfast every day or not to keep a candy dish on your desk or cookie jar in the kitchen.

Just as we have personal policies, restaurants, schools, grocers, and workplaces also have policies. Some are written down, and some are simply rules of thumb, like the customer is always right, or always put a bread basket on the table. These policies are all flexible. If a company's policy caused it to lose money or customers, it could be changed overnight (Wansink, 2014).

This is where consumers fit in. If changing these policies means enough to enough consumers, they can help encourage these places to make profitable changes that make it even easier for families, neighborhoods, and communities to be slim by design. The best policies are the ones that are win-win. They are the ones that let restaurants, companies, grocery stores, and schools benefit—and us as well (Wansink, 2014).

This chapter provides an outline of how small, consumer-driven changes can help change the institutions that feed us and that can help make us slim by design. One of the inhibitors of making such changes lies in our reliance on public policy and the outdated and often irrelevant toolbox that is used in the food environment. Following this, a basic outline is provided as to how we can go from an approach of focusing on what consumers cannot do to an approach to focusing instead on what they CAN. This allows us to move away from the resistance and reactance generated by laws, bans, and taxes and to move toward CAN efforts—efforts that make healthier foods more convenient, attractive, and normal to purchase and consume.

The low-cost, win-win success of the CAN framework is then illustrated in the context of how it has been implemented in the Smarter Lunchroom movement. Finally, the implications of this in the larger context in our communities and in our personal food radius is outlined along with a model for the new form of public policy that can best address related issues in a productive and promising way.

The Public Policy Toolbox

Our food environment has evolved to provide food that is highly available, affordable, and attractive. Food is highly available within a short distance of most places the average person visits at any time in a typical day—gas stations, vending machines, office supply checkouts, and probably desk drawers. Food is highly affordable—the average American family spent 24% in 1960 and spends only 7% today. And food is highly attractive, coming in more brands, more flavors, and more sizes than ever before.

Although available, affordable, and attractive food has helped to make us overweight, the solution is not to make food less available, less affordable, and less attractive. Not even the most extreme critics of the food supply would want to resort to growing maize and hunting buffalo to feed their family, nor would they want to pay five times more for bread or ice cream so they would eat less.

There needs to be another solution.

There is a classic observation that if the only tool you have is a hammer, everything looks like a nail. The warning is that any efforts one makes to build a better mousetrap or garage will be severely handicapped by the use of the wrong tool. Public policy efforts generally involve a limited number of tools—bans, regulations, taxes, and subsidies. While not as limiting as having only one tool, policy limits how resourceful, creative, and successful it can be outside of a limited number of contexts or problem areas.

As we just discussed, our food environment has evolved to become available, affordable, and attractive because that is what almost 300 million US consumers want. It is what our market system organically evolved to give us (Just, 2006). To try and reverse our preferences with taxes or subsidies, or restrict our choices with bans or regulations, is unlikely to provide the quick fix to what a more finely tuned food system has evolved to provide.

A German word, *Verschlimmbesserung*, resonates with many well-intended, but inexperienced handymen. It roughly translates to "Trying to fix something but making it worse." Public policy is a well intended, but inexperienced handyman in the food environment. Although policy has achieved some success in the tobacco environment, the food environment is different—just as fixing your car is different from fixing your home.

The Problem With Can't

Many efforts to change eating behavior focus on nutrition education or restrictive policy changes. Strategies based upon behavioral economic and social psychology theory may provide a way to encourage healthier behavior without inducing the resistance and reactance often associated with restrictive policies (Just, Mancino, & Wansink, 2007; Just & Wansink, 2009). Rather, behavioral policies offer the potential of creating long-lasting habits and attitudes. Institutions—restaurants, grocery stores, workplaces, and schools—can exert considerable control over the "choice architecture" even in simply changing how foods are offered and presented. Behavioral economics theory suggests several possibilities to structure environments in ways that noncoercively encourage healthier choices.

Consider a recent study wherein corporate wellness trainers at a conference retreat were invited to a free hot breakfast buffet. On one series of tables, the food items were arranged from healthiest to least healthy. After picking up their plate, they first saw cut fruit, low-fat yogurt, and low-fat granola, and the buffet ended with bacon, fried potatoes, and cheesy eggs. The other series of tables ordered the food in the exact opposite order. After picking up their plate, the people who had been randomly sent to this line first saw cheesy eggs, fried potatoes, and bacon, and they only saw low-fat granola, low-fat yogurt, and fresh cut fruit at the end of the line, after they had already filled their plate. Regardless of what they saw first, the first three items comprised two thirds of the different food they took (Wansink & Hanks, 2013). As Figure 9.1 indicates, if those items were healthy, two thirds of the items they took were healthy. If those items were unhealthy, two-thirds of the items they took were unhealthy.

When only bans and taxes are used, they often ignore a basic understanding of consumer behavior. Instead of banning bacon from the

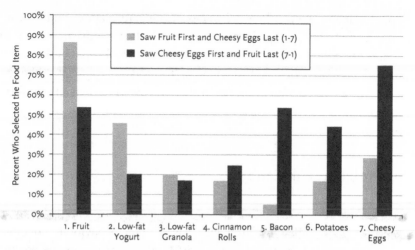

FIGURE 9.1 Food presentation order influences the percentage of diners who selected healthy or unhealthy foods. NOTE: The percentages are predicted percentages of individuals selecting an item in one of two buffet lines. These percentages were generated from a nonlinear estimation procedure using the logistic density function.

buffet, all one would have to do is put it at the end. As with the example of the buffet line, tremendous opportunity is lost for using wiser, less reactance-generating solutions. Consider two examples: chocolate milk bans and soft drink taxes.

When Chocolate Milk Attacks

Whether to remove flavored milk from school cafeterias has been actively debated as a measure to reduce childhood obesity. The predominant view of nutrition and medical researchers is that milk has nutrients essential for bone growth and development. Although low-fat chocolate milk contains over twice as much sugar as low-fat white milk, some school districts take the position that any milk is better than no milk while others have begun to limit or omit the sale of flavored milk in hopes of reducing children's total caloric and sugar intake from dairy. What is not known, however, is how changing the availability of flavored milk would influence other behaviors, such as what students might otherwise select, and what potential economic implications, such as impacts on participation in the school lunch program and milk waste, may result.

With an estimated two thirds of participating students in the National School Lunch Program (NSLP) choosing chocolate over white milk, reducing availability of flavored milk may lead many children to change what they drink and eat. Because most children drink flavored milk for its taste, as opposed to its nutritional content, its removal may not lead to a complete substitution of white milk, though students who select white milk instead are not consuming the added sugars. There is, however, strong evidence that removal or limitation of flavored milk in schools leads to a decrease in overall milk consumption, thus eliminating milk-specific nutrients, such as calcium and vitamin D, from children's diets.

Other similarly paternalistic policies, such as requiring that students take a fruit or vegetable with their lunch, have led to more waste while making lunches more expensive for cafeterias to serve. It is possible that restrictive policies related to milk, such as eliminating flavored milk, could have similar ramifications. Given students' documented preference for chocolate over white milk, eliminating it may have an impact not only on total milk sales but also the amount of milk students consume.

A natural experiment was afforded by 11 elementary schools, which made a clean transition from offering flavored milk to only white milk. Although the results are limited by the absence of control schools—and may not be generalizable in magnitude to middle schools and high schools—the consistency of these results offers important preliminary insights related to possible economic consequences of eliminating flavored milks. Among these schools, the elimination of flavored milk was associated with a 10% decrease in average daily milk sales, a 10% increase in the cost of milk, and a 30% increase in milk waste (Hanks, Just, & Wansink, 2014). Yet eliminating flavored milk reduced the amount of sugar and calories available in a student's lunch. As the infographic in Figure 9.2 illustrates, this set of findings demonstrates that removing flavored milk from a cafeteria can be accompanied with unintended consequences, which must be considered before such a decision is pursued.

An alternative approach is to simply make white milk more attractive than chocolate. When white milk is made more convenient by moving it to the front of the cooler, sales typically increase by 30%–40%. If at least one third of all milk is white, sales increase another 35%. No complaints. No front-page stories.

Beverage Taxes: From Coke to Coors

Taxes on energy-dense foods have been proposed to address the growing obesity problem (e.g., Brownell et al., 2009; Brownell & Frieden, 2009; Institute of Medicine, 2009; Jacobson, 2004). In the United States, the tax that has received the most attention is a tax on sugar-sweetened beverages,

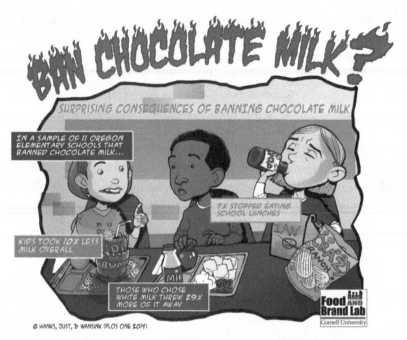

FIGURE 9.2 Surprising consequences of banning chocolate milk.

often referred to as a "soda tax" or "soft drink tax," which has been proposed by the Institute of Medicine (IOM), the Centers for Disease Control and Prevention (CDC), and several state and local governments (IOM, 2009; Paterson, 2008; Roehr, 2009; Rudd Report, 2009). The aim of such a tax would be to reduce calorie intake, improve diet and health, and generate revenue that governments could use to further address obesity-related health problems (Brownell & Frieden, 2009; Duffey et al., 2010; Jacobson & Brownell, 2000; Powell & Chaloupka, 2009; Smith, Lin, & Lee, 2010).

These reports and the subsequent policy debates have had two curious omissions (Campbell, 2011; Kuchler, Tegene, & Harris, 2004; Mytton, Clarke, & Rayner, 2012; Mytton, Gray, Rayner, & Rutter, 2007). First, they have omitted any discussion of consumer behavior and marketing responses other than simply assuming that if the price increases people will buy less. Indeed, no marketing or consumer behavior research from the *Journal of Marketing*—or any leading marketing journals—was cited in the reports by the IOM or by the CDC. Second, they lacked empirical evidence as to how people would respond to a tax on food—instead relying on epidemiological models of tobacco taxes (Adda & Cornaglia, 2006). This tobacco-food parallel may not be accurate. In 2011, Denmark imposed a tax on foods with 2.3% or more saturated fat (Zafar, 2011), increasing the cost of foods, such as butter, meats, and desserts, by as much as 30% (Press Association, 2011). After 1 year, they repealed it, claiming it did not improve health, and it hurt many small businesses because it merely led people to buy lower priced food or to make a stockpiling drive to Germany—which was foreshadowed in Grether and Holloway's (1967) *Journal of Marketing* article nearly half a century ago (Chouinard, Davis, Lafrance, & Perloff, 2007). The purpose of this research is to empirically investigate the impact of a soft drink tax in a way that can introduce both the consumer and marketing into important policy debates in this area and in other areas such as portion sizes (Mohr, Lichtenstein, & Janiszewski, 2012), advertising regulation (Kolsarici & Vakratsas 2010; Parsons & Schumacher 2012), deceptive marketing (Tipton, Bharadwaj, & Robertson, 2009), and fast-food restrictions (Dhar & Baylis, 2011).

Up to this point, two principal techniques have been used to assess the effectiveness of a tax on sugar-sweetened beverages (SSBs). The first relies on the natural variation in current soft drink taxes across states to identify responses in demand (Beasley & Rosen,1999; Fletcher, Frisvold, & Tefft, 2010; Powell, Chriqui, & Chaloupka, 2009; Zheng & Kaiser, 2008). The second estimates price elasticities for beverages and uses these elasticities to estimate responses to increases in prices of SSBs. A complement to these two methods is a controlled field experiment. A controlled field experiment could more cleanly provide within- and between-subject variation, household-specific demographic information, and a semicontrolled environment where the salience of the tax is not a concern (Harrison & List, 2004; Levitt & List, 2009; List, 2009, 2011). Furthermore, if conducted over a period of time, it would also provide household-level insights related to effectiveness, substitution, and decaying impacts of a tax (Chetty, Looney, & Kroft, 2009).

To examine this, we conducted a controlled field experiment in three major grocery stores in a small city (population: 62,000) in the eastern United States. In the study, 113 households in their shopper rewards program were randomly assigned to either face a 10% tax on SSBs or to be in the control group, and their individual household purchases were recorded over a 7-month period (Hanks et al., 2013).

Our initial results indicate that the tax had no significant impact on fluid ounces purchased of soft drinks. Among frequent buyers of soft drinks, we find evidence of a strong preference for soft drinks, such that households prefer calories from this beverage relative to other full-calorie beverages that may have more nutrients (sugar-sweetened fruit juice and whole and flavored milk). Yet, in a rather startling set of results, we also find that the tax drives frequent buyers of beer to purchase more beer than they would have without the tax. Even though there are other substitutes available, frequent beer buyers seem to prefer the trade-off of soft drinks for beer over trade-offs for other beverages.

We also found that the interaction between purchase frequency—which we use to proxy for preferences for soft drinks and beer—and the tax treatment suggests a significant correlation between frequent beer buyers in the tax treatment and fluid ounces of beer purchased over fluid ounces of soft drinks (Hanks et al., 2013; Wansink, Hanks, & Just 2015). This is not the substitution that was expected (i.e., Fletcher et al., 2011b). Specifically, the data suggest that the more frequent buyers of beer respond to the tax by purchasing 31.5 more fluid ounces of beer each month, translating into an additional 352 calories ($p < .01$ for both). Not only did the tax increase the amount of alcohol purchased by beer-drinking households, it also increased the amount of calories purchased as well. To public health officials and policy makers, this presents an important empirical result and more generally points toward wide-ranging contributions that consumer behavior research can make in their decisions.[1]

Moving From Can't to CAN

Consumer psychologists have been generating, testing, and publishing an increasing number of powerful insights in the area of food choice and consumption. Curiously, however, few of these insights seem to have made their way into effective public health interventions or treatments (Wansink, 2004), and most are unknown by the researchers, practitioners, and policy makers in these fields (Johnson, 2006).

Part of this lack of impact has to do with consumer psychology's focus on internal validity over external validity (lab studies versus randomized controlled trials) and on theory building and mediation over behavioral outcomes (interactions versus behavior-related main effects). Another part of consumer psychology's lack of impact also has to do with structural differences in where we publish (PsychInfo-indexed journals versus PubMed-indexed journals) and the search terms that are used (manipulations versus interventions, consumption versus intake, and so on).

Yet a third impact barrier is one that is much easier for us to address. It relates to how consumer psychology has not been able to provide public health with a systematic way to use all of the wide array of insights we have discovered (Wansink, 2015). Across consumer psychology and health psychology, findings often appear Balkanized. This is partially because they focus on different dependent variables (choice, affect, memory, behavioral intentions, and so on) and the use of vague or somewhat unwieldy independent variables (such as need for cognition or eating restraint) that cannot clearly be identified or manipulated in practice (Wansink & Chandon, 2014).

What is needed is a basic categorization system that can help us systematize our findings in a way that makes them useful to both public health researchers and practitioners. This basic framework focuses on interventions that can change choice and do so by making healthy choices more convenient (physically and cognitively), more attractive (comparatively and absolutely), and more normative (actual and perceived). Consider the acronym CAN: *c*onvenient, *a*ttractive, and *n*ormative.

Education and cognition are overrated when it comes to changing eating behavior. There is a very unreliable link between knowledge and behavior, and relying only on education, knowledge, cognition, or willpower to change eating behavior is frustratingly unsuccessful. Fortunately, there is an alternative.

Most people have a choice of what and how much they eat. Even if given only a bowl of gruel from the Oliver Twist cookbook, they have the choice of whether to eat any of it or whether to eat it all and ask for more. The key to changing eating behavior is not in convincing a person that an apple is better for him than a cookie. Instead, the key is to make sure that the apple is the more convenient, attractive, and normative food to choose (Figure 9.3).

Even though the typical person believes she makes about 20–30 decisions regarding food each day, she makes closer to 200 food decisions (Wansink & Sobal, 2007). About 90% of these decisions we are not fully aware of because they do not involve reason and deliberation. They involve quick, instinctive actions. This gives us a great opportunity to set up eating environments so a person's quick, instinctive actions are biased toward the healthier foods—biased toward the apple rather than the cookie.

In 2006, the New York State Department of Health raised the question, "How much would the government need to subsidize whole fruit in school lunchrooms so that children would take 5% more fruit?" A quick visit to five schools would have shown that these fruits were being sold in metal chafing dishes, under sneeze shields, in a dim corner of the line. The fruit's 50¢ price was probably not the problem, and it probably would not be the solution. Instead, the fruit needed to be put in nice bowls and placed in a

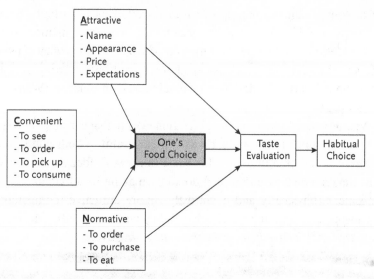

FIGURE 9.3 The CAN approach to changing one's food choice.

well-lit part of the line. When this was done, fruit sales increased an average of 103% for the entire semester (Just & Wansink, 2009).

Putting the fruit in an attractive bowl in a well-lit part of the line accomplished three goals. First, it made the fruit *convenient* to select. Second, it made the fruit appear more *attractive*. Third, it made the fruit appear *normative*, typical, or reasonable to take—partly because it was convenient and attractive. (See Table 9.1) This CAN approach to changing behavior is outlined in detail in the book *Slim by Design* (Wansink, 2014).

In dozens of different eating behavior studies in homes, grocery stores, restaurants, and schools, using this CAN approach—making healthy foods more convenient, attractive, and normative—has been shown to be much more effective than taking favorite foods away from people or artificially restricting what someone can order (Wansink, 2014). Doing this creatively and effectively can not only alter a person's food choice, but it can change expectations, which can alter taste evaluation (Wansink et al., 2012) and eventually lead to habitually healthier choices. Although these downstream ripples of one's food choices are critical to changing habits and health, a key focus should be on changing that choice in the first place, regardless of whether it is in the home, in restaurants, grocery stores, where we work, or where our children go to school (Table 9.2).

TABLE 9.1 Sample Findings Using the CAN Framework of Behavior Change

CONVENIENT	ATTRACTIVE	NORMATIVE
• *Convenient to see*: A fruit display near the cash register increased sales 35%, even when product was not discounted (Van Kleef, Otten, & van Trijp, 2012)	• *Attractively named*: Giving descriptive names to vegetables increased sales among elementary schoolers by 18% (Wansink et al., 2012)	• *Normative to order*: Placing a sticker of a vegetable on a tray increased the number of school children selecting vegetables by 61% (Mann & Redden, 2011)
• *Convenient to order*: Healthy "Grab and Go" lines in cafeterias led to a 82% increase in healthy food sales (Hanks et al., 2012)	• *Attractive appearance*: Placing nonedible garnish on a vegetable side dish increased sales and taste evaluation (Wansink, Payne, & Painter, 2014)	• *Normative to purchase*: Visually dividing a shopping cart in half and suggesting that half should be used for fruits and vegetables increased their sales by 27% (Wansink et al., 2014)
• *Convenient to pick up*: Conference goers fill 68% of their plate with the first three foods they encounter on the breakfast buffet (Wansink & Hanks, 2013)	• *Attractively priced*: Proportional pricing decreased market share for only the largest packaging (Vermeer et al., 2010)	• *Normative to serve*: Changing a container size decreased snack intake independent of portion size (Marchiori, Cornelle, & Klein, 2012)
• *Convenient to consume*: Large sip sizes increases increase food intake by 12% (Bolhuis et al., 2013)	• *Attractive expectations*: Altering the height of a package increased choice and perceptions of a product's healthfulness (Chandon & Ordabayeva, 2009)	• *Normative to eat*: 44% of the variation in the amount a woman serves herself in a buffet line is determined by what the woman ahead of her served herself (Wansink & Just, 2014)

Increasing Convenience

As Table 9.2 illustrates, a healthy choice needs to be made to be the convenient choice—convenient to see, to order, to pick up, and to consume. Consider what happens in schools that have adopted a behavior change program called the Smarter Lunchroom movement. In one study, when one of the food lines in a school cafeteria was redesigned to be a convenient line that only offered prepackaged healthy entrées and foods (such as salads), sales of these healthy foods increased 77% within 2 weeks (Hanks, Just, Smith, & Wansink, 2012).

Convenience can relate to the way food is offered. If one were to ask children why they don't eat more apples or pears, 5- to 9-year-old children say

TABLE 9.2 The CAN Approach to Changing Behavior in One's Food Radius

	1. MAKE IT MORE CONVENIENT	2. MAKE IT MORE ATTRACTIVE	3. MAKE IT MORE NORMATIVE
A mother who wants to eat better at home . . .	Puts precut vegetables on the middle shelf of the fridge and the bread out of sight	Buys more tempting salad dressings with cool names and less tempting bread	Sets salad bowls on the dinner table every day, even if they aren't being used, and gets rid of the butter dish
A restaurant owner who wants to sell more high-margin shrimp salads . . .	Makes it easy to find on the menu by putting it on the first page and in a bold font	Gives it a catchy name or one that appeals to the senses— "Scrumptious Savory Shrimp Salad Bonanza," anyone?	Describes it as a Special or a Manager's Favorite
A grocery store manager who wants to sell more fish at full price . . .	Places fish in a center cooler at the end of the vegetable section	Offers easy, appealing fish recipe ideas on notecards next to the fish that people can take with them	Put floor decals near it or have a green dashed line pointing toward the fish
An office manager who wants her workers to leave their desks and eat in the new healthy cafeteria . . .	Adds a $5 Grab & Go line filled with healthier foods, and maybe an honor system cash box	Has a more attractive cafeteria, break room, or brown bag series	Posts notices and news on bulletin boards in the cafeteria, break room, or fitness room, and not in the work area
A school lunch manager who wants to get more kids to take and eat fruit . . .	Puts it within easy reach in two different parts of the line—beginning and end	Puts it in a colorful bowl and/or gives it a colorful sign	Puts it in front of the cash register with a sign saying, "Take an extra one for a snack"

it is too big for their mouths or it gets stuck in their braces. Adolescent girls say they don't eat more fruit because it is messy and it looks unbecoming or unladylike. One solution to both problems would be to provide children with cut fruit. Indeed, when we put fruit sectionizers in school lunchrooms, children ate 70% more fruit (Wansink, Just, Hanks, & Smith, 2013).

Consider why 100-calorie packages have been so effective at reducing how much of a food most people consume in one sitting (Wansink, Payne, & Shimizu, 2011). One posited reason partially has to do with the inconvenience of opening a second or third bag, and the convenience of being able to pause and ask, "Am I really that hungry?" (Geier, Wansink, & Rozin, 2012). Making healthy food the more convenient choice leads to greater choice. Making less healthy food the less convenient choice leads people to consider more mindfully how hungry they are and whether it is worth the extra effort (Painter et al., 2002).

Convenience can be in the form of saving physical effort, but it can also take the form of saving cognitive effort. One often-cited technique to change behavior is to change defaults. For instance, if people are automatically given water with their combo meal unless they explicitly ask for a soft drink, water consumption would dramatically increase. While part of this might be explained by water being perceived as a more normative choice, another part of it is that it is the cognitively convenient choice to make.

Increasing Attractiveness

The second principle of the CAN approach is that the healthy choice needs to be made more attractive relative to what else is available. This includes more attractively named, more attractive in appearance, more attractively priced, and more attractive expectations. Fruit that is served in a steel chafer pan or stored in the bottom drawer of a refrigerator is not as attractive as fruit in a colorful bowl. Even simply giving food a descriptive name makes it more attractive and increases a person's taste expectations and enjoyment of it (Wansink, Just, Payne, & Klinger 2012). For instance, Dinosaur Trees are more exciting to a child and taste better than broccoli, and a Big Bad Bean Burrito tastes better and is more exciting than when it is called a Vegetarian Burrito. Even putting an Elmo sticker on apples led 46% more daycare kids to take and eat an apple instead of a cookie (Wansink, Just, & Payne 2012).

Making a food more attractive by altering its price relative to other options is a popular but overused tool of behavioral economists. Still, it has potential if more creatively employed for it can involve not only altering the price of the target product (decreasing the price of fruit) but also altering the price of nontarget products (increasing the price of cookies). Making a healthy food more attractive by adjusting price has creatively been done by offering people either a discount on a meal or a price premium on a less healthy one.

As Figure 9.3 illustrates, in addition to changing the name of a food and enhancing expectations of taste or enjoyment, making a healthy food more attractive can involve making it or its surroundings more visually attractive. Putting fruit in a nicer bowl leads children to take more, and putting garnish near a salad makes people rate the taste as better (Wansink, 2014).

Increasing Normativeness

Finally, many consumers often like what is popular; that is, they like what they think is normal. This includes being more normative to order, to purchase, to serve, and to eat (see Table 9.1). Efforts that make the healthy choice appear to be the more normal or normative choice appear to make it more. For instance, when 50% of the milk in a cooler is white (versus chocolate), middle school students are nearly three times as likely to take a white milk than when only 10% is white (Hanks et al., 2014). It seems like the normative choice. The same applies at home. When healthier food is placed on the front or middle shelf in a cupboard or refrigerator, it is more frequently taken and is rated as the more normative food to take—otherwise it wouldn't be so convenient (Chandon & Wansink, 2002).

Until now, much of this discussion has focused on how convenience, attractiveness, and normativeness influence choice. Also of interest is how they influence how much one consumes. In many cases there is a wide range to how much of a product a person can consume. A person may be quite content eating from 3–5 pieces of pizza for lunch and drinking 12–16 ounces of cola without feeling overly hungry or overly full (Wansink, 2006). Without a norm for how much pasta or potato chips one should consume, some people may unknowingly rely partly on past experience and partly on implied norms or consumption cues around them to determine the quantity or a range that is acceptable to consume. Regardless of one's gender or country of origin, all adults are members of the Clean-plate club, and they eat an estimated 92% of any food they serve themselves (Wansink & Johnson, 2015a). Fortunately, children consume only 60% of what they self-serve (Wansink & Johnson, 2015b). It is important to note that even with children, any cue that causes them to overserve, will cause them to overeat (van Ittersum & Wansink, 2014).

For instance, one category of cues that is often used to determine how much to serve is the cue that is provided by the package size or by the plate or bowl size (Wansink & van Ittersum, 2014; Wansink, 1996). Consumption norms—particularly those resulting from implicit visual cues coming from physical dimensions (Table 9.3)—hold tremendous promise for researchers for three reasons: (1) Their reach is farther than has been appreciated, (2) they can be found in an endless number of forms, and (3) their perceptual nature makes consumers more vulnerable than they believe. From an intervention standpoint, changing the size of a cafeteria tray or the size label on a restaurant menu can change consumption in an automatic way that does not necessitate willpower or an expensive public health education campaign.

TABLE 9.3 Physical Dimensions of Consumption Norms

PHYSICAL DIMENSIONS OF CONSUMPTION NORMS	ILLUSTRATIONS OF NORMS AND APPROXIMATE MAGNITUDE OF INCREASE
Package, serving, or dinnerware size	Doubling package size increases consumption by 22% (Wansink, 1996) Doubling serving size increased daily intake by 26% and is sustained over 11 days (Rolls, Roe & Meengs, 2006, 2007) Doubling dinnerware size increased food consumption with both bowls (37%) and serving spoons (14%) (Wansink, van Ittersum, & Painter, 2006)
Visual salience	Candies in clear dishes are consumed 37% more frequently than those in opaque dishes (Wansink, Painter, & van Ittersum, 2005)
Cognitive convenience	Bundles and "buy-on-get-one-free" promotional packs reduce perceived cost, which increases consumption (Chandon & Wansink, 2002; Wansink, 1996)
Attractiveness	Improving taste imagery facilitates the acceptance of downsizing (Cornil & Chandon, 2013)
Labeling	Adding a smaller or larger size shifts selection and consumption (Sharpe et al., 2008) Renaming regular size items as double-size decreases how much people consume by 29% (Just & Wansink, 2013)
Sequence of exposure	Altering the order of food in buffet lines leads people to fill 64% of their plate with the first three items on the buffet (Hanks, 2013)

Of initial value would be to more fully define the dimensions of implicit consumption norms. This would provide a way to determine which features of these norms led them to have the greatest impact on consumption volume. Knowing this would prove useful in directing research toward that which was most relevant, and directing interventions toward that which was most useful. One area where this is particularly important is when dealing with nutrition and children.

Case Study: The Smarter Lunchroom Movement

To see how behavioral science can effectively be used as a tool to change choices and eating behavior, consider the challenge of encouraging children to make smarter choices in school cafeterias. Rising obesity rates among children have led to harsh criticisms of school lunch programs.

Local school lunch administrators feel tremendous pressure from parents and activists to drop higher calorie items from the menu, such as cookies, french fries, or ice cream. Proponents of these measures argue that if children cannot buy it, they will not consume it, thus reducing the child's total intake of calories. Additional pressure on the USDA's subsidized school lunches has pushed for substituting familiar, favorite foods such as pizza and hamburgers with foods that are organic or vegetarian.

Yet introducing ultra healthy products into the lunchroom requires a significant increase in spending while reducing unit sales and total participation levels. Furthermore, banning popular items because of their content also directly reduces sales and participation. Suppose, however, that rearranging, repositioning, and reframing the currently offered food items could instead encourage children to buy more of the healthy foods and less of the rest. Such a strategy costs little, and it would provide a way for school districts to demonstrate an increase in the overall health content of their meals as well as in their popularity and participation.

Recent interventions in policy have experimented with behavioral economics (Johnson, 2006). The resulting success has helped establish various choice architectures that can sometimes guide or encourage people to make healthier decisions, without eliminating the freedom they have to make less healthy decisions (for instance, to purchase a cookie on Monday or french fries on Friday). Two features of school lunches make it an ideal candidate for using behavioral economics. First, there is substantial evidence that environmental and psychological influences can bias food selection and consumption (Just, 2006; Shiv, Carmen, & Ariely, 2005; Sunstein & Thaler, 2008). Second, while institutional food services focus on profit, they also have the noneconomic goal of encouraging people to make nutritious food choices (Oliveira & Variyam, 2003).

This research has two objectives relevant to making school lunchrooms smarter. First, it describes a new study that underscores that giving people a choice can result in higher intake and taste ratings of vegetables than if given no choice except for what they would have otherwise selected anyway. That is, junior high students who selected carrots over brownish celery ate more carrots and rated them as tastier than those who were simply given the carrots without a choice. Second, it summarizes recent field study findings that illustrate how small, "low cost, no-cost" changes in lighting, salience, convenience, and payment systems can result in unexpectedly large changes in the healthfulness of meal selections. The implications for local food service policies and for health and wellness boards are then outlined.

The Unexpected Power of Constrained Volition

Constrained volition refers to a person believing that she made a decision based on free will—with her own volition—without realizing the extent to which she was influenced by the artificial constraints placed on her. Constrained volition occurs when a decision context is engineered (or has accidently evolved) to guide the way in which people consider options, without being overtly perceived as doing so. Framing studies and studies on choice contexts may result in constrained volition. That is, their results frequently lead to changes in choice without a commensurate awareness of how they were guided toward a particular selection.

Constrained volition involves misinterpreting one's behavior as less constrained than it actually was. While the results would appear similar to an "opt in or opt out" scenario (Sunstein & Thaler, 2007), it could lead to very different inferences about behavior. This behavioral effect is disproportionate to one's level of awareness. In the case of a student's food selections, it would involve not fully acknowledging the larger set of constraints (such as the restrictions of a debit card) that might have led to this change.

With school lunches, as with all meals, there is a subjective dimension to food that makes people equally susceptible to environmental influences. Small environmental cues—such as the name of a food or how many others are eating it—can alter how one interprets its flavor, calorie content, and healthfulness (Wansink, 2004). If an invisible hand were to lead people to choose one food over another, it might also alter how they interpret their behavior and evaluate their choices.

Consider three situations: (1) Fruit is made more salient by buying a new bowl and shining a light on it, (2) a salad bar is moved so it breaks up foot traffic patterns, and (3) a vegetable option is provided of either baby carrots or brownish celery. If these interventions were to lead students to select foods (fruit, salad, and carrots) they might not have otherwise selected, there is psychological precedence that one may not even acknowledge their influence. Over 90% of the people involved in food intake studies routinely claim they were not influenced by the environmental cues such as package sizes or glass shapes (Vartanian et al., 2008). Because of either an unawareness of these environmental cues or an unwillingness to acknowledge their influence, there is a fundamental attribution error that occurs.

In this broad area of constrained volition, one area that has not been widely examined is the role that these small interventions can make in guiding particularly routine or automatic behavior such as lunchtime food selections. Such small, low-cost, no-cost interventions could lead people to pause their behavior—even for just a moment—and perhaps rethink their next action.

To illustrate how behavioral economic concepts can help increase the healthy content of foods without harming the bottom line, a few examples from the field may be helpful. Some of the tools are extremely simple to implement and can provide a big bang for the buck. For example, simply closing the lid on the freezer that contains the ice cream can reduce the number choosing ice cream from 30% to 14%. Similar results can be obtained by simply moving vending machines further from the cafeteria.

Lighting Up the Fruit

There are unexpectedly large responses to moving food or to moving the traffic flow patterns. In one Minnesota school, cash registers were found to be a bottleneck in the system. While students waited to pay, they were faced with a wide array of grain-based snacks, chips, granola bars, and desserts. This appeared to generate a number of impulse purchases. While one option would have been to move these temptations, this option would have almost assuredly decreased revenue. A better option was to replace these snacks with an array of fruits. This way, when students were waiting to check out, the impulse temptations were healthier options. Fruit sales increased, snack food sales decreased, and total revenue did not significantly decrease. Part of the increase in fruit sales may have also been aided by the inclusion of a wider variety of fruits (plums and peaches) in addition to the standard trio of apples, bananas, and oranges.

In order to obtain the USDA subsidy for a school meal, the meal must contain at least three separate food items and at least one must be from the protein food group. Being aware of this financial incentive, the food service staff person operating the cash register will often inspect a meal and if the meal has only two items, she will suggest that the student take an extra item. In many schools, because milk is kept right next to the cash register, it is often suggested as an option to complete the meal. When visiting one school where this setup prevailed, we quickly noticed that a number of the students taking milk were taking it because they had been asked. They did not intend to consume it. As a result, the trash bins contained many unused milk cartons.

Instead of milk, suppose this school placed fruit next to the cash register and milk at the front of the line. Several studies have shown that suggesting a student take fruit will increase the number of students *eating* (not just taking) the fruit by as much as 70%. Further, while milk can go bad or become unappetizing when warm, fruit may be easily carried out of the lunchroom and eaten later in the day. Finally, most fruit costs substantially less than a lunch-sized carton of milk. Thus, it could be that placing fruit at the end of the lunch line would maintain the level of USDA subsidy, increase the health content of the food consumed, and reduce the costs of providing the foods. Such simple solutions can make a nice addition to both health and financial goals.

Moving the Salad Bar

Consider the problem of a middle school in Corning, New York. Their lunchroom consists of two lunch lines feeding into two cash registers. A portable salad bar was initially introduced and situated against the wall just 3 feet to the east of the easternmost lunch line, and parallel to that line. Purchasing a salad would require students to walk to the salad bar, place their salad on a plate, and then go to the end of the lunch line to wait for the cash register. Sales of salad were rather sluggish. By rotating the salad bar 90 degrees and moving it 8 feet to the middle of the lunch room, it became something students had to walk around, not something they could mind-lessly walk by. Bulk sales increased 200%–300% after the move and con-tinued to increase as it became a part of the lunchtime routine for students.

Rather than gutting sales as many healthy measures may tend to do, this move increased overall sales and profitability. The level of visibility was increased; this increased their desire for the food, and the level of convenience was increased as one could wait through the line while get-ting a salad. Most important, children chose the salad without prodding or heavy-handed measures. This move makes it much more likely that chil-dren will begin to develop a healthy habit of choosing the salad at lunch when it is available. Indeed, in one high school of 1,000 students, simply introducing a salad bar increased average reimbursable lunch participation by 21% from one year to the next.

Keep Your Tray?

The type of tray used for carrying the food can also play heavily into the food decisions of the individual. Relevant to some high schools, there is a recent trend in college dining halls that might be of interest. To reduce waste, many colleges are phasing out the use of trays—especially in all-you-can-eat, buffet-style cafeterias—forcing students to carry individ-ual plates and glasses. This move was made in the hopes that they might reduce waste. That is, people might take less and eat more of what they do take. One key question this does not ask is this: If they take fewer foods, what do they leave behind—salads or desserts?

In an investigation of trayless cafeterias, we found not having a tray made students much more reluctant to take side dishes. Unfortunately, most of the fruit and vegetable content of meals is in these side dishes. Our matched-meal study of a 1,200-person dining hall at Cornell found that 26% fewer salads were taken, but only 8% fewer bowls of ice cream (Wansink & Just, 2013). Strangely, there was even more waste without the trays. Without trays, students took larger portions of things they liked. With larger portions and less variety, we found they tended to take more than they ended up eating. Cafeterias with fixed portion sizes may have less waste. Nevertheless, in the context of trayless serve-yourself cafeterias, going trayless reduced nutrition without reducing waste.

The Limitation of Changing Defaults

In fast-food restaurants and food courts, the default options offered in the meal—soft drinks and fries—tend to be what most order, even though milk, salads, or apple slices are also available at no added cost. The potential power of these options leads us to question what would happen if restaurants—or school lunchrooms—were to change the defaults. What if instead of putting tater tots on a tray, they put peas on the tray and gave students the option of substituting tater tots for peas if they wanted?

In one study with elementary school–aged students in a summer 4-H program, we examined how changing food defaults would work. On one day we gave these students a lunch where they were given french fries as the default but asked if they wanted to trade their french fries for apple fries (prepeeled, presliced apples) with caramel dip, commonly available at fast-food restaurants. Of the 21 students, 20 (95%) wanted to stay with the french fries default. Two days later we did the reverse; we gave these students a lunch were they were given apple fries as a default but asked if they wanted to trade them for french fries. Of the 22 students in class that day, 21 (96%) wanted to switch to french fries. What initially appeared to be a strong case for food defaults ended up being overwhelmed by overriding preference for french fries. While defaults might work well in cases where preferences are ambiguous or where people do not care (Johnson & Goldstein, 2003), they might not be the solution in the school lunchroom.

Of all of the different food psychology and behavioral economic tactics we have introduced so far into schools, the one that may have the largest success at the lowest cost is requiring high school students to pay cash for desserts and soft drinks. We do not take their desserts away, we just say, "If you want that cookie bad enough, you can pay cash for it." They cannot mindlessly put it on their debit card or on their pin account; instead, they have to take out the dollar they might otherwise spend on an iTune and ask themselves how bad they want the cookie.

In our experiments and in our analysis of the USDA's School Nutrition Dietary Assessment (SNDA) data, we find this change does not hurt revenue or participation and it leads to greater sales of more nutritious items and lower sales of the less nutritious items. Figure 9.3 presents some summary statistics for sales of healthy foods from the SNDA national sample of schools offering different payment methods. Those in the schools allowing cash purchases see higher sales of healthy foods. A seemingly modest adjustment to the existing school lunch payment systems or size label (medium versus large; half-size versus regular-size) could have a surprising influence on food choice (Just & Wansink, 2013). Over the years, this could significantly impact the weight and health of children.

Every school district that participates in the National School Lunch program is required to have a local school wellness policy—this is a tool that can be used to promote healthier eating through smarter lunchrooms. These nascent wellness policies are to be determined by, monitored by, and altered by a school district wellness board comprised of local citizens. Many of these boards are uncertain of the steps they can take to make a positive difference in their schools. Being able to champion a restricted debit card system would be an easy, high visibility initiative for a wellness board.

Policy Considerations for School Health and Wellness Boards

Food is not nutrition until it is eaten. We should not judge the quality of a school lunch by what is offered. We should judge it by what is eaten. Overly restricting a student's options is like forcing a child to eat his vegetables. In the end, we might win the in-school battle but lose the after-school war. We might condition them for food choices as a high school student but leave them unprepared for the battle of the Freshman-15 that awaits them afterward.

A seemingly modest adjustment to the existing school lunch payment systems could have a sizable influence on food choice. Over the years, this could significantly impact the weight and health of children. Restricting the use of prepaid debit cards to healthier foods would also allow parents to reclaim some control over their child's food choice set, without unfairly restricting them or without decreasing the revenue for school cafeterias.

Every school district that participates in the National School Lunch program is required to have a local school wellness policy—this is a tool that can be used to promote healthier eating and physical activity through changes in school environments. These nascent Health and Wellness policies are to be determined by, monitored by, and altered by a school district Health and Wellness board comprised of local citizens. Many of these boards are uncertain of the steps they can take to make a positive difference in their schools. Being able to champion any of the low-cost, no-cost changes would move them far ahead of peer schools (see Figure 9.4). Such changes can be an easier alternative than fighting against food service directors, waiting for federal policies to change, or readjusting the organic food supply. They can be accomplished quickly, easily, and between semesters.

For some Health and Wellness boards, the next step might be a cautious one that would require results from randomized controlled trials at a wide range of schools in their district. Yet such expense and caution may not be necessary. Given the strength of the effect reported here during one occasion, the ease of implementation, and the immediacy of the results, there are wellness boards who may simply want to implement a trial version of Smarter Lunchroom changes and gauge its acceptance by students, parents, and lunch staff.

Behavioral economics has a powerful potential to change behavior. By broadening their commonly used set of tools—beyond discounting—there is an increased opportunity to explain more of the variation in troubling behavior and to generate creative, scalable policy solutions. Because of reactance and compensation, direct approaches to behavioral change may be more effective in theory than in practice. Constrained volition offers a more frictionless nudge.

Creating a Self-Assessment Scorecard

Some people have a hard time believing that simply moving a fruit bowl or the white milk can change what kids eat overnight. But when they do it

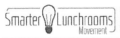
Since its founding in 2009 the Smarter Lunchrooms Movement has championed the use of evidence-based, simple low and no-cost changes to lunchrooms which can simultaneously improve participation and profits while decreasing waste. This tool can help you to evaluate your lunchroom, congratulate yourself for things you are doing well and and identify areas of opportunity for improvement.

Instructions

Read each of the statements below. Visualize your cafeteria, your service areas and your school building. Indicate whether the statement is true for your school by checking the box to the left. If you believe that your school does not reflect the statement 100%, do not check the box on the left. After you have completed the checklist, tally all boxes with check marks and write this number in the designated area on the back of the form. This number represents your school's baseline score. The boxes which are not checked are areas of opportunity for you to consider implementing in the future. We recommend completing this checklist annually to measure your improvements!

Important Words

Service areas: Any location where students can purchase or are provided with food

Dining areas: Any location where students can consume the food purchased or provided

Grab and Go Meals: Any meal with components pre-packaged together for ease and convenience – such as a brown bag lunch or "Fun Lunch" etc.

Designated Line: Any foodservice line which has been specified for particular food items or concepts – such as a pizza line, deli line, salad line etc.

Alternative entrée options: Any meal component which could also be considered an entrée for students - such as the salad bar, yogurt parfait, vegetarian/vegan or meatless options etc.

Reimbursable "Combo Meal" pairings: Any reimbursable components available independently on your foodservice lines which you have identified as a part of a promotional complete meal – For example you decided your beef taco, seasoned beans, frozen strawberries and 1% milk are part of a promotional meal called the, "Mi Amigo Meal!" etc.

Non-functional lunchroom equipment: Any items which are either broken, awaiting repair or are simply not used during meal service – such as empty or broken steam tables, coolers, registers etc.

Good Rapport: Communication is completed in a friendly and polite manner

Focusing on Fruit

☐ Fruit is available in all food service areas

☐ Daily fruit options are available in two or more locations on the service lines

☐ At least one daily fruit option is available near all registers (If there are concerns regarding edible peel, fruit can be bagged or wrapped)

☐ At least two types of fruit are available daily

☐ Whole fruit options are displayed in attractive bowls or baskets (instead of chaffing/hotel pans)

☐ A mixed variety of whole fruits are displayed together in bowls in all service areas

☐ Sliced or cut fruit is available daily

☐ Daily fruit options are displayed in a location in the line of sight and reach of students (Consider the average height of your students when determining line of sight)

☐ Daily fruit options are bundled into all grab and go meals available to students

☐ All available fruit options have been given creative or descriptive names

☐ All fruit names are highlighted on all serving lines with name-cards or product IDs daily

☐ All fruit names are highlighted and legible on menu boards in all service and dining areas

☐ Fruit options are not browning, bruised or otherwise damaged

☐ All fruit options are replenished so displays appear "full" continually throughout meal service and after each lunch period

☐ All staff members, especially those serving, have been trained to politely prompt students to select and consume the daily fruit options with their meal

Promoting Vegetables & Salad

☐ Vegetables are available in all food service areas

☐ Daily vegetable options are available in two or more locations in all service areas

☐ At least two types of vegetable are available daily

☐ Daily vegetable options are displayed in a location in the line of sight and reach of students (Consider the average height of your students when determining line of sight)

☐ Daily vegetable options are bundled into all grab and go meals available to students

☐ A salad bar is available to all students

☐ All available vegetable options have been given creative or descriptive names

☐ All vegetable names are highlighted on all serving lines with name-cards or product IDs daily

☐ All vegetable names are highlighted and legible on menu boards in the service and dining areas

☐ Vegetables are not wilted, browning, or otherwise damaged

☐ All vegetable options are replenished so displays appear "full" continually throughout meal service and after each lunch period

☐ All staff members, especially those serving, have been trained to politely prompt students to select and consume the daily vegetable options with their meal

Moving More White Milk

☐ White milk is available in all service areas

☐ White milk is in two or more locations in all service areas

☐ All beverage coolers have white milk available

☐ White milk represents 1/3 of all visible milk in the lunchroom

☐ White milk is placed in front of other beverages in all coolers

☐ White milk is eye-level and within reach of the students (Consider the average height of your students when determining eye-level)

☐ White milk crates are placed so that they are the first beverage option seen in all milk coolers

☐ White milk is bundled into all grab and go meals available to students as the default beverage

☐ White milk is highlighted on all serving lines with a name-card or product ID daily

☐ White milk is highlighted and legible on the menu boards in all service and dining areas

☐ White milk is replenished so all displays appear "full" continually throughout meal service and after each lunch period

Entrée of the Day

☐ A daily entrée option has been identified to promote - a targeted entrée in each service area and for each designated line (deli-line, pizza-line etc.)

FIGURE 9.4 Smarter Lunchroom Self-Assessment Scorecard.

and see that it works, they become huge converts and want to know what to do next. It is good to get advice, but once we get rolling, people—just like school lunch directors—pretty much know what will work best for them and what won't.

To help schools figure out how smart of a lunchroom they have and what they can do next, we have designed a do-it-yourself scorecard (from Slim by Design) that lunchroom staff, parents, or students can use. All it takes is the scorecard, a pencil, and a lunchroom—you can even skip the pencil and download the free app (Smarter Lunchroom Scorecard). Each lunchroom can get as many as 100 points because there are 100 tasks or changes that help kids choose better and eat better. The more changes your school makes, the higher the score. Most schools first score around 20 to 30, but they can quickly move up to 50 within a couple weeks if they really focus.

These are all research-based changes we have found help kids make smarter choices. We are still discovering new changes, so every school year there are a few new ones we rotate in and a few less effective ones we rotate out, but a school that got a 75 last year will probably get about a 75 this year if it has not made any changes or regressed.

Conclusion

Consumption is a context where understanding fundamental behavior has immediate implications for consumer welfare. People are often surprised at how much they consume, and this indicates they may be influenced at a basic level of which they are not aware or do not monitor. Similar to the fundamental attribution error, this explains why simply knowing these environmental traps exist does not typically help one avoid them (Vartanian et al., 2008). Relying only on cognitive control and on willpower is often disappointing. Furthermore, consistently reminding people to vigilantly monitor their actions around food is not realistic. Continued cognitive oversight is already difficult for people who are focused, disciplined, and concentrated. It is nearly impossible for those who are not.

The studies reviewed here illustrate how an individual can alter his or her personal environment so it does not have unintended effects on how much is eaten. We did not fully discuss the individual differences that would make some of these changes or "nudges" more effective than others. For some, this might involve repackaging food into single-serving containers, storing tempting foods in less convenient locations, and preplating one's food prior to beginning a meal. For others, simply using narrow glasses and smaller plates might be all that is required to make their environment less conducive to overeating.

Note

1. Although some price manipulation interventions found that hiking the price of beer might reduce cafeteria demand (Block, 2009), the tax level was extreme (35%) and was not in a retail shopping environment (Nederkoorn et al., 2011).

References

Adda, J., & Cornaglia, F. (2006). Taxes, cigarette consumption, and smoking intensity. *American Economic Review*, *96*(4), 1013–1028.

Beasley, T., & Rosen, H. (1999). Sales taxes and prices: An empirical analysis. *National Tax Journal*, *52*(2), 157–178.

Block, J. (2009). Point-of-purchase price and education intervention to reduce consumption of sugary soft drinks. *American Journal of Public Health*, *100*(8),1427–1433.

Bolhuis, D. P., Lakemond, C. M. M., de Wijk, R. A., Luning, P. A., de Graaf, C. (2013). Consumption with large sip sizes increases food intake and leads to underestimation of the amount consumed. *PLoS ONE*, *8*(1), e53288. doi:10.1371/journal.pone.0053288

Brownell, K., & T. Frieden. (2009). Ounces of Prevention—the Public Policy Case for Taxes on Sugared Beverages. *N. Engl. J. Med.* 360: 1805–1808.

Brownell, K., Farley, T., Willett, W., Popkin, B., Chaloupka, F., Thompson, F., . . . Ludwig, D. (2009). The public health and economic benefits of taxing sugar-sweetened beverages. *New England Journal of Medicine*, *361*(16), 1599–1605.

Campbell, D. (2011, December 12). Experts call for 10% 'fat tax' on soft drinks to prevent obesity. *The Guardian*. Retrieved July 2012, from http://www.guardian.co.uk/society/2011/dec/21/sugary-soft-drinks-obesity-tax?INTCMP=SRCH

Chandon, P., & Wansink, B. (2002). When are stockpiled products consumed faster? A convenience—salience framework of postpurchase consumption incidence and quantity. *Journal of Marketing Research*, *39*(3), 321–335.

Chetty, R., Looney, A., & Kroft, K. (2009). Salience and taxation: Theory and evidence. *American Economic Review*, *99*(4), 1145–1177.

Choi, J. J., Laibson, D., Madrian, B. C., & Metrick, A. (2003). Optimal defaults. *American Economic Review*, *93*(2), 180–185.

Chouinard H., Davis, D., Lafrance, J., & Perloff, J. (2007). Fat taxes: Big money for small change. *Forum on Health and Economic Policy, 10*(2), Article 2.

Dhar, T., & Baylis, K. (2011). Fast-food consumption and the ban on advertising targeting children: The Quebec experience. *Journal of Marketing Research*, *48*(5), 799–813.

Duffey, K., Gordon-Larsen, P., Shikany, J., Guilkey, D., Jacobs, D., Jr., & Popkin, B. (2010). Food price and diet and health outcomes: 20 years of the CARDIA study. *Archives of Internal Medicine*, *170*(5), 420–426.

Fletcher, J., Frisvold, D., & Tefft, N. (2011a). Are soft drink taxes an effective mechanism for reducing obesity? *Journal of Policy Analysis and Management*, *30*(3), 655–662.

Fletcher, J., Frisvold, D., & Tefft, N. (2011b). Soda taxes and substitution effects: Will obesity be affected? *Choices*, *26*(3), 1–4.

Geier, A., Wansink, B., & Rozin, P. (2012), Red potato chips: Segmentation cues can substantially decrease food intake. *Health Psychology*, *313*(May), 398–401.

Grether, E. T., & Holloway, R. J. (1967). Impact of government upon the market system. *Journal of Marketing*, *31*(2), 1–5.

Hanks, A. S., Just, D. R., Smith, L. E., & Wansink, B. (2012). Healthy convenience: Nudging students toward healthier choices in the lunchroom. *Journal of Public Health*, *34*(3), 370–376.

Hanks, A. S., Just, D. R., & Wansink, B. (2014). Chocolate milk consequences: A pilot study evaluating the consequences of banning chocolate milk in school cafeterias. *PLoS One*. doi: 10.1371/journal.pone.0091022.

Hanks, A. S., Wansink, B., Just, D., Cawley, J., Kaiser, H., Smith, L., ... Schulze, W. (2013). From Coke to Coors: A field study of a fat tax and its unintended consequences. *Journal of Nutrition Education and Behavior*, *45*, 4S, 40.

Harrison, G., & List, J. (2004). Field experiments. *Journal of Economic Literature*, *42*(4), 1009–1055.

Institute of Medicine (IOM). Report Brief September 2009. Local government actions to prevent childhood obesity. Available at http://www.iom.edu/Reports/2009/Local-Government-Actions-to-Prevent-Childhood-Obesity.aspx. Accessed (June/01/2015).

Jacobson, M. (2004). Steps to end the obesity epidemic. *Science*, *305*(5684), 611.

Jacobson, M., & Brownell, K. (2000). Small taxes on soft drinks and snack foods to promote health. *American Journal of Public Health*, *90*(6), 854–857.

Johnson, E. J. (2006). Things that go bump in the mind: How behavioral economics could invigorate marketing. *Journal of Marketing Research*, *63*, 337–340.

Johnson, E. J., & Goldstein, D. G. (2003). Do defaults save lives? *Science*, *302*, 1338–1339.

Just, D. R. (2006). Behavioral economics, food assistance and obesity. *Agricultural and Resource Economics Review*, *35*, 209–220.

Just, D. R., & Wansink, B. (2009). Better school meals on a budget: Using behavioral economics and food psychology to improve meal selection. *Choices, Choices*, *24*(3), 1–6.

Just, D. R., & Wansink, Brian (2013). One man's tall is another man's small: How framing of portion size influences food choice. *Health Economics*, *23*, 776–791. doi:10.1002/hec.2949.

Just, D. R., Mancino, L., & Wansink, B. (2007). Could behavioral economics help improve diet quality of nutrition assistance program participants? Economic Research Service Number 43. Washington, DC: US Department of Agriculture.

Kolsarici, C., & Vakratsas, D. (2010). Category- versus brand-level advertising messages in a highly regulated environment. *Journal of Marketing Research*, *47*(6), 1078–1089.

Kuchler, F., Tegene, A., & Harris, J. (2004). Taxing snack foods: Manipulating diet quality or financing information programs? *Review of Agricultural Economics*, *27*, 4–20.

Levitt, S., & List, J. (2009). Experiments in economics: The past, the present, and the future. *European Economic Review*, *53*, 1–18.

List, J. (2009). An introduction to field experiments in economics. *Journal of Economic Behavior and Organization*, *70*, 439–442.

List, J. (2011). Why economists should conduct field experiments and 14 tips for pulling one off. *Journal of Economic Perspectives*, *25*(3), 3–15.

Marchiori, D., Corneille, O., & Klein, O. (2012). Container size influences snack food intake independently of portion size. *Appetite*, *58*, 814–817.

Mohr, G. S., Lichtenstein, D. R., & Janiszewski, C. (2012). The effect of marketer-suggested serving size on consumer responses: The unintended consequences of consumer attention to calorie information. *Journal of Marketing*, *76*(1), 59–75.

Mytton, O., Gray, A., Rayner, M., & Rutter, H. (2007). Could targeted food taxes improve health? *Journal of Epidemiology and Community Health*, *61*(8), 689–694.

Mytton, O., Clarke, D., & Rayner, M. (2012). Taxing unhealthy food and soft drinks to improve health. *British Medical Journal*, *344*, e2931.

Nederkoorn, C., Havermans, R. C., Giesen, J. C., & Hansen, A. (2011). High tax on high energy dense foods and its effects on the purchase of calories in a supermarket. An experiment. *Appetite*, *56*(3), 760–765.

Oliveira, V., & Variyam, J. N. (2003). *Childhood obesity and the role of USFDA*. Food Assistance and Nutrition Research Report Number 34-11. Washington, DC: US Food and Drug Administration.

Painter, J. E., Wansink, B., & Hieggelke, J. B. (2002). How visibility and convenience influence candy consumption. *Appetite, 38*(3), 237–238.

Parsons, A. G., & Schumacher, C. (2012). Advertising regulation and market drivers, *European Journal of Marketing, 46*(11/12), 1539–1558.

Powell, L., & Chaloupka, F. (2009). Food prices and obesity: Evidence and policy implications for taxes and subsidies. *Milbank Quarterly, 87*(1), 229–257.

Powell, L., Chriqui, J., & Chaloupka, F. (2009). Associations between state-level soft drink taxes and adolescent body mass index. *Journal of Adolescent Health, 45*(3), S57–S63.

Reicks, M., Redden, J., Mann, T., Mykerezi, E., & Vickers, Z. (2012). Pictures in lunch tray compartments and vegetable consumption among children in elementary school cafeterias. *Journal of the American Medical Association, 307*, 784–785.

Roehr, B. (2009). US soda tax could help tackle obesity, says new director of public health. *British Medical Journal, 339*(7715), 316.

Rolls, B. J., Roe, L. S., & Meengs, J. S. (2006). Larger portion sizes lead to sustained increase in energy intake over two days. *Journal of the American Dietetic Association, 106*, 543–549.

Rudd Report. (2009). *Soft drink taxes: A policy brief*. New Haven, CT: Rudd Center for Food Policy and Obesity, Yale University.

Sharpe, K. M., Staelin, R., & Huber, J. (2008). Using extremeness aversion to fight obesity. Policy implications of context dependent demand. *Journal of Consumer Research, 35*, 406–422.

Smith, T., Lin, B-H., & Lee, J-Y. (2010). *Taxing caloric sweetened beverages: Potential effects on beverage consumption, calorie intake, and obesity*. ERR-100. Washington, DC: US Department of Agriculture, Economic Research Service.

Thaler, R. H., & Sunstein, C. R. (2008). *Nudge*. New Haven, CT: Yale Press.

Tipton, M. M., Bharadwaj, S. G., & Robertson, D. C. (2009). Regulatory exposure of deceptive marketing and its impact on firm value. *Journal of Marketing, 73*(6), 227–243.

Van Ittersum, K., & Wansink, B. (2013). Extraverted children are more biased by bowl sizes than introverts. *PLoS One, 8*(10), e78224.

Van Kleef, E., Otten, K., & van Trijp, H. (2012). Healthy snacks at the checkout counter: A lab and field study on the impact of shelf arrangement and assortment structure on consumer choices. *BMC Public Health, 12*, 1072.

Vartanian, L. R., Herman, C. P., & Wansink, B. (2008). Are we aware of the external factors that influence our food intake? *Health Psychology, 27*(5), 533–538.

Vermeer, W. M., Alting, E., Steenhuis, I., & Seidell, J. C. (2010). Value for money or making the healthy choice: the impact of proportional pricing on consumers' portion size choices. *The European Journal of Public Health, 20*(1), 65–69.

Wansink, B. (1996). Can package size accelerate usage volume? *Journal of Marketing, 60*, 1–14.

Wansink, B. (2004). Environmental factors that increase the food intake and consumption volume of unknowing consumers. *Annual Review of Nutrition, 24*, 455–479.

Wansink, B. (2006). *Mindless eating—Why we eat more than we think*. New York, NY: Bantam Dell.

Wansink, B. (2013). Convenient, attractive, and normal: The CAN approach to making children slim by design. *Childhood Obesity, 9*(4), 277–278.

Wansink, B. (2014). Slim by design—Mindless eating solutions for everyday life. New York, NY: William-Morrow.

Wansink, B. (2015). Change their choice! Changing behavior using the *CAN* approach and activism research. *Psychology and Marketing, 24*(3), 413–431.

Wansink, Brian, Koert van Ittersum, & James E. Painter. (2006). "Ice Cream Illusions: Bowl Size, Spoon Size, and Serving Size," *American Journal of Preventive Medicine, 145*(5), 240–243.

Wansink, Brian and Payne, Collin R. and Painter, & James E. (2014). What is Beautiful Tastes Good: Visuals Cues, Taste, and Willingness to Pay.

Wansink, B., & Chandon, P. (2014). Slim by design: Redirecting the accidental drivers of mindless overeating. *Journal of Consumer Psychology*, forthcoming.

Wansink, B., & Hanks, A. S. (2013). Slim by design: Serving healthy foods first in buffet lines improves overall meal selection. *PLoS One, 8*(10), e77055.

Wansink, B., & Johnson, K. A. (2015a). What percentage of self-served food is eaten? A preliminary investigation of how serving size and other factors influence intake. *International Journal of Obesity, 39*, 371–374.

Wansink, B., & Johnson, K. A. (2015b). Adults only: Why don't children belong to the Clean-plate Club? *International Journal of Obesity, 39*, 375.

Wansink, B., & Just, D. R (2013). Trayless cafeterias lead diners to take less salad and relatively more dessert. *Public Health Nutrition*, doi:10.1017/S1368980013003066.

Wansink, B., Hanks, A. S., & Just, D. (2015). From Coke to Coors: A field study of a soft drink taxes and its unintended consequences on beer purchases, under review.

Wansink, B., Just, D. R., Hanks, A. S., & Smith, L. E. (2013). Pre-sliced fruit in schools increases selection and intake. *American Journal of Preventive Medicine, 44*, 477–480.

Wansink, B., Just, D. R., & Payne, C. R. (2012). Can branding improve school lunches? *Archives of Pediatric and Adolescent Medicine, 166*, 967–968.

Wansink, B., Just, D. R., Payne, C. R., & Klinger, M. Z. (2012). Attractive names sustain increased vegetable intake in schools. *Preventive Medicine, 55*, 330–332.

Wansink, B., Payne, C. R., & Shimizu, M. (2011). The 100-calorie semi-solution: Sub-packaging most reduces intake among the heaviest. *Obesity, 19*(5 Spring), 1098–1100.

Wansink, B., & Sobal, J. (2007). Mindless eating: The 200 daily food decisions we over-look. *Environment and Behavior, 39*, 106–123.

Wansink, B., & van Ittersum, K. (2003). Bottoms up! The influence of elongation on pouring and consumption volume. *Journal of Consumer Research, 30*, 455–463.

Wansink, B., & van Ittersum, K. (2014). Portion size me: Plate size can decrease serving size, intake, and food waste. *Journal of Experimental Psychology: Applied, 19*(4), 320–332.

Wansink, B., van Ittersum, K., & Painter, J. E. (2006). Ice cream illusions: Bowls, spoons, and self-served portion sizes. *American Journal of Preventive Medicine, 31*, 240–243.

Zafar, A. (2011). Denmark institutes first-ever 'fat tax.' *Time NewsFeed*. Retrieved January 2012, from http://newsfeed.time.com/2011/09/30/denmark-institutes-first-ever-fat-tax/

Zheng, Y., & Kaiser, H. (2008). Advertising and U.S. nonalcoholic beverage demand. *Agricultural and Resource Economics Review, 31*(2),147–159.

10 | Applying Behavioral Economics in a Health Policy Context

DISPATCHES FROM THE FRONT LINES

MICHAEL SANDERS AND MICHAEL HALLSWORTH

RICHARD THALER, ONE OF THE founding fathers of behavioral economics and a standard bearer in the fight to see its lessons applied to public policy, memorably wrote that "As a general rule, the United States government is run by lawyers who occasionally take advice from economists. Others interested in helping the lawyers out need not apply" (Thaler, 2012). In the UK Government things are a little different. At the time of writing, 11 of the 22 members of the British Cabinet (the group of the heads of the most senior departments of the British government, including the Prime Minister and Deputy Prime Minister) are economists, or have university-level qualifications in economics; just three are lawyers or have law degrees (UK Government, 2014; calculations by the authors). At the same time, the dominant analytical force in the British Civil Service, whose role it is to advise ministers on policy and its consequences, is the Government Economic Service.

It is therefore perhaps fairer to say that, as a general rule, the British government is made up of economists who occasionally take advice from other economists. The prevalence of the economic approach makes it particularly important to understand how it contributes to, and detracts from, good policy making.

The purpose of this chapter is not to pour scorn on the efforts of economists to understand the world, or on their contributions to government, for a few reasons. First, one of its authors is an economist by training and inclination. Second, as we will see, there are many times when economics offers up perfectly good solutions to policy problems. Finally, a thriving market for critiques of economics already exists, and it may well be saturated.

Instead, the goal of this chapter is to describe the context under which we are writing, beginning with the origins of the Behavioural Insights Team in the United Kingdom, and concluding with the broad public health policy context in both the United Kingdom and across much of the developed world. We then give examples of areas of health policy where the lessons of behavioral economics may prove useful, followed by practical examples from randomized controlled trials of where these lessons have been applied. Finally, we discuss the use of randomized controlled trials in public policy from a practical perspective.

The Behavioural Insights Team

In May 2010, the United Kingdom experienced a rare event in its political history: the formation of a coalition government. None of the three major parties had secured enough seats in parliament to form a majority government, and so the Conservative party, which had won the most seats, entered a coalition with the Liberal Democrats. Prior to the election, British parties produce manifestos that detail their planned policies if they are elected. When the coalition was formed, a "Coalition Agreement" document was written to set out the policies to be pursued by the new coalition—a mixture of the two parties' agendas. In addition to electoral reform, deficit reduction, and decentralization, the coalition agreement contained a commitment to "help people to make better decisions for themselves" (Cabinet Office, 2010, p. 8). This commitment in many ways embodied the common ground between the two parties—the small-state Conservative party and the classical liberal heritage of the Liberal Democrats. It was also intended to mark a contrast with the previous Labor administration, which was seen (at least by the parties in the new coalition) as favoring increased intervention in social and economic life.

A part of this agenda to "help people to make better decisions for themselves" was the creation of a small Behavioural Insights Team, based jointly in Number 10 Downing Street and the Cabinet Office. The team was set up to apply the lessons of behavioral science to public policy; indeed, the Coalition Agreement makes specific reference to "harnessing the insights from behavioural economics and social psychology" (p. 12). Known by some as the "Nudge Unit," the foundation of the team was inspired by the interest of the Prime Minister and several of his senior advisors in behavioral economics, and in particular by the book *Nudge* by Richard Thaler and Cass Sunstein (2008). Sunstein was working at the time in the Office of Information and Regulatory Affairs in the Obama administration, while Thaler had met the Prime Minister prior to the formation of the new government.

In the 4 years since the team was formed, it has worked across the policy spectrum, from healthcare to tax compliance, and from charitable giving to employment policy. Although the team does provide policy advice based on existing research, its core approach has been to test interventions using randomized controlled trials in the field. These interventions have been based on insights drawn from a wide range of fields, including economics (behavioral and otherwise), psychology, political science, and sociology. To respond to the demand for its services, the Team has now become a separate social purpose company, owned in part by government, the employees, and the innovation charity Nesta.

The team was able to find opportunities in so many policy areas partly because of the fiscal climate. Government spending was being cut significantly, leaving officials searching for ways to maintain services while spending less money. At the same time, many of the ideas proposed by the team were cheap or even free to implement. Therefore, they attracted more attention than they would have done in times of budgetary comfort. For example, using social proof (evidence that other people, particularly "people like you" are engaged in a behavior) to encourage tax payments (reported in Hallsworth et al., 2014) was particularly attractive because it was costless, unlike traditional enforcement policies like court action. Although not all the team's proposals have been of this kind, its general approach highlighted how departments could improve performance through apparently minor changes to the way they do things.

Nevertheless, the team also had to overcome several barriers. As discussed earlier, governments are traditionally advised primarily by economists, who exhibit some scepticism about the applicability of many of these behavioral insights to government. Many (perhaps most) economists in government will openly admit the failings of economics as a discipline, and/or that a university economics course ill-prepares its students for practicing economics in government. They are also, however, sceptical that apparently minor cues in the decision environment can cause decisions of great importance to be made differently, and reluctant to accept that government should take note of them when making policies. Moreover, there is often a tendency for officials to perceive a new approach that attracts large claims as a transitory "fad," which can draw attention away from the core business of governing.

This background of scepticism is important for understanding why the Behavioural Insights Team needed to evaluate its work robustly. Randomized controlled trials, or field experiments, are seen as the gold standard of evidence for evaluating a policy and determining causal effect (Gerber & Green, 2012). When enough participants are randomly assigned to treatment and control group, the expected outcome for both groups is the same. Hence, if half are treated and half are not, any differences between the two can be said to have been caused by the treatment, and not by other factors, such as selection bias. The use of randomized controlled trials to evaluate programs and policies in the developing world has been pioneered by organizations such as the Jameel Adul Lateef Poverty Action Lab (J-PAL), in particular by the US academics Esther Duflo, Abhijit Banerjee, and Dean Karlan, but they are less common in the developed world.

Randomized controlled trials are not perfect: There have been criticisms of the extent to which their conclusions can be generalized (Cartwright & Hardie, 2012). Nevertheless, they have major advantages over other evaluation methods, and their use of experimentation encourages a cycle of continuous testing and improvement in government. By demonstrating that its work has been robustly evaluated, and acknowledging that success cannot simply be assumed, the Team has been able to convince sceptics in government and beyond that behavioral science can improve policy making.

Public Health Policy Context

From an economic perspective, the intervention of governments in individual decision-making processes is only easily justifiable where there is a clear market failure. In public health, the most obvious source of market failure is externalities, such as social cost or social benefit.

Externalities occur, crudely, when the benefits (or costs) to an individual and the benefits (or costs) to society diverge. An individual (i) makes decisions about his consumption based on his utility function, an example of which is Equation 1. Society (s), meanwhile, faces a different utility function, specified in Equation 2.

$$U_i = f(x_i) + g(h_i) + \sum_{j=0}^{N-1} l(h_j) \tag{1}$$

$$U_s = \sum_{i=1}^{N} \left(f(x_i) + g(h_i) \right) + \sum_{j=0}^{N-1} l(h_j) \qquad (2)$$

Here an individual's utility depends on his consumption of health-affecting goods or activities (h_i), his consumption of other goods (x_i), and the consumption of all other agents in the economy of health-affecting behaviors (h_j).

Each individual chooses his own behaviors (subscripted i), to maximize his own utility, given any constraints he is under. Because he does not choose the behaviors of others (subscripted j), he must accept the consequences of their action for his own utility. At the same time, the effect of his behavior on others does affect his own utility and so will not influence his decision making. Hence, his behaviors impose an externality on all other agents in the economy.

A benign central planner might attempt to maximize the social utility function found in Equation 2. This central planner tries to maximize the utility of the entire economy and so takes into account both the private benefits of an action taken by individual i and the effects of that action on everyone else in the economy (the full set of j's). Needless to say, the level of consumption of health-affecting behaviors chosen by a benign central planner will be different from the sum of all the decisions chosen by individuals. The difference between the two will depend on whether the externality is positive or negative.

An example of a health behavior with a positive externality might be getting vaccinated against measles. There is a benefit to the individual getting vaccinated—she dramatically reduces her likelihood of contracting measles—but there is also a benefit to society, as the number of possible carriers to transmit the disease to other people is reduced. A behavior with a negative externality might include smoking. The risks to the smoker in terms of increased cancer and mortality risk are well documented (Ezzati & Lopez, 2003), and this risk is at least partially transmitted to individuals in the vicinity of a smoker through passive smoke (Correa, Fontham, Pickle, Lin, & Haenszel, 1983). Where there are positive externalities, individuals (or firms) will tend to underconsume the health behavior compared to the social optimum, and the opposite will be true for negative externalities. Externalities and public good concerns are highly salient and important where health insurance risk is pooled between individuals, such as is the case with the British National Health Service.

It has been argued that intervention by governments may also be justi-fied when individuals fail to *internally* optimize their own behavior. This reason for intervention is more controversial than for externalities, as it assumes, at least under some circumstances, that governments are better at judging people's preferences than they are. There are several key find-ings in behavioral economics that suggest that individuals do not inter-nally optimize. When thinking about health outcomes, perhaps the most relevant finding is that of time-inconsistent preferences.

Under a classical model, individuals make decisions about their con-sumption of various goods over their lifetime in order to maximize their expected lifetime utility. Because the future is uncertain, future outcomes are discounted by some constant (but typically small) factor, denoted by ρ in our examples. Equation 3 shows a standard simple model of discounting.

$$E_t(U_i) = f(x_t) + \rho f(x_{t+1}) + \rho^2 f(x_{t+2}) + \cdots + \rho^n f(x_{t+n}) \tag{3}$$

Subscripts denote time periods, and the inclusion of E at the beginning of the equation shows that the equation is taken in expectation, that is, on average, based on an expected view of the world at time t. The effect of the discount factor is to make the future slightly less attractive than the present in terms of consumption. For example, if ρ is 0.98, consumption of a good in a year's time is (viewed from today) 98% as attractive as consuming the same good today. If we think about this in financial terms, this means that you would prefer £100 today to £100 in a year; be indifferent between £98 today and £100 in a year; and prefer £100 in a year to £96 today. If this model is correct, you will tend to save about enough for your retirement to keep your consumption roughly smooth over the rest of your life and thus to maximize your lifetime utility.

However, there are many situations where this model does not appear to hold in reality. For example, people tend to procrastinate. A simple for-malization of procrastination is reported by DellaVigna (2009), based on Laibson (1997) and O'Donoghue and Rabin (1999).

$$E_t(U_i) = f(x_t) + \beta \rho f(x_{t+1}) + \beta \rho^2 f(x_{t+2}) + \cdots + \beta \rho^n f(x_{t+n}) \tag{4}$$

This differs from the standard model by the addition of the β coefficient on all future time periods ($t + 1$ and greater). This creates a discontinu-ity in expected utility between the current period and the next, while the relative utility of all other future periods relative to each other remains the same. In a typical self-control-problem formulation, $\beta < 1$, while for the standard model $\beta = 1$. Intuitively, because people put their trust in their future self to make hard decisions, they are more pleasure seeking and less good at planning in the short run. This discontinuity need not produce undesirable outcomes when people can accurately predict their future ability to resist the temptation. However, if the agents are overconfident about their future abilities, they will tend to delay taking unpleasant or painful actions—such as quitting smoking or starting to diet—until tomorrow, as they believe it will be easier to exercise self-control then than it is today.

As DellaVigna (2009) shows, there are many situations where people do behave in line with the predictions of the procrastination model. If people have this kind of self-control problem, their lifetime utility will tend to be lower than optimal, as they will put off activities that are painful today but bring benefits in the future, and overconsume activities that are beneficial today but have negative long-term consequences. To the extent that they are naïve about their ability to overcome these self-control problems, or they lack the tools to do so, it may be justified for governments to intervene to help the public to make decisions more in keeping with their long-term interests. In many instances, the seeming divergence between people's stated preferences and their revealed behaviors, and their lived experience of the consequences of their actions, suggest that a case exists for intervention in this area. This remains a controversial area, however, because the question of whether long-term interests should be taken as "true" preferences is politically and philosophically contentious.

Interventions based on "nudges" have an appeal in this context because they usually do not alter an individual's choice set, allowing him to retain the option to continue unhealthy behaviors if he wishes. Nevertheless, the use of interventions inspired by behavioral economics and psychology to improve health outcomes is comparatively newer and less widely accepted.

Current Policy Problems and Traditional Tools

Taxonomies of government policy tools have been attempted from various academic perspectives (Hood 1983; Nuffield Council on Bioethics, 2007). Here we adopt a simple framework that captures much of the traditional government activity directed at influencing citizens' behavior: taxation, information, and regulation. These three approaches have been used to varying extents in the field of health.

Smoking, for example, is one of the leading causes of mortality worldwide, and it has been subject to considerable taxation in much of the developed world. Although these taxes are effective at reducing demand for cigarettes, the price elasticity of demand for these items is low, with Keeler et al. (1993) estimating it to be –0.5. As a result, taxes on cigarettes are at least partially sumptuary, producing revenue for governments without substantially reducing demand. Thus, while taxation is an important part of the policy mix, it is clearly not sufficient to eliminate smoking on its own.

Many countries and authorities have also used regulation to control smoking. New York has gone so far as to ban smoking in outdoor places likely to have high concentrations of the public, such as public parks, squares, and beaches. Smoking bans directly target the externalities caused by smoking by reducing the number of people subjected to passive smoking. Reviews of research conducted around the introduction of smoking bans have shown that health is indeed improved as a consequence (Hahn, 2010). More specifically, it appears that passive smoking is reduced by such a ban (Menzies et al., 2006; Mulcahy, Evans, Hammond, Repace, & Byrne, 2005). Therefore, this policy is clearly effective at reducing the externality component of smoking, but evidence for its effects on smoking prevalence and cessation is "mixed" (Hahn, 2010). Longo et al. (2001) investigate the effects of workplace smoking bans on quitting and find that people working in smoke-free workplaces are around twice as likely to quit as those in workplaces where smoking is allowed. Overall levels of relapse do not systematically differ between the two groups, however, and so longer term effects may be less substantial. Farkas et al. (1999) report more positive results, finding that workplace and household smoking restrictions increased quit attempts by more than 250%. They find that smoking cessation at 6 months also rose when both home and workplace bans on smoking were in place. For people only influenced at work, an effect of a 21% rise in quitting was observed, while for people affected at home the effect was more substantial, at 65%. These policies amounted to a total ban on smoking both at home and at work.

Finally (in terms of smoking), governments have conducted extensive information campaigns over the last few decades. On the one hand, the United Kingdom banned general tobacco advertising in 2003, with television cigarette commercials having been banned since 1965 (Wall, 2005). Evidence of the effectiveness of advertising bans at reducing smoking is mixed, however (Capella, Taylor, & Webster, 2008). On the other hand, governments have funded considerable marketing activities to discourage smoking (see Table 10.1 for an example), including health warnings placed on the packaging of cigarettes (Shiu, Hassan, & Walsh, 2009). However, a recent review found that the success of such warnings depended greatly on

TABLE 10.1 Interventions in an organ donation registration trial

1. Control			
2. Norm	Every day thousands of people who see this page decide to register.		Social norms (Elster, 1989)
3. Norm & Picture	Every day thousands of people who see this page decide to register.	Group of people	Salience (Bartrand, Karlan, & Mullainathan, 2010)
4. Norm & Logo	Every day thousands of people who see this page decide to register.	NHS logo	Salience (Bertrand et al., 2010)
5. Three Die	Three people die each day because there are not enough organ donors.		Loss aversion (Tversky & Kahneman, 1991)
6. Nine Lives	You could save or transform up to nine lives as an organ donor.		Self-efficacy (Bandura, 1977)
7. Reciprocity	If you needed an organ transplant, would you have one? If so, please help others.		Reciprocity (Fehr & Gachter, 2000)
8. Action	If you support organ donation, please turn you support into action.		Hypocrisy induction (Stone & Fernandez, 2008)

their means of presentation: Obscure text-only warnings had little impact, but prominent pictorial ones were much more effective (Hammond, 2011). In behavioral science terms, salience was the key factor in the policy's success (Dolan et al., 2012). Clearly, the combination of tobacco control policies based on taxation, regulation, and information have had a large effect on smoking prevalence. Our point is that behavioral science may offer new ways of enhancing the impact of these policies, as well as suggesting new routes of influence.

Another major health issue of concern to policy makers is obesity. In the United Kingdom, two thirds of adults are overweight, while a quarter are obese. This is a serious problem, and one that has increased over time, from one in six being obese 20 years ago (Public Health England, 2014). Obesity is also socially regressive, with people from low-income families being the most affected. Obesity has negative externalities, due to lost production and increased burden on health provision, but a large portion of the costs are borne by the individual. Obesity doubles the likelihood of dying prematurely, and it contributes to various health conditions, including type 2 diabetes, heart disease, and childhood asthma (National Obesity Observatory [NOO], 2013). Between a quarter and a third of cancers can be at least partially attributed to obesity (Vainio, Kaaks, & Bianchini, 2002). There are also substantive well-being costs, with obese people more likely to suffer from depression and anxiety (NOO, 2011).

The costs of obesity to the individual are large enough that a fully rational individual described by the standard model would certainly take steps to address it (or, more likely, never become obese in the first place). This clearly does not happen. Although there are many determinants of obesity, one major contributing factor is that, as Wansink and Sobal (2007) puts it, eating is "mindless": Generally speaking, people continue eating as long as there is food available. In broad terms, more calories have become available over the last 30 years. To the extent that "mindless eating" exists, there appears to be an important interaction between our psychology and our environment that can cause a serious self-control problem (DellaVigna, 2009) and have substantial long-term health costs.

Although this nonmaximizing behavior could offer grounds for intervention under the conditions outlined earlier, the case is more controversial than that for government interventions to reduce smoking. Each cigarette causes clear and instant health consequences; the same is not true of unhealthy food, which can be enjoyed in moderation without worsening health. Nevertheless, governments have used the basic set of policy tools to address this problem.

Most regulation has focused on ensuring that food items are not contaminated with materials or organisms that cause direct harm to humans. Laws to limit the supply of food for indirect reasons are less common. However, the line between direct and indirect harms to health is not clear: "Trans fats" have been shown to contribute to cardiovascular disease over time, and New York City has accordingly banned restaurants from using them (New York City Health Code, 2006).

Taxes to address obesity have been periodically suggested but rarely implemented due in part to a lack of broad public support (Friedman, 2009). Examples of successfully implemented schemes are taxes on fat in Denmark and Hungary and a tax on sugared carbonated drinks (soda) in France, although we note that the Danish tax was abolished soon after its implementation. Mytton, Clarke, and Rayner (2012), discussing the uses of "fat taxes," argue that the existing studies show that they can be effective at reducing fat consumption and promoting weight loss. A controlled experiment conducted by Block et al. (2010) found that a 35% tax on sugar-sweetened drinks reduced demand for those drinks by 26%. Systematic reviews of the literature on price effects on food consumption, for example by Shemilt et al. (2013) and Andreyeva et al. (2010), provide similar estimates of the effect size, as do analyses using primary data on both sides of the Atlantic, including Harding & Lovenheim's (2014) study of price elasticities in the United States and Tiffin et al.'s (2011) analysis for the Department for the Environment, Farming, and Rural Affairs in the United Kingdom. Although it appears there is little doubt that prices affect demand, policy makers must also be concerned with the extent to which demand falls when price rises—for example, what size of a tax would be required to reduce demand for a product by 10%.

Many estimates of price elasticity of demand (the proportional change in demand relative to a proportional change in price) suggest that fat consumption is responsive to changes in price, but that this response is inelastic (i.e., it has an elasticity of between 0 and –1). A tax of 10%, for example, would lead to a less than 10% fall in consumption. As a result, net spending on fatty products would rise, as the reduction in consumption is not enough to offset the rise in prices. One result of this rise is that both individuals and businesses are made worse off financially, with the government benefiting. As mentioned earlier, obesity and poor diet are negatively socially graded, and so the effects of these taxes may be felt most heavily by the poor (Leicester & Windmeijer, 2004). Although this argument makes fat taxes difficult to implement politically, it is noteworthy that the negative social grading means that poor diet affects the poor disproportionately compared to the rich, and so they could stand to gain the most in terms of health outcomes from this kind of policy.

To address health inequalities, it has been suggested that government could subsidize the consumption of healthy foods for poorer families (particularly those with new children). Healthy Start Vouchers in the United Kingdom, evaluated by Griffith and coauthors (unpublished data), are an example of such a policy. Although the effects of this campaign are positive, increasing consumption of fruit and vegetables, the longer term effects are ambiguous, and subsidies are often unpopular with politicians in times of austerity. Again, our purpose here is simply to point out that financial incentives are likely to need complementary measures to address the issue of obesity.

As is well known, governments have also used information campaigns to address poor diets. One route that has attracted recent attention is the provision of nutritional information in restaurants or on food packaging. These prompts may aim to resolve an information asymmetry, whereby consumers are unaware of what they are or should be consuming. This is in keeping with Laibson and Gabaix's model of shrouded attributes, in which individuals make choices about goods with some attributes that are obvious (salient) and others that are not (shrouded). When making food choices, individuals make decisions that are weighted toward the more salient characteristics (such as taste) and away from the others, such as the nutritional content. Indeed, there is much evidence that consumers are unskilled at assessing the caloric content of food, with their assessments being vulnerable to "halo effects" (so that a hamburger is seen as less caloric if it is presented with a salad; Chandon, 2013).

The effectiveness of providing information is unclear, however. Neuhouser et al. (1999) find that people who *use* nutritional information labels on packaged food consume less fat on average than those who did not, and that women, people under 35, and the more educated were more likely to make use of the labels when they were provided. How much of this can be attributed to the labels is unclear, however, because their use is likely to be endogenous—that is, people who use the labels may have been more diet conscious even in the absence of the intervention. Bollinger et al. (2010) find that posting calories in Starbucks cafes reduces calorie consumption per transaction by 6%, driven purely through changes in the choice of food (rather than beverages). They find that this effect is felt at the intensive and the extensive margin, as there is evidence that individuals switch from rival restaurants that are less healthy.

Yamamoto and coauthors (2005) conduct a within-subject experiment on 106 adolescents in fast-food restaurants, in which participants are asked to make choices from menus both with and without calorie and fat infor-mation. They find that most participants do not change their choice but, of those that do, 80% opt for a lower calorie meal, with the remainder choos-ing a healthier meal. However, this effect is weakest among the subset of participants who identify themselves as overweight or obese. There may also be a biasing effect, noted by Chandon and Wansink (2007), who find that when eating in restaurants that purport to be healthy, consumers decide to buy higher calorie side dishes, drinks, and desserts.

In this section, we have given an overview of how the three traditional policy tools can be used to affect health behaviors. Although these tools can be effective, they can also be unpopular, making them difficult to implement. Moreover, these tools can be applied without sufficient con-sideration of evidence about how citizens are likely to react, particularly evidence from psychology. The next section shows how the lessons of behavioral economics and psychology can be applied to enhance and com-plement more traditional policy tools.

Applications of Behavioral Science to Public Policy

As described earlier in this chapter, the UK government established the Behavioural Insights Team in 2010 to apply lessons from behavioral economics and psychology to public policy making. The current framework used by the team to analyze the behavioral roots of public policy problems, and thereby develop better policies, is the EAST framework (Behavioural Insights Team, 2014). EAST recommends that government officials and ministers should make policies *e*asy, *a*ttractive, *s*ocial, and *t*imely. The team's methodology for running randomized controlled trials in public policy is also summarized in the *Test, Learn, Adapt* document (Behavioural Insights Team, 2012).

In this section, we summarize some of the work done by the team that is either in the area of health or that might be applied to a health context. We want to stress that this is not a comprehensive account of the applications of behavioral science to public health. Not only are other studies by the team in progress or awaiting publication, but there are many other projects being implemented by other areas of the public sector (not least because public health is now the responsibility of local government). What follows should be considered a snapshot.

Organ Donation

Choosing to donate an organ to a stranger can be viewed as an act of substantial altruism, even when the donor is near death.[1] Through this lens, the practice of donating organs can be thought of as being a prominent example of a behavioral economics finding, falling under DellaVigna's (2009) definition of a nonstandard preference.

The medical science of human organ donation has come a long way since the first successful transplant of a cornea was carried out in what is now the Czech Republic in 1905 (Armitage et al., 2006). People willing to do so are able to donate their kidneys, heart, liver, small bowel, eyes, lungs, pancreas, or skin and tissue, or any combination of these (National Health Service Blood and Transplant [NHSBT], 2014). As a result, many lives can be saved, improved, or prolonged through organ donation. However, more needs to be done to increase the number of organs available. The United Kingdom has around 7,000 people in need of organ transplants and, on average, three people die every day waiting for a transplant.

There are obvious challenges to ensuring enough people have agreed to donate their organs. Contemporaneous consent may be difficult to obtain, because the donor is likely to be close to death. For this reason, many countries, including the United Kingdom and individual US states, maintain registers of organ donors who have given consent in advance. Both the United Kingdom and the United States use an opt-in system, whereby individuals are required to give explicit consent to donate their organs by joining the Organ Donor Register. Other countries, for example Austria, have an opt-out system, which means consent to donate organs after death is presumed unless individuals state otherwise.

Table 10.2 shows the registration rates for countries with an opt-in system, like the United Kingdom and the United States, compared to those countries that have an opt-out system, like Austria. Countries with opt-out systems have much higher registration rates than the countries with opt-in systems. However, the effects of the opt-out system are not totally clear.

TABLE 10.2 Effects of Treatments on Registration (Logistic Regression)

CONSTANT CONDITION	(1) CONTROL	(2) WOULD YOU
Norm	0.227***	−0.095***
	(0.024)	(0.023)
Norm & Picture	−0.061*	−0.383***
	(0.026)	(0.024)
Norm & Logo	0.242***	−0.080***
	(0.024)	(0.022)
Three People Die	0.287***	−0.035
	(0.024)	(0.022)
Nine Lives	0.223***	−0.099***
	(0.024)	(0.023)
Reciprocity	0.322***	
	(0.024)	
Action	0.209***	−0.113***
	(0.025)	(0.023)
Control		−0.322***
		(0.024)
Constant	−3.758***	−3.435***
	(0.018)	(0.016)
N	1,085,322	1,085,322

$^* p < .05,$ $^{**} p < .01,$ $^{***} p < .001$; beta values reported; standard errors in parentheses.

In countries such as Spain, which use an opt-out system but where the ultimate decision is made by close relatives of the potential donors, it has been argued that the higher number of donations can actually be explained by superior infrastructure, such as better marketing and information systems for identifying whether an individual is registered or not (NHSBT, 2014). Objections also exist to the use of defaults in many cases where individuals will not later have a chance to reverse their decision, such as organ donation, since these are viewed as violating an individual's right to self-determination.

An alternative to an opt-out is to require people to make a decision one way or another. This is called "mandated choice." When used in the United States, mandated choice has been shown to increase organ donation registration rates, bringing them much closer to individuals' stated preferences for organ donation (Thaler & Sunstein, 2008). Cotter (2011) suggests that the ethical superiority of mandated choice outweighs the loss in registration numbers compared with an opt-out system. This point about the "quality" of registrations outweighing their quantity should be taken seriously: Families appear to be more likely to refuse organ donation if the potential donor is on the organ donation passively (by dint of having not having unregistered) than if he or she is on it actively (by having chosen to be on the register).

These arguments highlight the importance of analyzing the ways in which the decision to register is presented. To address this point, the Behavioural Insights Team worked with the Department for Health (DH), the National Health Service Blood and Transfusion Service (NHSBT), and the Government Digital Service (GDS) to trial the effect of presenting different messages related to donor registration at the moment of decision. The decision point chosen was the moment directly after a citizen has finished renewing the vehicle tax or registering for a driving licence. At this point, the person is presented with a message that requests that he or she join the organ donor register (if he or she has not already done so) and then is provided with a Web link to online signup. The project team worked to test the impact of different theoretically informed messages on sign-up rates. Given that 17 million individuals use this page every year, even marginal improvements in the proportion signing up would represent large absolute increases in donor numbers.

Study Design and Treatments

The study participants were all visitors to the Web site who successfully completed the tax or licence process between June 24, 2013 and July 19,

2013. As mentioned earlier, these participants were shown a Web page that asked participants to sign up to the organ donation.

The experimental variation was that Web page visitors were randomly assigned to one of eight Web page variants. The control variant presents a simple request to "Please join the NHS Organ Donor Register." There is also a "Call to Action" button, labeled "Join," which takes users to the first page of the organ donor registration form, and a "Find Out More" hyperlink, which takes users to the NHSBT home page. The control condition has no additional information. The features stated earlier are common to all the experimental variations. Therefore, the three main options open to a participant are as follows: clicking on the "Call to Action" button; clicking the "Find Out More" button; or closing the Web page without any further action (because the main transaction is complete).

All the other Web page variants add a message between the request and the "Call to Action" button. These messages were informed by concepts from behavioral economics and social psychology, as set out in Table 10.1.

Data and Analysis

The total sample included more than 1,085,000 individuals, of whom around 135,000 were assigned to each condition. The dataset included the number of participants assigned to each Web page variant, the treatment assignment of individuals arriving at the organ donor registration page, and whether or not those individuals go on to register. Data were aggregated at the site-treatment-hour level and merged to form a treatment-hour aggregated list.

Table 10.2 gives the headline findings for the main outcome measure—whether or not a person joins the organ donor register, regressed on the Web page variant they saw. In the second column of Table 10.2, the best-performing variant is then respecified as the omitted category, which allows us to determine whether this variant performs better than the others. Table 10.3 reports the same regressions, changing the dependent variable to either clicking-through to the organ donation page or registering conditional on clicking through.

Although the absolute effects in Table 10.2 are small (less than 1 percentage point), the most effective message—labeled "Reciprocity"—produces a 39% increase in registration rates relative to the control group. Indeed, the second specification in Table 10.2 shows that the Reciprocity

TABLE 10.3 Effects of Treatment on Follow-Through (Logistic Regression)

OUTCOME MEASURE: CONSTANT CONDITION	CLICK THROUGH		CONVERT IF CLICK THROUGH	
	(1) CONTROL	(2) RECIPROCITY	(3) CONTROL	(4) RECIPROCITY
Norm	0.218*** (0.020)	−0.071*** (0.018)	0.034 (0.041)	−0.073 (0.038)
Norm & Picture	−0.128*** (0.022)	−0.418*** (0.020)	0.189*** (0.045)	0.081 (0.043)
Norm & Logo	0.174*** (0.020)	−0.115*** (0.019)	0.205*** (0.042)	0.097* (0.039)
Three People Die	0.284*** (0.020)	−0.005 (0.018)	0.019 (0.040)	−0.089* (0.037)
Nine Lives	0.211*** (0.020)	−0.079*** (0.018)	0.047 (0.041)	−0.061 (0.038)
Reciprocity	0.289*** (0.020)		0.108** (0.040)	
Action	0.185*** (0.020)	−0.104*** (0.019)	0.081* (0.041)	−0.027 (0.039)
Control		−0.289*** (0.020)		−0.108** (0.040)
Constant	−3.307*** (0.015)	−3.017*** (0.013)	0.586*** (0.030)	0.693*** (0.027)
N	1,085,322	1,085,322	44,875	44,875

* $p < .05$, ** $p < .01$, *** $p < .001$; beta values reported; standard errors in parentheses.

variant performs significantly better than all other treatments except for the "Three Die" variant. The study authors also isolate a backfire effect from one element of the variants. Although the social norm message produces a significant increase in registrations, the "Norm & Picture" variant—which is identical except for the addition of a picture showing a crowd of people—actually reduced registrations compared with the control (significant at the 5% level). It appears that it was this specific picture, rather than the addition of an image per se, that produced the backfire, since the addition of the transplant service logo ("Norm & Logo") did not cause any such adverse effect.

The results reported in Table 10.3 illuminate the causal mechanisms at work in this experiment. The study authors can estimate with some confidence that the difference in click-throughs between the two most successful treatments ("Three People Die" and "Reciprocity") is zero. However, conditional on commencing signup (i.e., clicking through), participants in the "Reciprocity" group are significantly more likely to register than participants in the "Three People Die" condition. This result suggests that both treatments are equally powerful at overcoming the friction costs associated with registration, but that the "Reciprocity" message is more effective at increasing motivation overall. It is also noteworthy that the negative impact of the "Norm & Picture" treatment is driven entirely through initial clicks (in other words, once people arrive at the registration page, they are not any less likely to sign up if they saw this message). Different specifications do not substantively alter these results.

Conclusions

The results from this experiment show that a short, timely message can lead to an increased number of people joining the organ donor register. The study authors calculate that, although the effect sizes are modest, the marginal improvement would mean 95,000 additional potential donors joined the register over the course of a year. Cost-benefit analysis suggests that an extra six lives per year could be saved by these donors. The experiment also shows the importance of testing insights in the field. Although the most successful variant is likely to save lives, the least successful variant performed significantly worse than the control, and it could lead to increased fatalities if it had been rolled out widely. This is a particularly important point because there were no a priori reasons to suspect that this variant would be less effective than the others.

Smoking-Cessation Campaign

As noted earlier, smoking is a major source of both public and private health problems, and it is a behavior that government has been trying to discourage for several decades.[2] Although government policies have been effective in reducing smoking prevalence, a major obstacle remains the addictive nature of nicotine, which makes quitting difficult.

Large-scale campaigns that encourage and support smokers to quit have the advantage of being voluntary and of not substantially changing the incentives of smokers to quit, making them difficult to object to on paternalistic grounds. Moreover, there is evidence that such campaigns contribute to successful tobacco control strategies (Bala, Strzeszynski, Topor-Madry, & Cahill 2013). For example, the UK government ran a high-profile "Stoptober" initiative in 2012 and 2013, which encouraged people to "sign up" to not smoke for 28 days in October. A recent study found that the 2012 Stoptober campaign led to 350,000 quit attempts, saving 10,400 discounted life years at £415 each (Brown et al., 2014). Increasing participation in such a campaign could create substantial public health improvements.

One way of maximizing participation is to use effective messages and presentation tactics. However, while some studies present general conclusions about effective messages for such campaigns (Durkin, Brennan, & Wakefield, 2012), many studies focus on attitudes (rather than actual behavior) or cannot provide a counterfactual. To address these issues, Public Health England worked with The Behavioural Insights Team to test various aspects of the design of the main Web site for Stoptober 2013. Focusing on a digital environment allows for rapid testing and rollout of successful, low-cost interventions. The study team took advantage of these low costs to test multiple Web site variants.

The authors' main hypothesis was that "including a Web site feature intended to increase visitors' motivation to register will lead to a higher registration rate than if that feature were absent" (Hallsworth et al., 2014). The features selected were as follows: messages about the consequences of quitting; a short testimonial from a previous participant; a picture of the participant to accompany this testimonial; and a rotating "carousel" of images and text.

The study team created Web site variants that were feasible, appropriate, and were in line with the main hypothesis. The messages developed were based on social norms ("160,000 people completed the challenge, join them!") and health benefits ("Live 10 years longer") (Pirie, Peto, Reeves, Green, & Beral, 2013). The final message was based on the expected economic benefits of quitting ("Save £200 in 28 days"), based on the evidence that financial incentives can increase quit success (Volpp et al., 2009).

The testimonial presented was a real participant's comments on her positive experience during the previous year's campaign. The "carousel" was placed at the top of the Web site to aid orientation, and it automatically rotated between four images. The first read "Stoptober, it's like October but without the cigarettes"; the second, "Stop for 28 days and you're five times more likely to stay smokefree"; the third, "There's lots of free support to help you"; and the fourth, "Last Stoptober over 160,000 people stopped smoking for 28 days. Join them!"

The study made use of a factorial design, in which each combination of Web site features was seen by some participants. This design provided

24 variants on the main Web site in which almost every combination of elements was represented, including a control condition that featured none of these elements.[3]

The trial period lasted for 9 days in September 2013, during which time 345,469 unique visits to the Web site occurred, with 56,273 resulting in a registration. Binary variables for each of the 24 conditions were derived.

The authors' primary analysis, which considered each treatment individually, found that the 11th variant (no carousel, health benefits message, testimonial, no picture) increased registrations by 0.9 percentage points compared to the control. Another intervention, with carousel, health benefits message, testimonial, and no picture, decreased registrations by 1.2 percentage points.

The authors also conducted an analysis aggregated at the Web site–feature level, These analysis show that the base registration rate was 16.4% of visits (when no Web site elements were active). The carousel reduced registrations by 0.5 percentage points ($p < .001$), while the other factors did not have a significant effect.

This initial analysis was followed, by analysis that investigated how "complex" the Web site was; that is, how many of the four Web site elements were shown to the user. By itself, the authors find that each additional element of "complexity" reduced registrations by 0.5 percentage points, although this was not significant at the 0.05 level ($p = .10$). However, the complexity variable did eliminate the negative effect of the carousel and reveal a positive effect for the message variable ($p < .020$).

To test for the impact of visit timing on registration decisions, the authors created a binary variable that represented whether a visit occurred before or after 12.00. When this variable was added to the model, it indicated that visiting before 12.00 was associated with a 3.8 percentage point reduction in registrations compared to visiting after this time ($p < .001$). In addition, the authors found a significant interaction between the "complexity" variable and time of visit. For morning visits each additional Web site element reduced registrations by 0.3 percentage points ($p = 0.028$)—people are particularly put off by complexity in the morning.

These findings show two main points of interest. First, they reinforce the message that small changes can make a big difference—the changes made to the Web site during the remainder of the campaign, although seemingly insubstantial, are estimated to have saved an additional 79.4 discounted life years. Second, they underline the value of testing through nimble but rigorous trials. The conventional wisdom at the time of designing the Web site, and indeed the authors' initial hypothesis, was that the

Web site elements would be broadly beneficial, and that the findings would reflect a matter of degree; instead, the opposite was found.

Reciprocity in a Health Context

The final example in this section is not an application or a randomized trial, but a striking finding. Missed appointments in doctors' surgeries and hospitals are a widespread and costly problem for healthcare providers. To compensate for this lost time, most hospitals and general practices overbook appointments, expecting some people not to attend. When too many people attend, and patients' appointments are either delayed or canceled by the hospital for other reasons, this causes considerably inconvenience for patients. For a risk-neutral hospital, this makes perfect sense. If a hospital wants to maximize its utilization, it wants to make sure that every appointment slot is attended. If the average likelihood of an appointment being missed by a patient is 20%, the hospital will want to book 125 appointments for every 100 slots available. Twenty percent of these will on average not show up, and so on average the hospital's utilization rate will be 100%. This strategy is optimal if the hospital dislikes the inconvenience for patients as much as it dislikes having empty appointment slots. In reality, hospitals may prefer keeping patients waiting to having empty slots, because having too many appointments per clinic is cheaper for the hospital than idle clinician time. If this is the case, they may tend to book more appointments and expect at least some patients to suffer delays.

This kind of demand management assumes that patients' behavior is not influenced by the hospital's behavior toward them. This may not be realistic. Many of our interactions with other people, and other organizations, are governed by implicit social contracts, or social norms of the society we are in. Evidence from behavioral economics suggests that people can be highly reciprocal (Alpizar et al., 2008; Charness, 2004; Falk, 2007). Reciprocity occurs when people respond to a positive action from one party with a positive action of their own, either directed at the first person (direct reciprocity) or a third party (indirect reciprocity). People have also been shown to punish negative actions by others (negative reciprocity). In their theory of reciprocity, Falk and Fischbacher (2006) argue that reciprocal relationships are based on the perceived motives of the first mover. The same act could attract positive reciprocity if it is viewed as being performed altruistically, and negative reciprocity if it is being performed selfishly. Where people are entered into a social contract with their hospital, and that hospital cancels their appointment, this could be argued to lead to

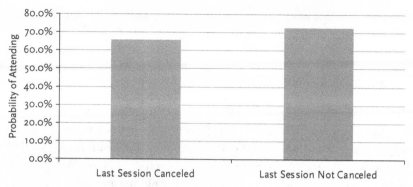

FIGURE 10.1 Attendance of hospital appointments and prior cancellations.

much the same effect: Their relationship with the hospital is harmed and they may be less cooperative in the future.

Looking at data on patients who have two appointments over a 3-month period at one hospital in London, this is exactly what we see. Overall, 18,000 appointments are accounted for by repeat appointments by the same period. This means we can compare the likelihood of attending a second appointment, depending on whether or not the first appointment was canceled by the hospital. We find that patients whose first appointment is canceled are roughly 10% less likely to attend the second appointment than people whose first appointment was not canceled (shown in Figure 10.1)—and these differences are statistically significant, remaining so when other factors are controlled for.

Of course, this result is not drawn from a randomized trial, and so we cannot be sure of what is driving these outcomes. It may be, for example, that patients are more willing to accept rearranged times that are less convenient to them but that they do not attend in the end. Nevertheless, there is a plausible case that reciprocity may play a role in patients' attendance at hospital appointments. If this finding stands up to more robust testing, it could substantively change our understanding of how public services should be delivered.

Running Trials in the Policy Field

In the final section of this chapter we discuss some of the practical considerations that need to be taken into account when running a randomized controlled trial in a policy environment. Successful implementation of this kind of trial will depend greatly on the *context* in which you are aiming to run the trial and on your own position. In some instances it can be easier to approach a government department to run a trial from outside; in others, practitioners can find it much more straightforward.

The practicalities of running a trial have been covered extensively elsewhere, for example by Green and Gerber (2012), Glennerster and Takavarasha (2013), or Behavioural Insights Team (2012). We can think of these practicalities as falling into two types: research and political. We now briefly outline each of these.

Research

When designing a field experiment or randomized controlled trial, the Behavioural Insights Team follows a "Test, Learn, Adapt" process. The Learn and Adapt components are covered under the political section that follows, while the Test component is more explicitly concerned with the process of conducting research.

Outcome Measures: What Do You Want to Achieve?

Establishing the intended outcome of a trial is the first vital component in trial design. Almost all government policies have an objective, and so it is easy to assume that this will lead to a natural outcome measure for a field experiment. Sometimes this is the case—for example, if the policy objective is "Reduce smoking prevalence by 10% in the next 10 years," then a reduction in official smoking rates might be the natural main outcome measure for the trial. Things may not be that simple, however—policies may have a broader aim ("improve outcomes for elderly patients") or present measurement difficulties (as in the debate between body mass index and waist size for measuring obesity and overweight). Before an intervention can be developed, much less trialed, it is important to determine what we mean by "outcomes." For example, the policy goal of an antiobesity drive may be clear, but the appropriate outcome variable for a trial within that policy may not be. Government may be interested in intermediate goals, such as diet, in which case the outcome measure might be calories consumed or number of pieces of fruit eaten. With an ambitious policy agenda like this, it is unlikely that any intervention is going to solve the entire problem.

Intervention Design: What Do You Want to Test?

Having established what you are trying to achieve, it is then crucial to work out what you want to test. Although the academic partner in a randomized controlled trial may have a detailed understanding of the broad policy area, and of behavioral science, the precise issues at play in any given context will vary. There are a large number of theoretical concepts that could be called upon but that may be in conflict with each other. For example, licensing effects (whereby doing something good at one juncture makes participants feel that they can behave poorly later on) are at odds with theories of self-perception, in which one act increases the extent to which they identify with that act and so increases the probability of future good behavior. The continued existence of both concepts in the academic literature suggests that there are at least some circumstances when each is true.

At the same time, trials should pay careful attention to the environment in which policies are being delivered. There may be some academic concepts that are simply inappropriate for the policy issue at hand or that cannot easily be translated into practice. Furthermore, any intervention should seek to minimize the burden on the people delivering the service. A complex and onerous change to existing practices increases the risk of unreliable implementation and subversion of randomization procedures. Where such a change is being introduced, a significant amount of time will be required for training and coalition building (see "Political Considerations").

Insights from the academic literature are therefore useful, but they can only take you so far. Spending time in the field and looking for behavioral biases and bottlenecks increases the chances that an intervention will be appropriate for a particular policy problem, and hence that it will be successful. Spending time listening to practitioners and policy makers, and engaging in a truly collaborative attempt to improve their policy or practices, also makes it more likely that your interventions will be welcomed and implemented.

Trial Design: How Do You Want to Test It?

Constructing this section in sequence is perhaps misleading. Often, the nature of an environment will dictate the way in which a trial must be run. For example, the scale of the trial is likely to be larger if the trial partner is a large group of hospitals or a government department or agency, rather than a single hospital or general practice.

If you have space for a large-scale trial, there are more options available. For example, it may be possible to run a small number of relatively minor interventions and still detect an effect or to run a larger number of potentially more powerful interventions. Alternatively, interventions that are likely to have social or spillover effects can be cleanly tested with large trials by making use of cluster randomization, which prevents spillovers within hospitals from contaminating your control group (at the cost of statistical power). In a smaller scale environment, such as a single hospital, the options are fewer. Clustered randomization may not be possible, either for practical reasons (there are no clusters), randomization reasons (randomization cannot be successful across a small number of clusters), or statistical reasons (the loss of power from clustering is too great). If this is the case, and interventions are to be randomized at the level of the individual, the interventions chosen to be tested will need to be ones for which there is no/less risk of spillovers.

Political Considerations

Promoting the use of behavioral economics through running trials is not simply a technical endeavor. To have a sustained impact, there are both tactical and strategic elements that must be considered. These may be of particular importance if you are interested in forming a longer term relationship with a partner organization.

Organizational Fit

This has many similarities to the establishment of a suitable outcome measure mentioned earlier. It is sensible to choose a topic that clearly fits with the organization's stated priorities—or which is capable of being presented in line with them. Senior officials generally know the criteria by which they will be judged and will be more supportive of research that allows them to show success. In the longer term, you will find it advantageous if the officials who are supportive of running trials become professionally successful.

Identifying the Right Point in the System to Intervene

A useful strategy is to get general clearance to act from a high-level official, but then establish your main relationship with someone who "owns" a system within the department—for example, the official responsible for sending letters to patients or for designing information campaigns. Buy-in from senior figures gets you a "foot in the door" and a good sense of the organization's overall objectives. Subsequently engaging more with middle-ranking officials is likely to give greater insight into the details of a policy and how to make a trial happen in practice.

Timing

When first working with an organization, there is obviously pressure to deliver results. Therefore, it is a good strategy to construct a trial that will give you results quickly (and to choose "low-hanging fruit" where it is easy to show improvements). However, there is a danger that this focus may lead to major, long-term issues being neglected. A good strategy is to have a mix of quick results and longer term investment. From an academic point of view, it is often better to have a relationship that produces five trials, of which the first is not terribly interesting from an academic standpoint, than to produce one interesting trial that closes the door to future collaboration.

Commitment and Cost

Many of the means for applying insights from behavioral science are inexpensive and require little investment (changing the wording of letters, for example). Even where interventions are costly, for example using lottery incentives, these may be achievable by a simple repurposing of money that was already going to be spent on incentives that do not make use of behavioral insights. Naturally, these are the projects to focus on first. The main response you want to engender in your trial partner is "why not?" If you can show that there are likely benefits (by referencing the academic literature on a given topic or intervention), and that the intervention is cheap and will fit in around their day job (many interventions, such as sending text messages rather than letters, are actually easier for practitioners), and that they will experience minimum disruption, then this response is more likely to be achieved.

Tactical Aspects

In addition to these strategic considerations, the success of a trial may come down to apparently minor details about how it is presented and managed. In other words, the tactics employed by the people responsible for the trial make a big difference. Some useful tactics include the following.

Be Personally Persuasive

Members of the Behavioural Insights Team who run many trials like to say that 80% of the effort they expend actually goes into practical tasks like working through details, reassuring collaborators, and solving problems. When dealing with colleagues in this way—particularly if they are sceptical—one's personal persuasiveness makes a big difference. If you can clearly explain why a particular task is necessary or address a colleague's concerns effectively, then the trial is much more likely to come to fruition. Considering the problems that a trial partner is likely to have with a trial before meetings, and being ready to assuage his or her concerns should they arise, or even to address them before they are mentioned, can also help to reduce the social distance between you and the partner and to elicit reciprocity.

Show Commitment

In our experience, this tactic is one of the most important when dealing with sceptical partners, particularly those on whose goodwill the trial is dependent. You may well be in a situation of asking partners to change their work patterns for the purpose of a trial—and usually you will be relying on their voluntary cooperation for the successful implementation of the intervention, as well as adherence to the trial itself. To help ensure they cooperate, you should show your commitment to the project as well; in other words, be "on site" regularly, in order to help them and deal with any problems. This show of commitment is likely to trigger feelings of reciprocity, leading to increased cooperation.

Emphasize Feedback

One useful tactic we have found is to emphasize that you will come back to the officials with whom you are collaborating and present them with the results—regardless of what they are. Doing this increases trust because it introduces an element of honesty, humility, and fairness.

Be Humble

If we don't know the answer to the question our research is intending to answer, we should say so, and be open about this. In fact, if we *do* know the answer to the question, we shouldn't be conducting the research. Acknowledging your lack of knowledge of every single detail of the environment you are conducting the research in can also go a long way to getting practitioners to help. As much as possible, the process should feel like a collaboration between researchers and practitioners, and not a lecture.

Compromise

Adhering inflexibly to a set design does not often lead to success. Usually it is necessary to compromise in order to fit in with day-to-day demands and developments. Therefore, it is necessary to be aware of backup options that retain the essential elements of the trial design but sacrifice less important ones. For example, it may be possible to adopt a "stepped wedge" (Hussey & Hughes, 2007) design, wherein everyone receives an intervention, but the *order* in which they receive it is randomized (and measurements are taken in the interval). Such a design can address concerns from practitioners about denying participants a potentially beneficial intervention. It is, however, crucial that the person running the trial identifies the key elements that should not be sacrificed. The main element that should be protected, we propose, is robust randomization.

Summary

In this chapter we have summarized the origins of, and arguments for, the use of behavioral economics in public policy making (and particularly in public health), through the lens of the UK Behavioural Insights Team. We have reported the results of a few of the trials that have been run using behavioral economics interventions in this area.

Evidence suggests that not only can behavioral economics be useful in making and shaping public health policy in the United Kingdom and abroad but also that policy makers are increasingly aware of this fact. Randomized controlled trials, previously primarily used to test the efficacy of drugs or the usefulness of an international aid program, have also become more widely used and accepted in government policy making. Despite this enthusiasm, strategic considerations in the design of both behavioral interventions and their evaluation remain vital if this trend is to continue and academic-practitioner collaborations are to be successful.

Acknowledgments

We are grateful to the Behavioural Insights Team for assistance in this work, in particular to Hugo Harper, with whom many of the studies described have been conducted. We are also grateful to colleagues at the Department of Health and Public Health England, including Dan Berry, Tim Chadborn, and Anna Sallis; to Dominic King at Imperial College London; and to Olivia Maynard from the University of Bristol. Sanders is especially grateful to Ariella Kristal for excellent research assistance. The views expressed here are those of the authors and not of the Cabinet Office or the UK government.

Notes

1. The trial reported here is also being published as an academic paper (Harper, Sanders, and Sallis, unpublished data), which is drawn upon for the following sections.
2. This section draws on Hallsworth et al. (2014), which gives full details of the study. We are grateful to our coauthors for their assistance in this paper.
3. The study authors point out that their design was not fully factorial, since not every combination of features was actually included, for practical reasons. More details are available in the full paper.

References

Alpizar, F., Carlsson, F., & Johansson-Stenman, O. (2008). Anonymity, reciprocity, and conformity: Evidence from voluntary contributions to a national park in Costa Rica. *Journal of Public Economics*, *92*(5), 1047–1060.

Andreyeva, T., Long, M. W., & Brownell, K. D. (2010). The impact of food prices on consumption: A systematic review of research on the price elasticity of demand for food. *American Journal of Public Health*, *100*(2), 216.

Armitage, W. J., Tullo, A. B., & Larkin, D. F. P. (2006). The first successful full-thickness corneal transplant: A commentary on Eduard Zirm's landmark paper of 1906. *British Journal of Ophthalmology*, *10*(90), 1222–1223.

Bala, M. M., Strzeszynski, L., Topor-Madry, R., & Cahill, K. (2003). Mass media interventions for smoking cessation in adults. *Cochrane Database of Systematic Reviews*. doi:10.1002/14651858.CD004704.pub3

Bandura, A. (1977). Self-efficacy: toward a unifying theory of behavioral change. *Psychological Review*, *84*(2), 191.

Behavioural Insights Team (2012). Test, Learn Adapt: Developing Public Policy with Randomised Controlled Trials.

Behavioural Insights Team (2014). EAST: Four Simple Ways to Apply Behavioural Insights. *Policy Paper*.

Bertrand, M., Karlan, D., Mullainathan, S., Shafir, E., & Zinman, J. (2010). What's Advertising Content Worth? Evidence from a Consumer Credit Marketing Field Experiment. *Quarterly Journal of Economics*, *125*(1), 263–306.

Block, J. P., Chandra, A., McManus, K. D., & Willett, W. C. (2010). Point-of-purchase price and education intervention to reduce consumption of sugary soft drinks. *American Journal of Public Health*, *100*(8), 1427.

Bollinger, B., Leslie, P., & Sorensen, A. (2010). *Calorie posting in chain restaurants* (No. w15648). Washington, DC: National Bureau of Economic Research.

Brown, J., Kotz, D., Michie, S., Stapleton, J., Walmsley, M., & West, R. (2014). How effective and cost-effective was the national mass media smoking cessation campaign 'Stoptober'?. *Drug and alcohol dependence*, *135*, 52–58.

Cabinet Office (2010). "The Coalition: Our Programme for Government" HM Stationary Office, accessed online 28/05/2015; https://www.gov.uk/government/uploads/system/uploads/attachment_data/file/78977/coalition_programme_for_government.pdf

Capella, M. L., Taylor, C. R., & Webster, C. (2008). The effect of cigarette advertising bans on consumption: A meta-analysis. *Journal of Advertising, 37*(2), 7–18.

Cartwright, N., & Hardie, J. (2012). *Evidence-based policy: a practical guide to doing it better.* Oxford University Press.

Chandon, P. (2013). How package design and packaged-based marketing claims lead to overeating. *Applied Economic Perspectives and Policy, 35*(1), 7–31.

Chandon, P., & Wansink, B. (2007). The biasing health halos of fast-food restaurant health claims: Lower calorie estimates and higher side-dish consumption intentions. *Journal of Consumer Research, 34*(3), 301–314.

Charness, G. (2004). Attribution and reciprocity in an experimental labor market. *Journal of Labor Economics, 22*(3), 665–688.

Choi, J. J., Laibson, D., & Madrian, B. C. (2011). $100 bills on the sidewalk: Suboptimal investment in 401 (k) plans. *Review of Economics and Statistics, 93*(3), 748–763.

Correa, P., Fontham, E., Williams Pickle, L., Lin, Y., & Haenszel, W. (1983). Passive smoking and lung cancer. *Lancet, 322*(8350), 595–597.

Cotter, H. (2011). Increasing consent for organ donation: Mandated choice, individual autonomy, and informed consent. *Health Matrix, 21,* 599.

DellaVigna, S. (2009). Psychology and economics: Evidence from the field. *Journal of Economic Literature, 47*(2), 315–372.

Dolan, P., Hallsworth, M., Halpern, D., King, D., Metcalfe, R., & Vlaev, I. (2012). Influencing behaviour: The mindspace way. *Journal of Economic Psychology, 33*(1), 264–277.

Durkin, S., Brennan, E., & Wakefield, M. (2012). Mass media campaigns to promote smoking cessation among adults: an integrative review. *Tobacco Control, 21*(2), 127–138.

Elster, J. (1989). Social norms and economic theory. *The Journal of Economic Perspectives, 3*(4), 99–117.

Ezzati, M., & Lopez, A. D. (2003). Estimates of global mortality attributable to smoking in 2000. *Lancet, 362*(9387), 847–852.

Falk, A. (2007). Gift exchange in the field. *Econometrica, 75*(5), 1501–1511.

Falk, A., & Fischbacher, U. (2006). A theory of reciprocity. *Games and Economic Behavior, 54*(2), 293–315.

Farkas, A. J., Gilpin, E. A., Distefan, J. M., & Pierce, J. P. (1999). The effects of household and workplace smoking restrictions on quitting behaviours. *Tobacco Control, 8*(3), 261–265.

Fehr, E., & Gächter, S. (2000). Fairness and retaliation: The economics of reciprocity. *The Journal of Economic Perspectives, 14*(3), 159–181.

Friedman, R. (2009) *Soft drink taxes: A policy brief.* New Haven, CT: Rudd Center for Food Policy and Obesity, Yale University.

Gallup Organization for the Partnership for Organ Donation. (1993). *The American public's attitude toward organ donation and transplantation.* Boston, MA: Gallup Organisation.

Gerber, A., & Green, D. (2012). *Field experiments: Design, analysis, and interpretation.* New York, NY: W.W. Norton.

Glennerster, R., & Takavarasha, K. (2013). *Running randomized evaluations: A practical guide.* Princeton, NJ: Princeton University Press.

Griffith, R., Scholder, S. V. H. K., & Smith, S. (2014). Getting a healthy start? Nudge versus economic incentives (No. 13/328). Department of Economics, University of Bristol, UK.

Hahn, E. J. (2010). Smokefree legislation: A review of health and economic outcomes research. *American Journal of Preventative Medicine, 39*(6), S66–S76.

Harding, M., & Lovenheim, M. (2014). *The effect of prices on nutrition: comparing the impact of product-and nutrient-specific taxes* (No. w19781). National Bureau of Economic Research.

Hallsworth, M., Sanders, M., Maynard, O., Amlani, A., Litson, H., Chadborn, T., & Harper, H. (2014). "Stoptober:" How a large randomised trial enhanced a nationwide stop smoking campaign, *working paper.*

Hallsworth, M., List, J. A., Metcalfe, R. D., & Vlaev, I. (2014). *The behavioralist as tax collector: Using natural field experiments to enhance tax compliance* (No. w20007). Washington, DC: National Bureau of Economic Research.

Hammond, D. (2011). Health warning messages on tobacco products: A review.*Tobacco Control, 20*(5), 327–337.

Hood, C (1983). Tools of Government. *London, Macmillan.*

Hussey, M. A., & Hughes, J. P. (2007). Design and analysis of stepped wedge cluster randomized trials. *Contemporary Clinical Trials, 28*(2), 182–191.

Keeler, T. E., Hu, T. W., Barnett, P. G., & Manning, W. G. (1993). Taxation, regulation, and addiction: A demand function for cigarettes based on time-series evidence. *Journal of Health Economics, 12*(1), 1–18.

Laibson, D. (1997). Golden eggs and hyperbolic discounting. *The Quarterly Journal of Economics, 112*(2), 443–477.

Leicester, A., & Windmeijer, F. (2004). *The 'fat tax:' Economic incentives to reduce obesity* (Institute for Fiscal Studies Briefing Paper, No. 49).

Longo, D. R., Johnson, J. C., Kruse, R. L., Brownson, R. C., & Hewett, J. E. (2001). A prospective investigation of the impact of smoking bans on tobacco cessation and relapse. *Tobacco Control, 10*(3), 267–272.

Menzies, D., Nair, A., Williamson, P. A., Schembri, S., Al-Khairalla, M. Z., Barnes, M., ... Lipworth, B. J. (2006). Respiratory symptoms, pulmonary function, and markers of inflammation among bar workers before and after a legislative ban on smoking in public places. *Journal of the American Medical Association, 296*(14), 1742–1748.

Mulcahy, M., Evans, D. S., Hammond, S. K., Repace, J. L., & Byrne, M. (2005). Secondhand smoke exposure and risk following the Irish smoking ban: An assessment of salivary cotinine concentrations in hotel workers and air nicotine levels in bars. *Tobacco Control, 14*(6), 384–388.

Musingarimi, P. (2008). Obesity in the UK: A review and comparative analysis of policies within the devolved regions ICLU-UK. Retrieved February 2015, from http://www.ilcuk.org.uk/images/uploads/publicationpdfs/pdf_pdf_45.pdf

Mytton, O. T., Clarke, D., & Rayner, M. (2012). Taxing unhealthy food and drinks to improve health. *BMJ, 344.*

National Health Service Blood and Transplant. (2013). Register for organ donation. Retrieved February 2015, from https://www.organdonation.nhs.uk/how_to_become_a_donor/registration/registration_form.asp?campaignCode=-1

National Health Service Blood and Transplant. (2014). *Opt in or opt out.* Retrieved November 2014, from http://www.organdonation.nhs.uk/newsroom/statements_and_stances/statements/opt_in_or_out.asp

National Obesity Observatory [NOO]. (2011). Obesity and mental health. Retrieved February 2015, from http://www.noo.org.uk./uploads/doc/vid_10266_Obesity%20 and%20mental%20health_FINAL_070311_MG.pdf

National Obesity Observatory [NOO]. (2013). *Health risks of adult obesity*. Retrieved February 2015, from http://www.noo.org.uk/NOO_about_obesity/ obesity_and_health/health_risk_adult

Neuhouser, M. L., Kristal, A. R., & Patterson, R. E. (1999). Use of food nutrition labels is associated with lower fat intake. *Journal of the American Dietetic Association, 99*(1), 45–53.

New York City Health Code, § 81.08, (2006). Retrieved February 2015, from http:// www.nyc.gov/html/doh/downloads/pdf/about/healthcode/health-code-article81. pdf

Nuffield Council on Bioethics (2007). Public Health: Ethical Issues. *Policy Paper*.

O'Donoghue, T., & Rabin, M. (1999). Doing it now or later. *American Economic Review, 89*(1), 103–124.

Pirie, K., Peto, R., Reeves, G. K., Green, J., & Beral, V. (2013). The 21st century hazards of smoking and benefits of stopping: A prospective study of one million women in the UK. *Lancet, 381*(9861), 133–141.

Pischon, T., Boeing, H., Hoffmann, K., Bergmann, M., Schulze, M. B., Overvad, K., & Riboli, E. (2008). General and abdominal adiposity and risk of death in Europe. *New England Journal of Medicine, 359*(20), 2105–2120.

Public Health England. (2014). Patterns and trends in adult obesity. *HM Stationary Office*.

Stone, J., & Fernandez, N. C. (2008). To practice what we preach: The use of hypocrisy and cognitive dissonance to motivate behavior change. *Social and Personality Psychology Compass, 2*(2), 1024–1051.

Thaler, R. H. (2012, July 7): Watching behavior before writing the rules. *The New York Times*. Retrieved February 2015, from http://www.nytimes.com/2012/07/08/ business/behavioral-science-can-help-guide-policy-economic-view. html?pagewanted=all&_r=0

Thaler, R. H., & Sunstein, C. R. (2008). *Nudge: Improving decisions about health, wealth, and happiness*. New Haven, CT: Yale University Press.

Tiffin, R., Balcombe, K., Salois, M., & Kehlbacher, A. (2011). Estimating Food and Drink Elasticities. *Reading: University of Reading*.

Tversky, A., & Kahneman, D. (1991). Loss aversion in riskless choice: A reference-dependent model. *The Quarterly Journal of Economics*, 1039–1061.

UK Government. (2014). Cabinet ministers. Retrieved from https://www.gov.uk/government/ministers on 31/03/2014.

Shemilt, I., Hollands, G. J., Marteau, T. M., Jebb, S. A., Kelly, M. P., Nakamura, R., . . . & Ogilvie, D. (2013). Effects of changes in the economic environment on diet-and physical activity related behaviours and corollary outcomes: A large-scale scoping review. *PLoS One, 8*(9), c75070.

Shiu, E., Hassan, L. M., & Walsh, G. (2009). Demarketing tobacco through governmental policies–the 4Ps revisited. *Journal of Business Research, 62*(2), 269–278.

Vainio, H., Kaaks, R., & Bianchini, F. (2002). Weight control and physical activity in cancer prevention: International evaluation of the evidence. *European Journal of Cancer Prevention, 11*, S94.

Volpp, K. G., Pauly, M. V., Loewenstein, G., & Bangsberg, D. (2009). P4P4P: an agenda for research on pay-for-performance for patients. *Health Affairs, 28*(1), 206–214.

Wall, A. P. (2005). Government demarketing: Different approaches and mixed messages. *European Journal of Marketing, 39*(5/6), 421–427.

Wang, Y. C., McPherson, K., Marsh, T., Gortmaker, S. L., & Brown, M. (2011). Health and economic burden of the projected obesity trends in the USA and the UK. *Lancet, 378*(9793), 815–825.

Wansink, B., & Sobal, J. (2007). Mindless eating: The 200 daily food decisions we overlook. *Environment and Behavior, 39*(1), 106–123.

Yamamoto, J. A., Yamamoto, J. B., Yamamoto, B. E., & Yamamoto, L. G. (2005). Adolescent fast food and restaurant ordering behavior with and without calorie and fat content menu information. *Journal of Adolescent Health, 37*(5), 397–402.

11 | From Choice Architecture to Policy Infrastructure
MULTILEVEL THEORY AND THE POLITICAL ECONOMY OF HEALTH BEHAVIORS

FREDERICK J. ZIMMERMAN

BEHAVIORAL ECONOMICS DEFINES ITSELF BY a collection of empirical results. In a recent review of the application of behavioral economics to health, Thomas Rice (2013) identifies the lack of a unifying theory as a major challenge facing behavioral economics. To the extent that behavioral economics can be said to have any theoretical content at all, it is two-system theory, which claims that our brains employ two distinct kinds of cognition: a System 1 that is intuitive, fast, effortless, and emotional; and a separate System 2 that is reasoned, slow, controlled, and rule governed (Kahneman, 2003). Two-system theory has its fullest presentation in Daniel Kahneman's book *Thinking Fast and Slow* (2011). Different scholars in the tradition of behavioral economics have slightly different formulations of this brain dichotomy, but the essential dichotomy is always present, either implicitly or explicitly.[1]

An essential part of this cognitive dichotomy is its normative valence: The reflective system makes better decisions than the intuitive system. Some writers explicitly assert that System 2 is rational (Thaler & Sunstein, 2008) while System 1 is not, although Kahneman is too much a psychologist to believe in the chimera of rationality, a concept that he clearly mistrusts. All the same, he writes, "only the slower System 2 can construct thoughts in an orderly series of steps" (Kahneman, 2011, p. 21). The unmistakable implication of dual-system theory is that whether or not it achieves the cognitive perfection that economists associate with rationality, the reflective System 2 produces better decisions than the impulsive System 1, albeit more slowly and with greater effort. Call it rational, deliberative, reflective, or effortful, there is no mistaking the presumption that System 2 produces the good decisions that elude System 1.

The intuitive system is characterized as one might describe a small child: intuitive, quick to judge, impressionable, and prone to systematic errors. For Thaler and Sunstein, "Brain scientists are able to say that the activities of the Automatic System are associated with the oldest parts of the brain, the parts we share with lizards" (Thaler & Sunstein, 2008, p. 20). The reflective system is clearly the grown-up in this pair: It is reflective, controlled, and rule based, and its job is to "monitor and correct" System 1. "One of the tasks of System 2 is to overcome the impulses of System 1" (Kahneman, 2011, p. 26).

Seen in this light, behavioral economics only partially replaces rational-choice theory. Its strong empirical results have put paid to the presumption that people behave rationally, but a nub of rationality is retained. The way to incorporate the reality of behavior inconsistent with rational choice has been to divide thinking into two parts: an irrational (or "intuitive") part and a rational (or at least "reflective") part. As Kahneman puts it, "Theories in behavioral economics have generally retained the basic architecture of the rational model, adding assumptions about cognitive limitations designed to account for specific anomalies" (Kahneman, 2003, p. 1469).

Although some behavioral economists eschew theory altogether, whenever behavioral economics needs a conceptual foundation, it turns to two-system theory. Yet this conceptual foundation has many cracks, and it may put the empirical gains of behavioral economics in danger when they come under stress. The three most significant problems are the lack of a conceptualization of growth or development in cognitive processing; the inattention to the process that selects whether System 1 or System 2 is engaged in any given decision; and the strong implication that System 2 produces better decisions than System 1.

Most work in behavioral economics seems to treat the quality of System 1 and System 2 as static and exogenous. The task has almost always been to create a short-term experiment that will manipulate the associations available to System 1, thereby changing behavior. The notion that System 1 can be trained to produce better decisions is recognized in the literature (Kahneman, 2011; Sloman, 1996) but has played almost no role in the empirical work. This failure is a problem because presumably public health could benefit from improving System 1 in general, rather than creating choice architectures that nudge System 1 one decision at a time.

The second problem is that no mechanism is specified for how System 2 is triggered. Yet this is perhaps the most interesting process of all, and it is arguably far more important than the distinction between System 1 and System 2. In describing the advantages of System 2 over System 1, Kahneman cites research by Walter Mischel (Mischel, Shoda, & Rodriguez, 1989) in which children were asked to wait patiently for cookies. Those who were most successful were able to distract themselves by singing, tapping their hands, or pretending to sleep. Are these actions part of System 1, System 2, or some other system? Nobody knows. If System 2 is in charge of monitoring and correcting System 1, then is it always paying attention? And, if so, how do mistakes happen? And for that matter, how can System 2, which is slow, keep up with System 1? How does System 2 even know when System 1 is making a mistake? If System 2 has to wait for System 1 to alert it to a mistake, how can System 1 know that it is about to commit an error? This theoretical failure represents a deep conceptual flaw in two-system theory that is rarely acknowledged, but potentially fatal.

This problem is dealt with imperfectly in the literature. Kahneman reports that "when System 1 runs into difficulty, it calls on System 2 to support more detailed and specific processing that may solve the problem of the moment," suggesting that it is up to System 1 to know when it is in over its head (Kahneman, 2011, p. 24). Yet at the same time, he writes, "one of the tasks of System 2 is to overcome the impulses of System 1," suggesting that System 2 initiates its own takeover of processing (Kahneman, 2011, p. 26). Elsewhere he suggests that errors occur not really because of either System 1 or System 2, but because the errors escape the detection of System 2 (Kahneman, 2003, p. 1468).

This conceptual problem creates circular reasoning in two-system theory. System 2 is said to avoid the biases of System 1, but, in the absence of observable differences in the activation of System 1 and System 2, how do we know that System 2 systematically produces better decisions? The answer seems to be that we know of the superiority of System 2 over System 1 because observed better decisions are said to be the outcome of System 2 and mistakes are said to reflect the shortcomings of System 1. For advocates of two-system theory, evidently, saying is believing.

Repeatedly we are warned against the "errors of intuitive judgments" (Kahneman, 2003, p. 1467) and the "quirks of System 1" (Kahneman, 2011, p. 413). These attributes of the two systems are occasionally allowed to adhere to individuals, with unambiguously moral overtones. Describing people who do poorly on a particular cognitive task, Kahneman writes, "System 2 is weak in these people ... they are prone to answer questions with the first idea that comes to mind and unwilling to invest the effort needed to check their intuitions. Individuals who uncritically follow their intuitions about puzzles are also prone to accept other suggestions from System 1. In particular, they are impulsive, impatient, and keen to receive immediate gratification" (Kahneman, 2011, p. 48).

It is this dichotomy that justifies the use of nudges in public policy: a rational, deliberative process among public decision makers is deployed to come up with ways of harnessing the biases of people's irrational brains in ways that will make those people better off. The justification for libertarian paternalism only works if the effortful decision making provided by System 2—and employed by public decision makers—is superior to the intuitive System 1 that influences the decisions of individuals. This assumption should be questioned.

In the end, Kahneman does not in fact seem to really believe in dual-system theory, but he is using it only as a heuristic. "System 1 and System 2 are so central to the story I tell in this book that I must make it absolutely clear that they are fictitious characters. Systems 1 and 2 are not systems in the standard sense of entities with interacting aspects or parts. And there is no one part of the brain that either of the systems would call home" (Kahneman, 2011, p. 29). The dual-system model has little to do with dual systems, and instead it boils down to the statement that we usually (not always) do better (but still not perfectly) when we pay more attention.

Fair enough. One can certainly understand the need to simplify reality when creating useful theoretical categories. But the way in which these categories are created has important framing effects, as any behavioral economist would have to concede. The question then is what are these framing effects, and how useful are they?

To replace rational choice with half-rational choice achieves nothing. When pressed, behavioral economists recognize that System 2 makes systematic errors, and that even deliberative thought over decisions with enormous economic consequences not only can go wrong but can go wrong in systematic ways that can be identified and predicted by behavioral economics—even when the stakes are high (Ariely, 2009).

Yet in this finding, its own frame is working against it. The idea that we have a rational brain and an irrational brain, or even that we have an intuitive System 1 that is watched over and corrected by a reflective System 2, suggests that we will get the big things right. Indeed, if not, the justification for libertarian paternalism falls apart.

While the results of empirical work in behavioral economics suggest that people can make cognitive errors that lead to lifelong regret, or that big financial meltdowns are possible, or that we can all commit collective suicide by global warming, the frame says otherwise. System 2 should catch and correct the biases and quirks that would lead to such choices long before the consequences ever become that large. But as the linguist George Lakoff has observed, "When the facts don't fit the frames, the frames are kept and the facts are ignored" (cited in Romm, 2012). Two-system theory accordingly destroys the insights created by behavioral economics. There must be a better way.

An important place to start is with the recognition that the brain is immensely sophisticated and is capable of a stunning variety of processes, most of which it does quite well, but rarely perfectly. There are patterns to these imperfections, but these patterns do not suggest in any way that some parts of the brain or some cognitive processes produce fewer mistakes than others. If two-system theory is retained at all, it must be with the recognition that both System 1 and System 2 are capable of surprising achievements and systematic biases. There is no quality difference between the two systems.

The Learning Brain

An alternative theory turns away from the economist's preoccupation with rationality toward an older psychological and institutionalist theory of instinct, habit, custom, and power. In this theory, thought is more like language than like math: Whereas math is algorithmic, thought, like language, builds on itself. At any point in time decisions can be good or bad, but they change—usually for the better—over time. The brain learns.

At stake are small decisions such as the placement of vegetables at lunch or the decision to offer chocolate milk in schools, and much larger decisions, such as those involving campaign finance and the nature of democracy itself.

This alternative theoretical paradigm offers a much stronger foundation for the contributions of behavioral economics than does the two-system paradigm. It is based on the notion that the brain learns both from experience and from others. This learning brain does a good job with decisions it has seen before, especially if it has experienced the consequences of those decisions. It can also do reasonably well with decisions that others in its social group have seen before. It tends to do poorly with novel decisions, and it can be tricked.

Because this alternative, called multilevel theory, has been presented in some depth previously (Zimmerman, 2013), it is described only briefly here. Multilevel theory holds that we have one brain, not two. This brain works using cognitive habits, built up one on another. Thought is inherently social and fundamentally emotional. Custom is the social manifestation of cognitive habits in the form of shared values, heuristics, and conceptual categories. Custom is a storage bank of ways of thinking that have proven beneficial to our forebears and will be passed along to our progeny. Customs, and with them the individual cognitive habits that constitute custom, evolve over time in response to selective pressure to improve. In making decisions based upon the cognitive habits we have inherited from others, we are able to achieve an optimality that our own limited rationality would not achieve.

Habit

Work in behavioral economics has led to widespread acceptance that people are cognitive misers, extensively using convenient and unconscious heuristics such as rules of thumb or following the examples of others to make conscious decisions. In this sense, behavioral economics sketches out a view of rationality that is idiomatic: Chunks of rationality make sense internally, and these chunks are used by analogy in novel situations, with varying degrees of success. While individuals do not directly engage in utility maximization, social structures have evolved a set of behavioral and cognitive patterns—or habits of mind—that typically serve the ends of individual decision making very well. These habits of mind, including heuristics, rules of thumb, cognitive frames, social references, and so on, do not involve any direct utility maximization but are quasi-rational or idiomatically rational in the sense that on average they produce choices that closely approximate those that would arise from individual utility maximization.

While the interpretive emphasis in the empirical behavioral economics literature has been on departures from the predictions of individual, rational-choice models, a reading of behavioral economists such as Herbert Simon, Gerd Gigerenzer, Daniel Ariely, and others shows that this idiomatic, quasi-rational decision making in fact performs surprisingly well. Heuristics are not mistakes or even cognitive shortcuts; they are the building blocks of thought itself. So far from separating thought into intuitive and reflective parts, the learning-brain paradigm recognizes that deliberation is mostly unconscious and that "Reason, even in its most abstract form, makes use of, rather than transcends, our animal nature" (Lakoff & Johnson, 1999, p. 4).

The role of cognitive habits has a long tradition in psychology, meriting a chapter in William James's *Principles of Psychology* (James, 1890/2007). The institutional economist Thorstein Veblen wrote extensively about habits of mind (Twomey, 1998), and the related concept of habitus is an essential component of Bourdieu's social theory (Bourdieu, 1992).

For these authors, habit means a full sequence of thoughts or actions that can be triggered by a single stimulus and, once triggered, continues to the end (Neal, Wood, & Quinn, 2006). The essential element of habit is accordingly not repetition, but cohesion. A habit is a group of thoughts or actions that hang together, not a single action that is repeated. The role of habit in decision making is discussed in greater detail in Chapter 3 by Rünger and Wood.

Each habit has both a trigger and a sequence of cognitions. Habits are productive in that the triggers can become more nuanced and the sequences longer and more refined with experience. Because brain activity is valuable, the chunking together of discrete cognitions into a cognitive habit represents efficiency in behavior and decision making (Desrochers, Jin, Goodman, & Graybiel, 2010; Wood, Quinn, & Kashy, 2002). An individual deciding how to cook Brussels sprouts for dinner relies on cognitive habits for these decisions. With practice, the cooking of the Brussels sprouts both becomes easier and produces better results. With feedback, decisions are made more competently and with less thought over time. A rational cook would cook the dish exactly the same way every time (perfectly from the beginning) and with exactly the same cognitive effort. By definition, the rational cook would be cognitively engaged and deliberative about all the decisions in the kitchen. In contrast, the learning brain learns to improve its cooking. It is—perhaps ironically—precisely the creature of habit who learns, whose habits can become more efficient over time.

The role of learning is one of the major differences between the cognitive-habits model and the rational-choice model. The rational-choice model assumes that people are "lightning calculators" (Twomey, 1998), with a memory and decision rule. Two-system theory supposes that people are lightning calculators . . . with imperfections. Or that they are lightning decision makers and perfect calculators, but not at the same time. By contrast, the cognitive-habits model assumes that people improve through trial and error.

One advantage of conceiving the brain as a learning brain, rather than as a rational or half-rational brain, is that the learning-brain paradigm places thought itself into the explanatory frame. Not only decisions but also thought can be more or less successful, that is to say, more or less suited to the environment and problems that face it.

Words like "social determinants," "confounding," or "elasticity" have particular meanings to the specialists who understand them, and these meanings are cognitive habits: complex chains of cognitions such as "the percent change in a dependent variable that is caused by a percent change in an independent variable" that are triggered by a single word, such as "elasticity." Heuristics are like subroutines that save us a lot of verbiage—and conscious thought. But, of course, it takes a long time to develop a cognitive habit like "elasticity," and it is worth it only if one is regularly facing situations that call for it. Expertise is accordingly the development of a large number of cognitive habits related around a theme.

Expertise can also delete the imperfect cognitive habits used by others. To an expert in land rights in Africa, for example—who understands that there are separate rights to use, abuse, rent, buy, bequeath, pledge, lend, take from, or modify land—the term "private property" has no meaning: It is just too vague to be useful anymore. Ask a land-tenure expert whether "private property" promotes economic development and you will get a blank stare. But ask a nonexpert the same question, and you are likely to get a woefully confident answer.

The paradigm of the learning brain accordingly provides a very different understanding of some of the core empirical findings of behavioral economics than does the paradigm of two systems. In an often-cited experiment (Frederick, 2005) participants were told that a bat and ball together cost $1.10 and that the bat cost $1.00 more than the ball. They were invited to report how much the ball cost. The answers tend to be bimodal, with many people providing the intuitive, but incorrect, answer that the ball costs 10¢, while others provide the correct answer that the ball costs 5¢. Very few people provide any other answer. Proponents of two-system theory suggest that these results illustrate the existence of separate intuitive and reflective cognitive processes. Yet two-system theory provides no explanation for how these different answers arise, other than to appeal to the black box of attentional control. The learning-brain theory, by contrast, provides a clear explanation: Most people have a cognitive habit already that $1.10 - $1.00 = 0.10. Those with more expertise have more sophisticated cognitive habits to the effect that the problem to be solved is the value of x for $(x + $1.00) + x = 1.10.

The experimental results showed that students at MIT answered this question correctly far more often than students at less illustrious universities (Frederick, 2005). Why is that? Two-system theory suggests that MIT students were better at suppressing the impulse to answer with the intuitive, but incorrect answer. That is to say, students at MIT have better self-control. The learning-brain theory suggests that MIT students have learned more than students at the other universities. There may be any number of reasons why the MIT students have more sophisticated cognitive habits at a similar age than the other students, including native intelligence, opportunity, the quality of their schools, or even self-control. But the two-system theory offers only the self-control explanation.

It should now be clear that the frame one uses to understand the empirical results of behavioral economics has extremely meaningful implications for public policy and political discourse. Two-system theory suggests that MIT students, having greater self-control, are able to make more rational decisions and in that sense are inherently superior morally and intellectually to others. Learning-brain theory suggests that MIT students may be intellectually or morally superior, *or* they may have had more opportunities. There is a world of difference between these two frames.

Cognitive habits are like subroutines that make all complex and abstract thought possible: "the 95 percent below the surface of conscious awareness shapes and structures all conscious thought" (Lakoff & Johnson, 1999, p. 13). However, because cognitive habits are built up, one upon another, in ever more complex and sophisticated chains, an incorrect or unproductive cognitive habit at a basic level can taint all the other cognitive habits of which it is a part. If one believes instinctively that $2 + 2 = 5$, one can never get the right answer for questions like $27 + 24$. It is therefore important to understand how cognitive habits develop and change, and what disciplining process makes them more likely to be helpful than harmful.

Evolution

The learning brain learns from experience. Cognitive habits that trigger unpleasant consequences are discarded, while those that trigger fun and joy are retained. While a habit is not a compulsion, a habit is reinforced and strengthened by repetition. The emotional consequence of the chain of cognitions is a part of the habit itself. While in many cases this emotional reinforcement is internal, in other cases there is no obvious emotional return from a given chain of cognitions ($2 + 2 = 4$). For these kinds of cognitive habits—where the benefit of the cognitive habit is not obvious and immediate—we learn from others.[2]

Cognitive habits exist in the brain (Zimmerman, 2013), but they also have a social manifestation. At the social level, cognitive habits are called custom and include norms, common assumptions, shared values, metaphors, language, and law.

Cognitive habits on their own are not subject to the constraints of logic. One can adamantly oppose government deficits and equally vigorously oppose tax increases and spending reductions. One can go broke saving money on large purchases. Although they are not subject to logic, cognitive habits are subject to an equally rigorous discipline—that of selective pressure. The development of cognitive habits, as well as their refinement, pruning, and alteration, occurs through evolution, a process that involves variation in habits, selective pressure, and replication (Cosmides & Tooby, 1994; Stoelhorst, 2008).

Part of the feedback process in this evolution relies on one's own assessment of the value of a habit, and it is one important way in which habits are trimmed, modified, expanded, and reproduced. Habits that are useful get used and therefore are reinforced. Habits that are not useful fall into disuse and in time are forgotten. Painful habits are actively extinguished.

Selective pressure is exerted by friends, family, coworkers, and strangers who either punish or reward actions and who either reinforce or dissipate mental associations. This pressure can be wholesome or hurtful. Parents who consistently say "no" to sugary snacks before dinner extinguish over time children's habit of asking for them. On the other hand, children who bring raisins as dessert in their school lunches may find that their peers make fun of their dessert.

Habits of mind are offered to us by our social environment as the bequest of previous generations. They are a bank of wisdom, deposits of common sense and discoveries that were earned by the toil and experience of those who lived long ago (Hodgson, 2004). Eggplant, fava beans, tapioca, and mushrooms—all foolhardy risks long ago—are ours only because of the legacy of habits of preparation.

When it works properly, the evolution of cognitive habits reveals the collective and historical wisdom of a social group, not only about methods and procedures but also about what has value (Stoelhorst, 2008). In this sense, rationality is collective, not individual (Bromley, 2006). Over time, the flow of selective pressure smoothes out the rough edges of our imperfect thinking. It is selective pressure that can make of individually predictable irrationality more optimal social custom.

A recent agent-based simulation model by Geoffrey Hodgson and Thorbjørn Knudsen (2004) shows the promise of this approach, as well as the value of cognitive habit and social custom in individual decision making. They simulate the evolution of the custom of driving on a particular side of the road in an environment of 40 agents driving around a ring road, half going in each direction. The agents begin by driving on either the left or right side of the road and then choose whether to change sides as they see oncoming traffic, hoping to avoid collision. As the simulation proceeds, agents develop a history of tending to drive on the right or the left. A parameter set exogenously at the beginning specifies how much weight they attach to their personal history—to what extent drivers are set in their ways. This parameter turns out to matter a great deal to both personal and collective outcomes of the system. Gradually a custom emerges to drive on either the right or the left. For a wide range of parameter values in the model, the importance agents attach to habit significantly improves the speed at which the agents collectively coalesce around a particular custom. What is more, the strength of habit is the single most important parameter to the efficiency of the system as a whole. While other parameters—such as desire to avoid hitting other cars or the distance ahead that a driver can see—were strong predictors of individuals avoiding harm, only habit had a strong influence on how rapidly the system as a whole converges to a solution. This research suggests that a paradigm of the learning brain, built upon cognitive habits, can provide a strong foundation for rigorous simulation modeling, and that important insights may emerge when it does. To date, such rigorous modeling has not been possible with two-system theory.

But while cognitive habits may improve outcomes for both individuals and systems, they need not always do so. Just as prices can be distorted, perverting the social optima of rational-choice models, so can the evolution of cognitive habits. Because our cognitive habits are so susceptible to influence, it is useful to understand how we can be led away from optimality by those with the power to do so.

Power

People loath thinking about power. The powerful prefer the sources of their power to be invisible, or, if visible, conferred by the magic of the market, or ordained by God. The powerless prefer not to see themselves as subject to forces beyond their control, and in any event are in no position to rock the boat. Neither side cares to dwell on what might have been.

Changing power relations is immensely difficult and can go badly awry, often making everyone worse off. For all of these reasons, a case can be made for taking existing power relations as given. Yet the social progress we value most has always come by spreading power more broadly, whether in expanding civil rights in the middle and late 20th century, expanding access to higher education after World War II, extending the franchise to women at the beginning of the 20th century, or through limiting the role of government in the economy in the 17th and 18th centuries. While the powerful try always to consolidate and enhance their power, social progress comes from diffusing power.

In public health the discussion of power is particularly important. As Nancy Krieger has written, "a society's economic, political, and social relationships affect both how people live and their ecologic context, and, in doing so, shape patterns of disease distribution" (Krieger, 2008, p. 223). Yet notwithstanding its obvious importance for population health outcomes, there are no CDC or NIH funding mechanisms for the study of power, and little emphasis on the role of power in public health. Instead, there are a handful of scholars who explicitly recognize the importance of power, treading water in a vast ocean of research that is methodologically individualistic and that takes power relationships as given. Why might this be? Why should one of the most important determinants of health receive so little attention? Perhaps one answer is that power is seen as too vague a concept to permit rigorous theoretical attention or quantitative empirical analysis. That need not be so.

An excellent overview of power is in Steven Lukes's *Power: A Radical View* (2004). This book stresses that power is a capacity, which must be understood as distinct from its results. A powerful person is still powerful, even if he fails to achieve his goals. Power can accordingly be defined as the capacity to cause pain or pleasure in others at relatively little cost to oneself.

Lukes identifies three faces, or dimensions of power. These are not distinct types of power, but rather three ways of understanding power. They are direct power; agenda-setting power; and power over ideas, or framing power.

Direct power is the capacity to directly hurt or help others and—in a sense—to get away with it.

Agenda-setting power is the capacity to keep items on or off the table for discussion. In the recent debate over improving health insurance coverage that resulted in the Affordable Care Act, the health insurance lobby was able to put a single-payer plan off the table.

In public health, this kind of power has been deployed to devastating effect. When a patient-outcomes research project determined that certain commonly used surgical procedures are ineffective for back pain, a group of orthopedic surgeons successfully lobbied to slash funding for the Agency for Healthcare Research and Quality, which had funded the research (Deyo, Psaty, Simon, Wagner, & Omenn, 1997; Rosenstock & Lee, 2002). Since then, any attempts to use the science of effectiveness to limit reimbursement to only procedures that actually work have been—first de facto and now de jure—off limits (Neumann & Weinstein, 2010).

Framing power is the capacity to make the outlandish seem reasonable and the unappealing seem desirable. Framing power derives from the quality and quantity of rhetoric. MLK's power came not from his evocation of civil rights or equality for African Americans. These ideas were already mainstream. His power came from his insistence that equality meant that tired African Americans should sleep in any hotel of their choosing, that African Americans should sit next to Whites on buses, and that Black and White children should attend school side by side, and from his refusal to believe that "the bank of justice is bankrupt." Those ideas were outlandish before King—almost as much in the North as in the South—but came to be seen as reasonable as people listened to King's rhetoric. That is framing power: It is power over the way we think.

Not so long ago it would have seemed outrageous to consume a large soda with every meal; now it is commonplace. This shift did not happen because a rational population suddenly came to believe they were better off drinking soda than water or milk. It came about because technological changes led to a massive increase in the power of marketers to exert selective pressure on the evolution of our cognitive habits (Zimmerman, 2011).

Because the learning brain learns not only from its own experience but also from others, it is susceptible to learning the wrong lessons. In a sense, access to our cognitive habits is nonexcludable: Anyone can influence our cognitive habits. While this insight is a core finding of behavioral economics, it has been couched primarily in terms of behaviors, but it is equally true for thought itself. Power resides in discourse (Kesting, 1998).

In all of these dimensions, power operates on the evolution of cognitive habits in ways that matter profoundly for ways of thinking about public policy and by extension for public health. One of the primary social determinants of health is the extent to which governments are willing to invest in spending on early childhood interventions, education, income support, public health, and low-income healthcare. Yet all of these expenditures have been stagnant or even trending downward for decades. One reason is the pervasive belief that taxes are too high. Yet taxes as a percentage of the economy are both lower than in any other OECD country and lower than they have been in the United States in four decades. Paul Krugman notes on his blog that he regularly receives mail accusing him of being communist and anti-American for arguing for higher taxes, yet as he points out, high taxes on the wealthy were invented in America, and were explicitly accepted as a means of keeping the rich from getting richer (Krugman, 2014). The evaporation of the social consensus around high taxes did not happen by accident but was actively promoted by the wealthy—with adverse affects for population health.

All the same it is unfashionable to speak of power, and that fact itself is a frame, a heuristic, or a cognitive habit that has not arisen by accident. It is useful to hide power, which can be accomplished by defining it in such a way as to make most kinds of power invisible—an example of the agenda-setting dimension of power. Two-system theory, in endorsing a rational brain (or even rational people) separate from an impulsive brain (or from impulsive people), participates in this veiling of power.

Lukes (2004) cites the example of Indian widows in terrible health, or Indian wives subjected to domestic violence, who "lacked any sense of being wronged" and saw their suffering as "natural and normal." He identifies such attitudes as the outcome of "lifelong socialization and absence of information." This way of thinking of their own status is not a quirk and has nothing to do with System 1 or System 2 thinking. Instead, these ways of thinking are reinforced through the selective pressure operating in the interests of the powerful. An evolutionary perspective is quite helpful here: Preferences can be both adaptive in that they help individual people in the short run to avoid useless struggle, but at the same time they can be damaging to that class of people and their interests overall (Laajaj, 2012).

Instead of two ways of thinking, one impulsive and one rational, we have one cognitive function, but it learns. The brain can learn from experience or from others, and when it learns from others, these others can prioritize learning that will help the learner or learning that will help the teacher. Power distorts the ways of thinking that underlie all thought. Where there are low-quality decisions, there are often power imbalances.

The differences between two-system theory and the learning brain can be described in terms of the systematic mistakes of thinking: In two-system theory, these mistakes are predictable biases, randomly distributed in the population, or perhaps along the lines of innate differences in self-control. In the learning-brain paradigm of multilevel theory, mistakes in thinking are distributed along lines of social and economic power imbalances.

Although nudging such behaviors back into place can be useful, a more effective public health would document, quantify, and reverse the power imbalances that shape unhealthy cognitive habits in the first place.

Having put forward an alternative paradigm, a case study of sugared milk in the Santa Monica School District is presented to illustrate the differences in the two theoretical frames of decision making.

Milk: A Case Study

Public health is the creation of social conditions in which people can choose to be healthy. Fulfilling this mandate ethically requires that decisions made in the public's interest be as close to optimal as possible. The observation that highly deliberative processes can produce suboptimal or even downright harmful decisions is therefore an exceptionally important observation for public health.

We have the automobile to thank for skim milk. In the first half of the 20th century, skim milk was a troublesome waste by-product of butter production (Smith-Howard, 2013). It was poured into the streams in rural areas around dairies, emitting a foul smell, soiling streams and spoiling the pristine landscape. Although unpleasant to rural inhabitants, the disposal of skim milk into waterways became a major marketing problem only when urban automobilists began to come to rural areas on their Sunday drives. Suddenly the noxious and disgusting sight of milky streams threatened milk's reputation as clean and wholesome. Something had to be done. After World War II, milk marketers discovered that they could sell previously useless skim milk by marketing it as a weight-loss wonder. Though no shred of scientific evidence ever existed to support this marketing claim, it seemed intuitive that a product that had much of its fat removed would help remove fat from those who consumed it. Call this belief an intuition arising from System 1 or a belief based on the simple cognitive habit that equates dietary fat with body fat.

Having discovered a useful marketing heuristic, the dairy industry pushed it as far as it could. Given the dairy industry's image of wholesomeness—the milk of human kindness and motherhood all wrapped up in a clean, white package—this was pretty far. In 1985 the USDA officially endorsed skim milk for the first time, and by 1988 low-fat and skim-milk sales exceeded whole milk for the first time (Green, 2013). Over time, the public health community has aggressively supported the dairy industry in its insistence on skim milk, steadily removing first whole milk and then 2% milk from dietary recommendations, public institutions, and—especially—schools.

Notwithstanding the consistency of these recommendations, there is no evidence that switching from whole milk to reduced-fat milk prevents obesity, and some evidence to the contrary (Barba et al., 2005; Scharf, Demmer, & DeBoer, 2013). Public health has developed a harmful custom—a dangerous, collectively held cognitive habit—not because of its own experience or analysis, but because the power of an interested party. Along the way, dietary recommendations have been subjected to tremendous expert deliberation. Surely it is not possible to develop expert recommendations without employing System 2.

The history of milk recommendations provides a useful test of two-system theory. If System 2 produces better decisions than System 1, then recommendations should be rational: They should withstand the test of time, and get better, not worse. Recommendations can change with new evidence, but in the absence of new evidence they should not change: A rational decision is rational for all time. However, if on the other hand, deliberation is built upon heuristics that may be faulty and are subject to the meddling of powerful outsiders, then recommendations will shift with the prevailing winds of power. With recommendations shifting markedly over the decades away from whole milk and toward ever lower-fat milk, this history provides strong evidence against two-system theory. Instead, the effortful deliberations that have produced these changing recommendations have increasingly relied on the simple heuristic that dietary fat = body fat, a heuristic consistently reinforced by a dairy industry keen to take the fat out of milk so that it could be sold separately as butter and cheese.

Of course, a more sophisticated heuristic recognizes that it is energy balance that determines weight gain, not dietary fat per se. This heuristic might argue that low-fat milk could be justified because it has lower caloric content. Yet this heuristic, too, is misguided. Both fat and sugar promote palatability, and foods that have neither fat nor sugar nor salt are unlikely to be palatable on their own, especially for children (Drewnowski, 1998). Skim milk and 1% milk are indeed unpalatable to children, so although the choice is often presented as whole milk versus unflavored low-fat milk, in fact when presented with this choice children choose neither, which is part of the reason that milk consumption has been declining in the United States and is regarded as inadequate (Dietary Guidelines Advisory Committee, 2010). Instead, it has been necessary to increase the palatability of low-fat milk by adding sugar. Now the choice is between whole milk and flavored low-fat milk. Flavored 1% milk has about the same number of calories as unflavored whole milk and flavored 2% has more (Dietary Guidelines Advisory Committee, 2010). In its drive to reduce obesity, the public health community has in effect promoted higher caloric intake.

Shooting oneself in the foot cannot be ascribed to System 1, and the dichotomy between the two systems is not helpful in understanding how such a mistake could arise. Multilevel theory provides a stronger theoretical frame for directing efforts to improve policy making and avoiding mistakes.

The Santa Monica School Board was motivated by a desire to sustain the calcium intake of its students. Although its process was clearly effortful and deliberative, it was also shot through with bias. The Board relied, for example, on evidence that removing the sugar from milk would reduce milk consumption. Yet the only studies showing a link between flavored milk consumption and total milk intake were funded by dairy groups (Frary, Johnson, & Wang, 2004; Murphy, Douglass, Johnson, & Spence, 2008). It may have been responding to perceived differences of opinion among parents, but while over 1,000 parents signed a petition to remove flavored milk, those arguing in favor of retaining milk were largely outside experts—but not independent ones. In a subsequent press release, the dairy lobby later boasted of defeating the Santa Monica initiative through an astroturf campaign, stating, with no apparent sense of irony, "Dairy Council launched a proactive grassroots effort" to persuade school districts to retain flavored milk (Dairy Council of California, 2012). Finally, the Board may have believed it was protecting the freedom of students in rejecting a ban on flavored milk. Yet although the language of a ban was frequently invoked, this was no ban akin to a weapons ban or a ban on bullying: Students would have been free to bring any beverage they chose. The language of banning, while inaccurate, serves the purpose of casting those who urged the schools to stop selling sugared milk as coercive. The hysterical opposition to Michelle Obama's food plate is part of the same irrational fear, and it participates in the same frame of government nutrition advice as coercive overreach.

By 2013 there was a growing scientific consensus that recommendations to replace whole milk with skim milk—sugared or not—were at variance with the evidence and likely do more harm than good, and that sugared milk in particular should be avoided (Ludwig & Willett, 2013). This consensus is exactly the opposite of both current USDA recommendations (Dietary Guidelines Advisory Committee, 2010) and the decision reached by the Santa Monica School Board.

But what makes this story particularly bemusing is that parents and the School Board were vigorously disputing the wrong issue. Instead of debating whether kids will drink less milk if sugary milk is replaced by unsugared skim milk or whether a teaspoon of sugar a day will make kids obese, they should have focused on the goal of improving bone health and how to educate children's palates for a lifetime of healthy eating. This issue switch has tremendous implications for the use of behavioral economics in public health and for libertarian paternalism in general.

The idea that parents who care about their children might improve their behavior when given new information seems never to have occurred to the School Board. Although it claimed that its primary purpose in retaining sugared milk was to maintain the calcium intake of students, the School Administration never bothered to inform parents of the importance of calcium in their children's diets. The whole debate over sugared milk would have been the ideal time to mention the importance of dairy in the diet, but it failed to do so. That any authority would try to encourage milk consumption by adding sugar to milk without ever troubling to inform people of the value of milk to health is surprising. That a deliberative body whose mandate is to educate children would forget to do so is stunning. But frames are powerful things.

There is a final irony. Two recent scientific reviews have found that the relationship between dietary calcium intake and bone health is slim to nonexistent (Lanou, Berkow, & Barnard, 2005; Winzenberg, Shaw, Fryer, & Jones, 2006). The justification for fostering milk consumption in children itself rests on a faulty heuristic: that because milk contains calcium, and because bone density relies on calcium in the bones, dietary calcium must promote bone density. At heart, this heuristic is little different than the Medieval belief that because walnuts resemble brains, walnuts must promote intelligence.

The problem with two-system theory is not so much that there are two different cognitive processes, one intuitive and one deliberative. That much is, well, intuitive. The problem is that in its formulation in both behavioral economics and in the popular imagination these two processes are distinct—they are alternative strategies for solving similar problems—and that one system produces better decisions than the other. This is a powerful heuristic, that we have two brains, a good, but slow one and a bad, but fast one. Instead, the learning brain paradigm of multilevel theory argues that we have one brain and that conscious, deliberative thinking is built up of unconscious, intuitive habits of mind. Accordingly, deliberative thought is not better than intuitive thought; it inherits all of its biases. There is a real danger that libertarian paternalism will make us worse off.

The Learning Brain and Behavioral Economics

At several junctures Kahneman recognizes the potential or even actual superiority of intuition over reasoning, and when he does it is because of the ways in which System 1 is similar to cognitive habits: "but intuitive thinking can also be powerful and accurate. High skill is acquired by prolonged practice, and the performance of skills is rapid and effortless" (Kahneman, 2003, p. 1450). Cognitive habits are useful because in linking long chains of what might otherwise be separate cognitions, they become faster and more available.

In fact, most of the main findings of behavioral economics might be expected from a learning brain that pieces together more sophistical reasoning from heuristics, or cognitive habits.

Automatic Behaviors

A great deal of population health depends on people's automatic behaviors: things they do or do not do without really thinking about it. Eating, physical activity, use of tobacco and alcohol, as well as seat belts and condoms. All of these behaviors are driven by cognitive habit: a particular environmental cue happens, and a set of cognitions and behaviors is triggered and continues to its end. Eating is among the most important and most intensively studied such automatic behavior (Cohen & Farley, 2008).

Behavioral economists and marketers have begun to explore the influence of cognitive habit on eating, demonstrating, for example, that people will eat more when in the presence of another person who eats a lot (Cohen & Farley, 2008; Wansink, 2004); that people will eat more when the portion size is larger (Wansink, 1996; Young & Nestle, 2002); that people will eat differently when exposed to the choices of others, including strangers (Ferraro, Bettman, & Chartrand, 2009), and to the cues of advertising (Harris, Bargh, & Brownell, 2009). For behavioral economists, these results are curiosities of behavior that can be exploited in highly context-specific ways to nudge people toward healthier choices, for example by placing the healthiest foods at the beginning of the lunch line (see Chapter 9 by Wansink).

In multilevel theory, though, these habits can be learned or unlearned, and the role of behavioral economics should not be to nudge people to better behaviors but to inculcate better cognitive habits (Zimmerman, 2009).

For food marketers, however, people's dependence on cognitive habit in food choices opens the gates of power. Product placement, aggressive marketing in schools, pouring rights contracts, improved packaging and food product engineering, more retail food points of sale, increased marketing at the point of sale—all these are either new or greatly expanded since 1980. It has been argued that the tremendous increase in obesity since about 1980 is largely due to a significant expansion in the power and scope of food marketing (Zimmerman, 2011).

Heuristics, Frames, and Rules of Thumb

Behavioral economics has done an excellent job popularizing an understanding of heuristics in decision making. What multilevel theory makes clear is that, as cognitive scientists have known for a long time, heuristics—that is, cognitive habit or habits of mind—influence not only our actions but our ways of thinking (Lakoff, 2004; Lakoff & Johnson, 1999).

Much of advertising works this way: by repetition to increase cognitive accessibility and by creating associations with pleasant things. Because of its importance to the political economy of public health and consequently as a determinant of population health, framing is addressed in greater detail in the next section.

Availability Bias, Default Options, and Anchoring

One of the deepest cognitive habits is the metaphorical association of seeing with understanding (Gilbert, 1991). Children learn the concept of understanding (which they cannot directly observe) through the concept of seeing (which they can). The phrase "seeing is believing" is therefore true in a literal sense and a conceptual sense. Behavioral economics has identified availability bias, the likelihood to rely on and trust information that comes easily to mind more than information that is not as available, in many studies. Availability bias underlies anchoring, status-quo bias, the pull of default options, and prospect theory. For Kahneman, availability bias is what underlies the distinction between Systems 1 and 2. System 1 depends on information that is readily accessible, while System 2 uses the information that is most relevant.

In multilevel theory, accessibility is also important, but theory is more comprehensive than two-system theory in two ways. First, cognitive habits are more accessible because they are reinforced by use. The phrase William James used is apt: "currents pouring in from the sense-organs make with extreme facility paths which do not easily disappear" (James, 1890/2007, p. 107). At first, these cognitive habits are perceptual, as Kahneman believes, but the fact that cognitive habits build upon one another means that as thinking becomes more sophisticated, it is no longer only the sense organs that are carving indelible paths but also other cognitive habits. Second, accessibility can be purchased by outsiders who have the capacity to reinforce certain associations in our brains. These differences explain why accessibility bias affects not only intuitions but also deliberative thought.

Social Referencing

In multilevel theory the learning brain learns both from its own experience and from others. The capacity to learn from others is completely reasonable given the wealth of experience others have to offer. If we each had to learn from our own experience, we would be a sorry race indeed. But in learning from others we can go awry.

In two-system theory, and in the lab, social referencing is a source of bias. So much so that people can be induced to endorse propositions that are obviously false (Sunstein, 2003). But in multilevel theory in the context of the real world, learning from others is an adaptive cognitive habit. Not only does it enable us to improve our own cognitive habits by leveraging the experience of others, but even in isolated, one-off situations it can improve our judgments. In one famous example, a crowd guessing the weight of a bull had a mean guess that was within 1 pound of the bull's measured weight, much closer than any of the individual estimates provided by the cattle experts present (Surowiecki, 2005).

Bounded Selfishness

Several experiments have shown that people are not as selfish as would be predicted by the rational-choice model. Even in repeated iterations of the prisoner's dilemma game, for example, in which people have an incentive to cooperate in one period to ensure cooperation in successive periods, rational-choice theory predicts less cooperation than is observed in practice. This empirical regularity is part of behavioral economics because of its departure from rational-choice theory. Yet it is primarily an issue of sociability and not one of System 1 or System 2 at all. However, multilevel theory gives a good reason for this behavior. Because people routinely interact with each other in ways that are analogous to the prisoner's dilemma, they have cognitive habits that permit them to cooperate beyond what a calculating agent would engage in. They have learned to cooperate. This cooperation is optimal in the real world, and it carries over into the laboratory.

In sum, the paradigm of a learning brain that assembles thoughts out of habits of mind provides at least as good a fit to the empirical findings of behavioral economics—and generally a much better fit—than two-system theory. Yet, if it is no worse, is it any better? What is to be gained by adopting a new cognitive frame for how we think? Before delving into this question it is worth reviewing the literature on framing in general.

Framing and Population Health

A cognitive frame is "a spatial and temporal bonding of a set of interactive messages" (Bateson, 1972) that serves the purpose of organizing information into a coherent package to make it meaningful (Ortiz, 2013). Behavioral economists have written extensively about framing effects. For example, it is well known that people fear losses more than they crave gains, and the effect has been estimated as high as 2:1—that is, people will forgo a gain of $20 to avoid a potential loss of $10 (Rice, 2013; see also Chapter 2 by White and Dow). Research on framing effects has revealed that loss avoidance can be triggered not just by the reality of potential losses but also by foregrounding potential losses in the way a question is framed. Telling people, "If you do not use energy conservation methods, you will lose $350/year" is more powerful than "If you use energy conservation methods, you will save $350/year" (Thaler & Sunstein, 2008). The underlying choice problem is precisely the same: It is only the framing of the problem that affects the results.

The effects of framing extend to highly consequential decisions in areas in which people have expertise and make deliberative decisions. In a well-known experiment, physicians—thinking consciously about issues in their area of expertise—are more likely to recommend an operation if "90 out of 100 are alive" than "10 out of 100 are dead" (Tversky & Kahneman, 1981).

A frame is a cognitive habit in action. The purpose of framing is to set up a decision problem in such a way as to make a particular cue, or trigger, particularly salient, so that it will trigger a particular kind of cognitive habit. For example, physicians have adopted the cognitive habit of "First, do no harm." Accordingly a problem that is phrased in such a way so as to make the possibility of harm especially salient will elicit decisions that focus on avoiding harm. Physicians will avoid a scenario in which "10 out of 100 are dead." But the same problem presented in a way in which the harm is not salient will not trigger the cognitive habit of "First, do no harm" and will encourage decisions that result in "90 out of 100 alive."

Results around framing effects have been replicated in the health-care setting many times using precise experimental designs (Perneger & Agoritsas, 2011). In results like these, behavioral economists are documenting not the existence of two systems but the powerful influence of cognitive habits on ways of thinking.

A frame works best when its trigger is most salient. An experiment involving African American women found that messaging about HIV testing was far more effective when it evoked specific aspects of the African American experience than a more generic message (Kalichman & Coley, 1995). A study of the promotion of dental flossing found that messages whose framing was congruent with the participants' personalities—approach oriented or avoidance oriented—were more effective than similar messages whose framing was not congruent (Sherman, Updegraff, & Mann, 2008).

Loss framing is one type of framing that has been extensively studied, but it is not the only type of framing, and it does not work universally. It has been proposed that loss framing may work best when the target is to detect illness, while gain framing may work better when the target is to encourage health-promotion behavior (Rothman & Salovey, 1997). These theoretical observations have been confirmed in experiments involving many health-related behaviors, including Pap-smear testing (Rivers, Salovey, Pizarro, Pizarro, & Schneider, 2005), HIV screening (Apanovitch, McCarthy, & Salovey, 2003), sunscreen use (Detweiler, Bedell, Salovey, Pronin, & Rothman, 1999), and prevention of gum disease (Rothman, Martino, Bedell, Detweiler, & Salovey, 1999). A recent meta-analysis has found that gain framing works best for health-promoting behaviors (as opposed to only attitudes or intentions), and that the effectiveness of loss framing remains unclear (Gallagher & Updegraff, 2012).

In these analyses, it is the relative riskiness of a choice—potential future gains or losses of one option versus another—whose framing is being manipulated. It is also possible to use framing to alter perceptions of the attributes of a choice on its own (Levin, Gaeth, Schreiber, & Lauriola, 2002; Levin, Schneider, & Gaeth, 1998). For example, college students were more likely to recommend a medical procedure to others that "was 50% effective" than if it had "a 50% failure rate" (Levin, Schnittjer, & Thee, 1988). Similarly, a study of the willingness to pay for a cancer screen was higher when the result was expressed in terms of cancers found than when it was expressed as cancers missed (Howard & Salkeld, 2009).

Many of the behavioral interventions discussed in this volume are in fact framing interventions. For example, a stoplight system to influence food choice (see Chapter 6 by Riis and Ratner) sets up a particular cognitive habit—that of stopping when cued with red and moving ahead when cued with green—that is universal and automatic. Guidelines on healthy eating and active living (see Chapter 8 by Lewis and Block) not only provide information but set up a frame in which behavior can be guided by a user's manual, as if active living is like assembling a piece of IKEA furniture. Conditional cash transfers (see Chapter 2 by White and Dow) seem to work even when the cash incentive is very low compared to the economic benefits involved. In these examples, the interventions work by highlighting the salience of a payment within an incentive frame.

Framing and Thought

While much of the work on framing in health has focused on behavior, an important emerging literature recognizes that how we think about public health and policy is sensitive to the way issues are framed (Dorfman, Wallack, & Woodruff, 2005). This work responds to work in political science and linguistics, which has identified a distinction between episodic framing (the framing of a human-interest story, in which an issue is presented in the context of its particulars) and thematic framing (the framing of social science, in which general rules and patterns are presented). Analyses of framing have shown that the popular media presents social problems like poverty, crime, and poor health in episodic frames (Gitlin, 1980; Iyengar, 1994). Individual people are portrayed with their individual problems being the result of their individual choices. Not surprisingly, this framing makes it difficult for the public to embrace policies that redress the structural barriers that shape people's choices.

Work in public health is beginning to suggest how public health messages can be framed in ways that make them more palatable to the general public. A recent report offers many suggestions for framing the social determinants of health for effective communication, suggesting that social factors do resonate with the public when explicitly raised; that explicit reference to social disparities in health can backfire; and that emotional and values-based appeals build support for public health policies, even among elites (Robert Wood Johnson Foundation, 2010). In the area of obesity, recent studies have shown that on television obesity is portrayed episodically, and that the solution to obesity is individual behavior change, while newspapers are more likely to follow expert opinion in framing obesity as having multiple causes, some of them structural (Barry, Jarlenski, Grob, Schlesinger, & Gollust, 2011; Ortiz & Zimmerman, 2014). These differences matter because those who employ the episodic frame that locates the causes of obesity within the individual are much less likely to support obesity-prevention policies than are those who employ the thematic frame that emphasizes the social structural causes of obesity (Barry, Brescoll, Brownell, & Schlesinger, 2009; Oliver & Lee, 2005). Emerging work now is beginning to explore the extent to which alternative frames—episodic or thematic—can be deliberately invoked to alter support for public health policies (Gollust, Lantz, & Ubel, 2009; Ortiz, 2013). This area will be one of rich research in the near future.

The problem for public health is that because episodic framing tells a personal story it is immediately relatable and easily understood, while thematic framing requires more advanced habits of mind. It is not possible to understand structural barriers if one does not have a history with the words "structural barriers." Unfortunately, for many people that which is unintelligible does not exist.

Abstract thinking is built upon concrete thinking, and it is more successful when more elaborate abstractions are readily available. An economic game called a "beauty contest" makes these abstract observations concrete. In this contest, participants are asked to submit a number between 0 and 100, and the person whose number is closest to one half of the average wins a prize. A concrete way of thinking would generate a guess of 25, which would be half of the mean if the numbers were submitted at random. A more sophisticated, and abstract, form of reasoning would suggest a guess of 12.5, which incorporates the insight that these numbers would not be submitted at random, but would instead have a lower average than the average of random numbers. A yet more sophisticated guess would be 0, because, if everyone is perfectly thoughtful, everyone would be trying to submit lower numbers than everyone else in a conceptual race to the bottom. Finally, the most sophisticated, elaborate, and abstract reasoning would recognize all of these features of the game but would also incorporate the insight that not everyone is particularly abstract. Empirical results (Nagel, 1995) show that about one third of the guesses are roughly 12.5; about one quarter are roughly 25; about one sixth are just under

50; and the rest are intermediate values. (The optimal guess turned out to be 13.5.)

The ability to engage in abstract thinking accordingly profoundly affects judgment and behavior. Several recent presidents seem to have been largely incapable of abstract reasoning. Ron Reagan junior has said of his father, "Tenderhearted and sentimental in his personal dealings, he could nonetheless have difficulties extending his sympathies to abstract classes of people" (Matthews, 2013, p. 127). When President Reagan was told about how his cutbacks in social spending would cause hardship for individual people, he would respond with great kindness and direct a staffer to solve the person's problem. But he could never understand the connection between the personal story and the larger policy. As one journalist wrote, "While Reagan could be made to take interest in, and even genuinely seem to care about a particular situation, he remained unmoved if the same hardship story was multiplied into a million similar ones" (Matthews, 2013, p. 127).

Because everyone has a tendency toward similarly concrete thinking, media reports of health issues focus on the concrete experience of individuals, which in turn cues an episodic frame of personal responsibility and hence a distrust of government programs that would lessen the consequences of personal actions. This is all an attempt to report more diplomatically John Stuart Mill's insight: "I did not mean that Conservatives are generally stupid; I meant that stupid persons are generally Conservative."

Frames can help to make the abstract concrete by embedding structural themes into a personal narrative. For example, a story about homelessness might begin, "The homeless shelter was full again tonight, as Jane Doe contemplated whether to sleep on the street or risk another night with her abusive boyfriend." Public health must learn to sell its potential and its achievements by framing them in ways that are concrete, yet emphasize structural factors.

Framing and Emotion

Chapter 4 by Ferrer and colleagues reviews a literature demonstrating the influence of emotion on decision making. A separate, but related, literature has shown that emotion itself is contingent on framing effects.

Properly constructed episodic framing can create emotions of sympathy for a character and increase support for policies that remove structural barriers. In an experiment involving mandatory minimum sentencing, an episodic frame that emphasized the accidental way in which a young woman came to assist her boyfriend, a drug dealer, elicited emotions of pity and mitigated support for mandatory jail time for drug offenses (Gross, 2008).

Emotions can be primed and trained as well (Todorov, Harris, & Fiske, 2006). An experiment showed that repeated exposure to threatening words heightened the salience of subsequent, unrelated threatening words in a disambiguation task, such as writing down "die" or "dye" after hearing the word (Grey & Mathews, 2000). An enormous literature has shown that children, adolescents, and adults who are exposed to violent television both think and behave more aggressively as a result, and this result holds in experimental settings as well as in long-term, longitudinal data (Anderson et al., 2003).

Two-system theory, which holds that processes governing emotion and reflection are inherently separate and exogenous, misses important public health opportunities—beginning, but not ending with social cognitive theory—that leverage the interactions between emotion and reflection.

This connection can also lead to serious public health problems, as when Andrew Wakefield was able to bottle a toxic stew of fear, misinformation, and Cherie Blair to sell the canard that the measles, mumps, and rubella vaccine causes autism (Goldacre, 2010). The point here is not that people act irrationally when they are afraid; it is that fear is surprisingly easy to create.

As Ben Goldacre so aptly puts it, "Without anybody's noticing it, bullshit has become an extremely important public health issue" (Goldacre, 2010, p. 254).

Frames clearly have enormous importance to public health. As public health begins to embrace behavioral economics more warmly, it is essential to do so in the right frame of mind. A two-system frame of decision making that opposes a rational brain to an irrational one—or worse, rational people to irrational people—will reify the individual, personal-responsibility frame, albeit with some indulgence. A learning-brain frame is more consistent with the historical mission of public health.

What Does a New Paradigm Have to Offer?

The human brain is an immensely complex organ, capable of a stunning variety of tasks. That we can find fault with some of its operations—even systematic biases—is not surprising, and it would be stunning if no such mistakes could be found. Trying to shoehorn everything the brain can do into a single model is probably a fool's errand. However, precisely because of its complexity, simplifying everything the brain does into a causal frame is useful in better understanding our decisions and what drives them. The question is to find the right simplifying frame—one that is internally logical, broadly consistent with empirical observations, and produces useful insights for policy and research. Rational choice is not that frame, and largely for the same reasons, dichotomizing the brain into a rational part and an impulsive part is also not that frame. This chapter offers an alternative frame, that of the learning brain.

The crucial difference between dual-system theory and cognitive-habit theory is that dual-system theory believes in two essentially distinct systems of cognition (thinking, fast and slow), and that System 2 produces better decisions—if more slowly—than does System 1. Cognitive-habit theory, by contrast, believes that conscious, deliberative thought is built up of heuristics and is therefore subject to all the biases and potential manipulations that afflict System 1. What is to be gained from a recognition that conscious, deliberative thought is subject to bias?

As the previous sections argued, there are no empirical results that can be explained by two-system theory than cannot be explained by multilevel theory. But multilevel theory provides several important theoretical insights that are missing from two-system theory.

To begin with, a credible theory is required. With rational-choice substantially undermined, many behavioral economists seem not to want to engage theoretically at all. This approach has the virtue of integrity, but into a theoretical vacuum people will pour all kinds of biases and superstitions, so that when experts endorse no theory, they might as well endorse the worst theory. Theoretical frames are important, a proposition that should not be a hard sell to behavioral economists.

Multilevel theory has the potential to be generative, like rational-choice theory, but unlike two-system theory, it can serve as the foundation for models that provide unexpected insights, nuanced representations, and testable predictions that go beyond existing empirical observations. A recent agent-based simulation uses the concepts of cognitive habits and social referencing—learning from others—to model dietary behavior in a variety of alternative policy scenarios in a population modeled on Pasadena, California (Zhang, Giabbanelli, Arah, & Zimmerman, 2014). This model shows that for a very wide range of empirically estimated parameter values, even very aggressive policies to provide greater access to healthy food (redressing food desserts) have virtually no effect on behavior. Taxes on obesigenic foods have a small effect. But changing the marketing environment either by restricting marketing of obesigenic foods or increasing marketing of fruits and vegetables would increase fruit and vegetable consumption by roughly 7%.

Although this kind of research is in its infancy, this model, like the model of a traffic convention described earlier (Hodgson & Knudsen, 2004) suggests that there could be important research insights to be gained from simulation modeling built upon multilevel theory.

As suggested earlier, multilevel theory, with its frame of the learning brain, provides a theoretical frame that is not at war with its own results. Daniel Ariely (2009) movingly recounts how other economists were tolerant and even interested in his results, but they thought they were minor intriguing quirks, well away from the serious work of economics. He had a hard time getting anyone to understand how fundamental these departures from rational-choice behavior were, until the major financial meltdown in the mid-2000s. Ariely seems convinced that this financial crisis has ended the notion that behavioral economics does not matter to real economics. But for many people he is wrong. One still hears many economists saying that behavioral economics produces cutsey results, but not substantial ones. One reason is no doubt the frame that says that our deliberative, effortful thinking will correct the quirks of our intuitive system. Learning says that reflective thought built out of erroneous cognitive habits will be biased. Big decisions can go awry with big consequences.

While behavior economics has pointed to quirks and biases, multilevel theory says that these biases are socially and economically patterned through inequalities in the distribution of power. It is no accident that low-income and minority borrowers were the most likely to fall prey to manipulative mortgages, or that low-income minority neighborhoods have roughly twice as much advertising as low-income White neighborhoods (and 50% more for obesigenic food) (Yancey et al., 2009). For two-system theory, such differences are uninteresting; for rational-choice theorists they can only be about selection; for multilevel theory they are at least in part about exploitation.

One of the most interesting features of behavioral economics is how the specter of exploitation is always present, but never fully engaged. Exploitation could be defined as using the insights of behavioral economics to structure context of choice so that the outcomes of the choice will benefit the structurer at the expense of the chooser. Senior citizens dislike the structure of Medicare Part D plans, and with good reason. The number of plans is so confusing to seniors that once they have a plan they stick to it rather than braving the thicket of options to choose again. Although it has been estimated that 43% of seniors would benefit from switching plans, less than 10% do so (Rice & Cummings, 2010). The cost to nonswitchers has been estimated at $500 per beneficiary per year. If libertarian paternalism is possible then—necessarily—so is exploitation.

In *Nudge* Sunstein and Thaler refer to the possibility of exploitation again and again: "markets often give companies a strong incentive to cater to (and profit from) human frailties, rather than to try to eradicate them or to minimize their effects." "The opportunity to fleece customers is valuable," they note, and remind us that African Americans, low-income Americans, and poorly educated Americans paid hundreds, and even thousands of dollars more for their mortgages than well-educated and White Americans, even controlling for credit risk. The central questions of choice architecture are Who uses? Who chooses? Who pays? Who profits? (Thaler & Sunstein, 2008, p. 99).

The only meaningful response to the possibility of exploitation is to place strict limits on the power of those who would engage in the exploitation. But more muscular regulation is not on Sunstein and Thaler's agenda. Instead, they commit to libertarian paternalism, suggesting, for example, that a good fix for the potential for abuse in mortgage lending would be to provide clearer information about interest rates in teaser-rate mortgages. That seems like a sensible, libertarian-paternalist alternative to regulatory restriction of such mortgages. And it is, at the individual level. But at a market level, this proposal will not work. If teaser-rate mortgages save money for every borrower who takes one out instead of a standard fixed-rate mortgage, the banks would lose money, and the mortgages would not be offered. If they are offered, it can only be the case that more borrowers lose than gain. The market for teaser-rate mortgages can accordingly only be a gamble, in which the house (the bank) takes a large cut. If borrowers on the whole had information about whether they would need the mortgage beyond the initial period, then the banks would not make money. If borrowers do not have such information, then in the best-case scenario they are simply gambling, and in the worst-case scenario their cognitive failings—of overconfidence, of trust in their relationship with their bank, of innumeracy—are being exploited. Whatever happened to Who pays and who profits? Sunstein and Thaler may believe that libertarian paternalism represents a third way in politics, but in fact it represents only a fig leaf to the old way: Let the buyer beware. Perfectly fine policy advice if you believe in rational-choice theory; terrible advice if you do not.

This third-way, libertarian paternalism, has been taken up both by the Obama administration in the United States and the Cameron administration in the United Kingdom, where it has taken the form of the

Behavioural Insights Team, or "Nudge Unit." An article in the *New York Times* reports that in its first 3 years of existence the Nudge Unit has saved the British government tens of millions of pounds, according to its director (Bennhold, 2013). Although such savings might not justify Prime Minister Cameron's claims of "a new age of government," it is an important set of successes. Never mind that many of the nudges—such as a program to reduce paperwork and improve counseling in unemployment offices or the use of evidence in policy making—look less like clever nudges and more like common sense. By putting old wine into new bottles, behavioral economics has been able to sell public health to some new customers, and that is a good thing. But it has also undermined traditional public health, and that is a bad thing.

Strong reservations have been raised about the use of nudges in public policy. Some have argued that nudges are an unacceptable interference with individual autonomy (Hausman & Welch, 2010), while others counter that people do not mind being nudged, especially when it really is in their best interest. What seems clear in this debate is that the legitimacy of libertarian paternalism is only as strong as the credibility of the entity doing the nudging. Yet this credibility cannot be taken for granted, and it is safe to say that behavioral economists and politicians who have embraced the nudge approach to public policy have undertheorized the role of government credibility. The same people who support the nudges of the IRS to get people to pay taxes on time might not be so supportive of nudges on the part of the NSA to get people to reveal private information.

The characterization of nudging as libertarian paternalism reads like an attempt to invoke a cognitive frame that may evoke sympathy in a population tired of stark left-right political divides (Bonell, McKee, Fletcher, Haines, & Wilkinson, 2011). Yet nudging is clearly not libertarian (Hausman & Welch, 2010), and neither is it necessarily paternalistic, in the sense of being in the nudgee's best interest. Instead, nudging is an example of the use of power to influence the thinking and decisions of others. This process is not inherently bad, but it must not be given a free pass from careful ethical review.

Nudging has been even more forcefully criticized for its potential to take attention and resources away from more traditional approaches to social policy, including health promotion, regulation, and pricing (Bonell et al., 2011; Loewenstein, Asch, Friedman, Melichar, & Volpp, 2012).

Beyond these concrete consequences, there is the role of the paradigm itself. People do not in general want to be treated as half-rational, in need of nudging. Replacing the two-system theory with multilevel theory emphasizes the learning brain and accordingly the role of education in improving behavior. While education can be a mutually respectful process, nudging cannot be, particularly when the nudge is justified on the basis of a rational brain disciplining the excesses of an irrational brain. Choice architecture can quickly come to seem like a euphemism for manipulation.

The Stakes for Public Health

Most experts agree that about 5%–6% of children across all societies suffer from an organic disorder of executive function that causes symptoms of attention-deficit/hyperactivity disorder (ADHD). Yet in the United States, 11% of children have been diagnosed with ADHD, and 70% of these take prescription medication for it (Hinshaw & Scheffler, 2014). The disjuncture between underlying need and diagnosis and prescription may seem odd, but it is explained in large part by an increase in diagnoses since the early 1990s, driven primarily by a huge increase in marketing (Schwarz, 2013). In the 10 years following 1993, sales of ADHD medication in the United States tripled in real terms (Scheffler, Hinshaw, Modrek, & Levine, 2007) and have more than tripled again since then (Schwarz, 2013). While there was once a consensus that ADHD involved both undertreatment and overtreatment, a consensus is now emerging that significant overtreatment is happening (Schwarz, 2013).

Medicating children is one of the most important health-related decisions that both physicians and parents undertake. While there may be some instances of slapdash prescribing, one hopes that in the vast number of cases, decisions are made with extensive deliberation. In two-system theory, these decisions should be relatively immune from the biases of System 1. It is true that, as Kahneman acknowledges (2011, p. 415), "Often we make mistakes because we (our System 2) do not know any better." Yet can overtreatment of a child behavioral disorder really occur simply because the physicians and parents involved don't know any better. No. This explanation—or rather, nonexplanation—is required by two-system theory, but it is not reasonable. The notion that bad decisions are made because we do not know any better flies in the face of the empirical results of behavioral economics.

In contrast, multilevel theory, with its paradigm of the learning brain, recognizes that we take our information and our ways of thinking from others. In this context, we are susceptible to influence by others and this influence can be both deliberate and self-serving. Overdiagnosis of ADHD has happened not because of random cognitive mistakes, but because of marketing of ADHD drugs. This marketing is an example of the enormous power held by pharmaceutical companies over parental decision making, and all of the most cherished tropes of family life—a successful student, a son happily taking out the garbage, a dad who is home in time for dinner—are invoked to sell stimulant medication (Hall, 2005; Schwarz, 2013). Pharmaceutical companies have for years aggressively marketed directly to parents and directly to teachers (Phillips, 2006), and these marketing efforts have been highly successful at boosting the number of children medicated—whether or not it is in their best interest. The marketing of ADHD drugs is an example of a nudge that is anything but paternalistic.

If multilevel theory only highlighted the health dangers of pharmaceutical marketing, it would be helpful but neither unique nor essential. The distortions of advertising have been recognized in academic work, if little acknowledged outside of academia. The courts and the general public continue to privilege the rational-choice frame: that we are all perfectly capable of making up our own minds and doing so, for the most part, optimally (Tesh, 1994). This deep belief in individual rational choice could be challenged by behavioral economics, except that frames are not displaced by facts: They are displaced by more plausible frames.

Three Frames That Matter

The case of overprescribing of stimulant medication illustrates that the stakes for public health are potentially high. Although a great deal of attention has been attached to healthy eating and physical activity, these areas, as important as they are, cannot by themselves account for all or even most differences in population health. Exposure to toxins and to psychosocial stress matters a great deal to public health, as does the functioning of the healthcare system, and public policy in areas as diverse as education, criminal justice, and macroeconomics. One study finds that 500,000 deaths per year are attributable to low education, low income, and income inequality, with an additional 300,000 deaths attributable to racial segregation and poor social support (Galea, Tracy, Hoggatt, DiMaggio, & Karpati, 2011). Altogether these 800,000 deaths per year are about double the deaths per year attributable to smoking. These social causes of disease are not easily amenable to nudging, if at all. Instead, they can only be understood through imbalances in power.

But the appeal to power imbalances raises important conceptual and practical questions. How, in a democratic society can power imbalances persist, especially if they have such large impacts on well-being? And, if power is meaningful, how can it be restrained when by definition the powerful hold such power?

To begin to answer these questions, it is useful to briefly mention three cognitive frames that change the way people think about public health policy and politics.

Rationality and Free Speech

Individual rationality is a powerful cognitive frame that assigns blame for poor health squarely on the individual. It frequently interferes with public health by delegitimating public attempts to promote health, even if those attempts are as modest as Michelle Obama's My Healthy Plate initiative.

Despite extensive evidence that all forms of marketing change behavior—including, for example, food advertising to children or small gifts to physicians by pharmaceutical companies (Dana & Loewenstein, 2003)—there is steady resistance to any attempts to limit such marketing. This opposition travels under the banner of free speech, but, of course, this speech is very much bought and sold.

Competition

A related cognitive frame holds that people will perform better in competitive environments than they do without the pressures of competition. The cognitive frame of competition's being beneficial is assisted by Darwinian selection in evolution, as in the phrase "the survival of the fittest." But Darwin was reluctant to employ this phrase, which was coined by Herbert Spencer, and which Darwin seems to have mistrusted (Hodgson, 2004). In fact, modern evolutionists have noted the sustainability of behaviors of coexistence and cooperation, even in settings in which competition might seem advantageous (Roughgarden, 2009). Nonetheless, the phrase "survival of the fittest" stuck, and along with it its implications that competition promotes performance. This belief then became a byword in economics, with equally shaky evidence. In fact, as Oliver Williamson has pointed out, there are many situations of economic exchange in which competition is disastrous, and cooperation essential.

The notion of the efficiency of competition has led to a reflexive presumption that markets are somehow better at providing social welfare than governments, and the result has been a steady erosion of support for government and all it does. Even as more money is spent on Social Security and Medicare, the total amount spent by government as a share of the economy has decreased for decades, resulting in stagnation of education and other essential services. Ideological opponents Stanley Fish and Noam Chomsky agree that educational reform is just "a euphemism for the destruction of public education" (Fish, 2013). With a quarter of a million lives lost annually due to low education, there can be no doubt that the antigovernment frame has been a damaging one for public health.

This damage is manifested in unexpected ways. After No Child Left Behind was implemented, diagnoses of ADHD went up—but only for kids below 200% FPL (Hinshaw & Scheffler, 2014). There was no increase in those states for kids above 200% of FPL. Because there was no change in the system for identifying kids with unmet need, a large proportion—possibly most—of the increase was likely to be overdiagnosis under pressure to meet educational targets. If so, any legal means that would restrict schools for pumping up ADHD diagnoses would have stopped the overtreatment. And indeed, in the five states passing laws prohibiting schools from pushing drugs, there was no increase in ADHD prescriptions.

Healthcare as a Human Right

The last frame is controversial. On the face of it, to assert that healthcare is a human right seems to favor social justice. The problem is that this frame has no limits—and neither does healthcare itself. And when an unstoppable force reaches an unlimited field, all bets are off. Healthcare in the United States currently accounts for 18% of GDP, and the amount is growing. While the United States has a particularly expensive system—combined with particularly poor coverage—its main peril is in its rate of growth. Already, money spent on healthcare has wiped out income gains for the middle class (Auerbach & Kellermann, 2011) and is crowding out educational expenditures (Emanuel & Fuchs, 2008), in a cycle that, given the importance of both income and education to health, may be injurious to health. Yet no one seems to be asking whether the resources currently spent on health might in fact promote health more effectively if they were spent on other things (McCullough, Zimmerman, Fielding, & Teutsch, 2012).

As this very brief overview hints, the main threats to public health are not in the myriad of small behaviors that can be redressed with a nudge here or there. Instead, population health will continue to suffer when people who think carefully and deliberately about problems do so using frames, heuristics, assumptions, and information that lead them to focus narrowly on individual decisions. Power imbalances persist and even grow in a democracy because people do not believe in them. And they do not believe in them because their cognitive habits—their ways of thinking—make them systematically blind to most kinds of power. That is not by accident, of course.

Reprise

In a midst of a London cholera epidemic, John Snow famously disabled a contaminated pump. This action was more than a nudge, and its decisiveness seemed to interfere with the natural order of things as perceived at the time. Today's natural order revolves around rational-choice theory. Behavioral economics has usefully poked holes in this theory, allowing us to peek at insights that had been previously hidden. But behavioral economics to date has been more about holes than about structure, and there is no theory of behavioral economics that can replace rational-choice theory. This chapter sketches out some elements of behavioral and institutional economics that could contribute to a theoretical alternative to rational-choice theory, and it discusses the implications of such a theory for public health.

The Santa Monica School Board's decision to continue selling sugary beverages to children is hardly the most important health issue facing its children. Yet in this small sketch of public life—with its manipulation of evidence, lobbying for guidelines, perverse framing, and attention to the wrong public health questions—are all the details and colors of the much bigger challenges posed by behavioral economics.

Behavioral economics has a frame that is at war with itself: either departures from rationality are not thematized at all, suggesting that they are really not that important, or they arise from the failure of a reflective brain to adequately discipline the intuitive brain, and therefore cannot be important.

The current framing of empirical results in behavior economics carries three dangers. It distracts, almost by design, from traditional regulation, education, and incentives. It obscures the fact that those in power might not actually have our best interests at heart. And it places power outside the discussion.

All of these dangers are attenuated when we recognize the true theoretical underpinnings of behavioral economics are not two brains, but one shared set of habits of mind.

In John Snow's era and for many years thereafter, public health was about the microscopic vectors that carry disease. By improving water and sanitation systems, these vectors would be eliminated, improving the health of the population. Today's vectors are just as difficult to see with the naked eye, and just as potent. And just as in John Snow's day, advancing public health will require controlling the spread of disease through these vectors in ways that balance important values of autonomy, justice, and beneficence.

Notes

1. The two-system theory of behavioral economics owes a great deal to dual-process theory in psychology, but there are differences. The focus in this chapter is on two-system theory as it has been articulated by various behavioral economists. Some, but not all, of the same critiques would apply to dual-process theory. See, for example, Frankish (2010), Evans (2008, 2012), Osman (2004), and Keren and Schul (2009).
2. Sloman (1996) makes the distinction between learning from experience and learning from others a primary distinction in his two-process theory of cognition.

References

Anderson, C. A., Berkowitz, L., Donnerstein, E., Huesmann, L. R., Johnson, J. D., Linz, D., . . . Wartella, E. (2003). Science, politics, and violence in the media. *Psychological Science in the Public Interest, 4*(3), 81–110.

Apanovitch, A. M., McCarthy, D., & Salovey, P. (2003). Using message framing to motivate HIV testing among low-income, ethnic minority women. *Health Psychology, 22*(1), 60.

Ariely, D. (2009). *Predictably irrational: The hidden forces that shape our decisions* (2nd ed.). New York, NY: Harper.

Auerbach, D. I., & Kellermann, A. L. (2011). A decade of health care cost growth has wiped out real income gains for an average US family. *Health Affairs, 30*(9), 1630–1636.

Barba, G., Barba, G., Troiano, E., Russo, P., Venezia, A., & Siani, A. (2005). Inverse association between body mass and frequency of milk consumption in children. *British Journal of Nutrition, 93*(1), 15–20.

Barry, C. L., Brescoll, V. L., Brownell, K. D., & Schlesinger, M. (2009). Obesity metaphors: How beliefs about the causes of obesity affect support for public policy. *Milbank Quarterly, 87*(1), 7–47.

Barry, C. L., Jarlenski, M., Grob, R., Schlesinger, M., & Gollust, S. E. (2011). News media framing of childhood obesity in the United States from 2000 to 2009. *Pediatrics, 128*(1), 132–145.

Bateson, G. (1972). *Steps to an ecology of mind: Collected essays in anthropology, psychiatry, evolution, and epistemology.* Lanham, MD: Chandler Press.

Bennhold, K. (2013, December 8). Britain's Ministry of Nudges. *The New York Times.* Retrieved February 2015, http://www.nytimes.com/2013/12/08/business/international/britains-ministry-of-nudges.html?pagewanted=all

Bonell, C., McKee, M., Fletcher, A., Haines, A., & Wilkinson, P. (2011). Nudge smudge: UK Government misrepresents "nudge." *Lancet, 377*(9784), 2158–2159.

Bourdieu, P. (1992). *The logic of practice.* (Richard Nice, Trans.) Stanford, CA: Stanford University Press.

Bromley, D. W. (2006). *Sufficient reason: Volitional pragmatism and the meaning of economic institutions.* Princeton, NJ and Oxford, UK: Princeton University Press.

Cohen, D., & Farley, T. A. (2008). Eating as an automatic behavior. *Preventing Chronic Disease, 5*(1), A23.

Cosmides, L., & Tooby, J. (1994). Better than rational: Evolutionary psychology and the invisible hand. *American Economic Review, 84*(2), 327–332.

Dairy Council of California. (2012). California fights back for flavored milk in schools. Retrieved February 2015, from the *AgWeb* website http://www.agweb.com/article/california_fights_back/

Dana, J., & Loewenstein, G. (2003). A social science perspective on gifts to physicians from industry. *Journal of the American Medical Association, 290*(2), 252–255.

Desrochers, T. M., Jin, D. Z., Goodman, N. D., & Graybiel, A. M. (2010). Optimal habits can develop spontaneously through sensitivity to local cost. *Proceedings of the National Academy of Sciences USA, 107*(47), 20512.

Detweiler, J. B., Bedell, B. T., Salovey, P., Pronin, E., & Rothman, A. J. (1999). Message framing and sunscreen use: Gain-framed messages motivate beach-goers. *Health Psychology, 18*(2), 189.

Deyo, R. A., Psaty, B., Simon, G., Wagner, E. H., & Omenn, G. S. (1997). The messenger under attack: An occupational hazard for health researchers. *New England Journal of Medicine, 336,* 1176–1180.

Dietary Guidelines Advisory Committee. (2010). Dietary guidelines for Americans, 2010. Washington, DC: US Department of Agriculture, *Agricultural Research Service.*

Dorfman, L., Wallack, L., & Woodruff, K. (2005). More than a message: Framing public health advocacy to change corporate practices. *Health Education and Behavior, 32*(3), 320–336.

Drewnowski, A. (1998). Energy density, palatability, and satiety: Implications for weight control. *Nutrition Reviews, 56*(12), 347–353.

Emanuel, E. J., & Fuchs, V. R. (2008). Who really pays for health care? The myth of "shared responsibility." *Journal of the American Medical Association, 299*(9), 1057–1059.

Evans, J. S. B. (2008). Dual-processing accounts of reasoning, judgment, and social cognition. *Annual Review of Psychology, 59,* 255–278.

Evans, J. S. B. (2012). Questions and challenges for the new psychology of reasoning. *Thinking and Reasoning, 18*(1), 5–31.

Ferraro, R., Bettman, J. R., & Chartrand, T. L. (2009). The power of strangers: The effect of incidental consumer brand encounters on brand choice. *Journal of Consumer Research, 35,* 729–741.

Fish, S. (2013, December 9). Scholarship and politics: The case of Noam Chomsky. *The New York Times.* Retrieved February 2015, from http://www.nytimes.com/2013/12/10/opinion/fish-scholarship-and-politics-the-case-of-noam-chomsky.html?pagewanted=all

Frankish, K. (2010). Dual-process and dual-system theories of reasoning. *Philosophy Compass, 5*(10), 914–926.

Frary, C. D., Johnson, R. K., & Wang, M. Q. (2004). Children and adolescents' choices of foods and beverages high in added sugars are associated with intakes of key nutrients and food groups. *Journal of Adolescent Health, 34*(1), 56–63.

Frederick, S. (2005). Cognitive reflection and decision making. *Journal of Economic Perspectives, 19*(4), 25–42.

Galea, S., Tracy, M., Hoggatt, K. J., DiMaggio, C., & Karpati, A. (2011). Estimated deaths attributable to social factors in the United States. *Americna Journal of Public Health, 101*(8), 1456–1465.

Gallagher, K. M., & Updegraff, J. A. (2012). Health message framing effects on attitudes, intentions, and behavior: A meta-analytic review. *Annals of Behavioral Medicine, 43*(1), 101–116.

Gilbert, D. T. (1991). How mental systems believe. *American Psychologist, 46*(2), 107.

Gitlin, T. (1980). *The whole world is watching: Mass media in the making and unmaking of the new left.* Berkeley, CA: University of California Press.

Goldacre, B. (2010). *Bad science: Quacks, hacks, and big pharma flacks.* New York, NY: Faber and Faber.

Gollust, S. E., Lantz, P. M., & Ubel, P. A. (2009). The polarizing effect of news media messages about the social determinants of health. *American Journal of Public Health, 99*(12), 2160.

Green, E. (2013). The controversial life of skim milk. *The Atlantic.* http://www.the-atlantic.com/events/archive/2013/11/the-controversial-life-of-skim-milk/281655/, accessed 3/10/15

Grey, S., & Mathews, A. (2000). Effects of training on interpretation of emotional ambiguity. *Quarterly Journal of Experimental Psychology: Section A, 53*(4), 1143–1162.

Gross, K. (2008). Framing persuasive appeals: Episodic and thematic framing, emotional response, and policy opinion. *Political Psychology, 29*(2), 169–192.

Hall, A. L. (2005). Welcome to ordinary? Marketing better boys. *American Journal of Bioethics, 5*(3), 59–60.

Harris, J. L., Bargh, J. A., & Brownell, K. D. (2009). Priming effects of television food advertising on eating behavior. *Health Psychology, 28*(4), 404–413.

Hausman, D. M., & Welch, B. (2010). Debate: To nudge or not to nudge. *Journal of Political Philosophy, 18*(1), 123–136.

Hinshaw, S. P., & Scheffler, R. M. (2014). *The ADHD explosion and today's push for performance: Myths, medication, and money.* Oxford, UK: Oxford University Press.

Hodgson, G. M. (2004). *The evolution of institutional economics: Agency, structure and Darwinism in American institutionalism.* London, UK: Routledge.

Hodgson, G. M., & Knudsen, T. (2004). The complex evolution of a simple traffic convention: The functions and implications of habit. *Journal of Economic Behavior and Organization, 54*(1), 19–47.

Howard, K., & Salkeld, G. (2009). Does attribute framing in discrete choice experiments influence willingness to pay? Results from a discrete choice experiment in screening for colorectal cancer. *Value in Health, 12*(2), 354–363.

Iyengar, S. (1994). *Is anyone responsible? How television frames political issues*: University of Chicago Press.

James, W. (2007). Habit. In *Principles of Psychology, Vol 1*. New York, NY: Cosimo Classics. (original work published 1890)

Kahneman, D. (2003). Maps of bounded rationality: Psychology for behavioral economics. *American Economic Review, 93*(5), 1449–1475.

Kahneman, D. (2011). *Thinking, fast and slow*. New York, NY: Farrar Straus & Giroux.

Kalichman, S. C., & Coley, B. (1995). Context framing to enhance HIV-antibody-testing messages targeted to African American women. *Health Psychology, 14*(3), 247.

Keren, G., & Schul, Y. (2009). Two is not always better than one: A critical evaluation of two-system theories. *Perspectives on Psychological Science, 4*(6), 533–550.

Kesting, S. (1998). A potential for understanding and the interference of power: Discourse as an economic mechanism of coordination. *Journal of Economic Issues, 32*(4), 1053–1055.

Krieger, N. (2008). Proximal, distal, and the politics of causation: What's level got to do with it? *American Journal of Public Health, 98*(2), 221.

Krugman, P. (2014, March 25). What America isn't—or anyway wasn't. *The New York Times*. Retrieved February 2015, from http://krugman.blogs.nytimes.com/2014/03/25/what-america-isnt-or-anyway-wasnt/?_php=true&_type=blogs&_r=0

Laajaj, R. (2012). *Closing the eyes on a gloomy future: Psychological causes and economic consequences*. Paper presented at the Pacific Development Economics Conference, University of California, Davis, March 17, 2012.

Lakoff, G. (2004). *Don't think of an elephant: Progressive values and the framing wars—a progressive guide to action*. White River Junction, VT: Chelsea Green.

Lakoff, G., & Johnson, M. (1999). *Philosophy in the flesh: The embodied mind and its challenge to western thought*. New York, NY: Basic Books.

Lanou, A. J., Berkow, S. E., & Barnard, N. D. (2005). Calcium, dairy products, and bone health in children and young adults: A reevaluation of the evidence. *Pediatrics, 115*(3), 736–743.

Levin, I. P., Gaeth, G. J., Schreiber, J., & Lauriola, M. (2002). A new look at framing effects: Distribution of effect sizes, individual differences, and independence of types of effects. *Organizational Behavior and Human Decision Processes, 88*(1), 411–429.

Levin, I. P., Schneider, S. L., & Gaeth, G. J. (1998). All frames are not created equal: A typology and critical analysis of framing effects. *Organizational Behavior and Human Decision Processes, 76*(2), 149–188.

Levin, I. P., Schnittjer, S. K., & Thee, S. L. (1988). Information framing effects in social and personal decisions. *Journal of Experimental Social Psychology, 24*(6), 520–529.

Loewenstein, G., Asch, D. A., Friedman, J. Y., Melichar, L. A., & Volpp, K. G. (2012). Can behavioural economics make us healthier? *British Medical Journal, 344*, e3482.

Ludwig, D. S., & Willett, W. C. (2013). Three daily servings of reduced-fat milk: An evidence-based recommendation? *Journal of the American Medical Association Pediatrics, 167*(9), 788–789.

Lukes, S. (2004). *Power: A radical view*. New York, NY: Palgrave Macmillan.

Matthews, C. (2013). *Tip and the Gipper: When politics worked*. New York, NY: Simon and Schuster.

McCullough, J. C., Zimmerman, F. J., Fielding, J. E., & Teutsch, S. M. (2012). A health dividend for America: The opportunity cost of excess medical expenditures. *American Journal of Preventive Medicine, 43*(6), 650–654.

Mischel, W., Shoda, Y., & Rodriguez, M. I. (1989). Delay of gratification in children. *Science, 244*(4907), 933–938.

Murphy, M. M., Douglass, J. S., Johnson, R. K., & Spence, L. A. (2008). Drinking flavored or plain milk is positively associated with nutrient intake and is not associated with adverse effects on weight status in US children and adolescents. *Journal of the American Dietetic Association, 108*(4), 631–639.

Nagel, R. (1995). Unraveling in guessing games: An experimental study. *American Economic Review, 85*(5), 1313–1326.

Neal, D. T., Wood, W., & Quinn, J. M. (2006). Habits—A repeat performance. *Current Directions in Psychological Science, 15*(4), 198–202.

Neumann, P. J., & Weinstein, M. C. (2010). Legislating against use of cost-effectiveness information. *New England Journal of Medicine, 363*(16), 1495–1497.

Oliver, J. E., & Lee, T. (2005). Public opinion and the politics of obesity in America. *Journal of Health Politics, Policy and Law, 30*(5), 923–954.

Ortiz, S. E. (2013). *Identifying alternative frames and values to increase public support for health policies that target obesity*. Unpublished Ph.D. dissertation, University of California, Los Angeles.

Ortiz, S. E., Zimmerman, F. J., & Gilliam Jr, F. D. (2015). Weighing In: The Taste-Engineering Frame in Obesity Expert Discourse. *American Journal of Public Health*, (0), e1–e6.

Osman, M. (2004). An evaluation of dual-process theories of reasoning. *Psychonomic Bulletin and Review, 11*(6), 988–1010.

Perneger, T. V., & Agoritsas, T. (2011). Doctors and patients' susceptibility to framing bias: A randomized trial. *Journal of General Internal Medicine, 26*(12), 1411–1417.

Phillips, C. B. (2006). Medicine goes to school: Teachers as sickness brokers for ADHD. *PLoS Medicine, 3*(4), e182.

Rice, T. (2013). The behavioral economics of health and health care. *Annual Review of Public Health, 34*, 431–447.

Rice, T., & Cummings, J. (2010). Reducing the number of drug plans for seniors: A proposal and analysis of three case studies. *Journal of Health Politics, Policy and Law, 35*(6), 961–997.

Rivers, S. E., Salovey, P., Pizarro, D. A., Pizarro, J., & Schneider, T. R. (2005). Message framing and pap test utilization among women attending a community health clinic. *Journal of Health Psychology, 10*(1), 65–77.

Robert Wood Johnson Foundation. (2010). A new way to talk about the social determinants of health. Princeton, NJ: Robert Wood Johnson Foundation. http://www.rwjf.org/content/dam/farm/reports/reports/2010/rwjf63023, accessed 3/10/15

Romm, J. J. (2012). *Language intelligence: Lessons on persuasion from Jesus, Shakespeare, Lincoln, and Lady Gaga*. North Charleston, SC: CreateSpace.

Rosenstock, L., & Lee, L. J. (2002). Attacks on science: The risks to evidence-based policy. *American Journal of Public Health, 92*(1), 14.

Rothman, A. J., Martino, S. C., Bedell, B. T., Detweiler, J. B., & Salovey, P. (1999). The systematic influence of gain-and loss-framed messages on interest in and use of different types of health behavior. *Personality and Social Psychology Bulletin, 25*(11), 1355–1369.

Rothman, A. J., & Salovey, P. (1997). Shaping perceptions to motivate healthy behavior: The role of message framing. *Psychological Bulletin, 121*(1), 3.

Roughgarden, J. (2009). *The genial gene.* Los Angeles, CA: UC Press.

Scharf, R. J., Demmer, R. T., & DeBoer, M. D. (2013). Longitudinal evaluation of milk type consumed and weight status in preschoolers. *Archives of Disease in Childhood, 98*(5), 335–340.

Scheffler, R. M., Hinshaw, S. P., Modrek, S., & Levine, P. (2007). The global market for ADHD medications. *Health Affairs, 26*(2), 450–457.

Schwarz, A. (2013, December 14). The selling of attention deficit disorder. *The New York Times.* Retrieved February 2015, from http://www.nytimes.com/2013/12/15/health/the-selling-of-attention-deficit-disorder.html?pagewanted=all

Sherman, D. K., Updegraff, J. A., & Mann, T. (2008). Improving oral health behavior a social psychological approach. *Journal of the American Dental Association, 139*(10), 1382–1387.

Sloman, S. A. (1996). The empirical case for two systems of reasoning. *Psychological Bulletin, 119*(1), 3.

Smith-Howard, K. (2013). *Pure and modern milk: An environmental history since 1900.* New York, NY: Oxford University Press.

Stoelhorst, J. W. (2008). The explanatory logic and ontological commitments of generalized Darwinism. *Journal of Economic Methodology, 15*(4), 343–363.

Sunstein, C. R. (2003). *Why societies need dissent.* Cambridge, MA: Harvard University Press.

Surowiecki, J. (2005). *The wisdom of crowds.* New York, NY: Random House.

Tesh, S. (1994). *Hidden arguments: Politics, ideology and disease prevention policy.* New Brunswick, NJ: Rutgers University Press.

Thaler, R. H., & Sunstein, C. R. (2008). *Nudge: Improving decisions about health, wealth, and happiness.* New Haven, CT: Yale University Press.

Todorov, A., Harris, L. T., & Fiske, S. T. (2006). Toward socially inspired social neuroscience. *Brain Research, 1079*(1), 76–85.

Tversky, A., & Kahneman, D. (1981). The framing of decisions and the psychology of choice. *Science, 211*(4481), 453–458.

Twomey, P. (1998). Reviving Veblenian economic psychology. *Cambridge Journal of Economics, 22*(4), 433–448.

Wansink, B. (1996). Can package size accelerate usage volume? *Journal of Marketing, 60*(3), 1–14.

Wansink, B. (2004). Environmental factors that increase the food intake and consumption volume of unknowing consumers. *Annual Review of Nutrition, 24,* 455–479.

Winzenberg, T., Shaw, K., Fryer, J., & Jones, G. (2006). Effects of calcium supplementation on bone density in healthy children: Meta-analysis of randomised controlled trials. *British Medical Journal, 333,* 775.

Wood, W., Quinn, J. M., & Kashy, D. A. (2002). Habits in everyday life: Thought, emotion, and action. *Journal of Personality and Social Psychology, 83*(6), 1281.

Yancey, A. K., Cole, B. L., Brown, R., Williams, J. D., Hillier, A., Kline, R. S., ... McCarthy, W. J. (2009). A cross-sectional prevalence study of ethnically targeted and general audience outdoor obesity-related advertising. *Milbank Quarterly, 87*(1), 155–184.

Young, L. R., & Nestle, M. (2002). The contribution of expanding portion sizes to the US obesity epidemic. *American Journal of Public Health, 92*(2), 246–249.

Zhang, D., Giabbanelli, P. J., Arah, O., & Zimmerman, F. J. (2014). Impact of different policies on unhealthy dietary behaviors in an urban adult population: An agent-based simulation model. *American Journal of Public Health, 104*(7), 1217–1222.

Zimmerman, F. J. (2009). Using behavioral economics to promote physical activity. *Preventive Medicine, 49*(4), 289–291.

Zimmerman, F. J. (2011). Using marketing muscle to sell fat: The rise of obesity in the modern economy. *Annual Review of Public Health, 32*, 285–306.

Zimmerman, F. J. (2013). Habit, custom, and power: A multi-level theory of population health. *Social Science and Medicine, 80*, 47–56.

INDEX

"f" indicates material in figures, "n" indicates material in endnotes, and "t" indicates material in tables.

advertisements (*Cont.*)
  positive affective appeals in, 8
  timing of, 189
  of tobacco industry, 4, 272
  vividness of, 187
advice taking, 111, 117
affect heuristic, 7–8
affective processing, 105, 122. *See
    also* heuristic processing; intuitive
    processing; System 1 thinking
affective states. *See also* emotions
  and alcohol use, 102
  and exercise, 124n.3
  and flexible thinking, 124n.6
  and overconfidence, 50
  pictures to prime, 121
  of providers, 118
  and smoking, 102
  triggering, 124n.6
Affordable Care Act (ACA), 171,
    224–226, 228–229, 310
African Americans, 321, 328
Agency for Healthcare Research and
    Quality, 311
agenda-setting power, 310, 312
agent-based simulations, 308, 326
alcohol
  abstaining from, 1, 39
  beer, 53, 84, 244, 260n.1
  drinkers (*see* alcohol users)
  glassware size impact on serving, 184
  payday effects on purchase of, 43
  taxes on, 63, 244
alcohol industry, 4, 20
alcohol users
  affective states and consumption
    by, 102
  binge drinking by, 15, 20, 115, 135
  bright-line rules for, 56
  discounting by, 37
  financial incentives for treatment of, 37
  NCD development after
    overindulgence by, 69
  peer norms and, 115, 135
  precommitment strategies for, 39
  present bias of, 10
  with self-control problems, 84

and social norms, 133
  soft commitments by, 56
  valuation and choice by, 110
American Medical Association, 142
amount of healthy choices, 184, 195–196
anchoring
  and availability bias, 318
  of eating behavior, 138, 140–141,
    152, 195
anger
  ATF on, 106t.
  graphic warning labels targeting, 8
  in health decision making, 108–114
  incidental, 103
  in medical decision making, 116–118
  mixed with other emotions, 122
  in policy making, 120–121
  projection bias with, 48
  of providers, 118
  risk perception with, 8, 104, 110,
    113–114, 116, 120
  and status quo bias, 117
  System 1 thinking in, 112
anorexia, 143
anterior cingulate cortex, 44–45
anticipated effort with emotions,
    106–107t., 108
anticoagulation therapy, 218–219
antimalarial bed nets, 57
anxiety, 111
appearance self-esteem, 141
appointments, missed medical, 285–286
appraisal dimensions, 106–107t., 108–109
appraisal tendency framework (ATF)
  description of, 8
  future research on, 122–123
  for health decisions, 105–115
  for medical decisions, 115–119
  for policy making, 119–121
  purpose of, 103–104
approach-oriented personalities, 321
Ariely, Daniel, 327
artificial neural network, 73
associative cortico-basal ganglia loop, 86
assortment of healthy choices, 182–184,
    193–195
asthma, 69, 217, 273

beverages
    alcohol (*see* alcohol)
    calorie warning signs for, 198
    cup size for, 195, 247t.
    default option for, 186, 249, 256
    location of, in coolers, 196, 241
    milk (*see* milk)
    NUVAL shelf labeling system for, 172
    and obesity, 150
    pop (*see* soft drinks and sodas)
    taxation of, 63, 240, 241–244
    traffic light labeling of, 172
    water (*see* water)
biases
    accessibility, 319
    availability, 318
    cognitive, 30, 55, 59, 61–62, 118
    optimism, 7, 50–51
    present (*see* present bias)
    projection, 10, 47–49, 61
    self-serving, 40
    status quo, 10–11, 60, 117, 186,
        209, 318
    in System 1 thinking, 5–8
    unit, 184
bikini bathing suits, 143
blame, 106–107t., 109, 111, 118
blood pressure, 2, 59
body-esteem, 142–143, 153
body image, 142
body mass index (BMI), 5, 6, 148
Body Shop's "Love Your Body"
    campaign, 142
body types, 139–145, 153
boomerang effect, 135, 170, 227
bounded rationality, 4, 51, 52
bounded selfishness, 319–320
breast cancer, 32, 116
bright-line rules, 56–57

cafeterias. *See also* dining halls;
    lunchrooms
    CAN framework on food in,
        247t., 248t.
    fruits in, 183, 241, 248t.
    at Google, 193–198

health express line in, 185, 247
portion sizes in, 256
prepackaged healthy entrées in, 247
pricing items in, 184
traffic light labeling system in, 14,
    172, 188
trays used in, 250, 255–256
USDA guidelines and menus for, 167
vegetables in, 241
calcium and bone health, 316
calories
    assessing, 276
    counting, in weight-loss programs, 5
    and environmental cues, 253
    financial incentives to lower, 205
    in hedonic foods, 114
    in Japanese cuisine, 11
    labels for menus, 6, 171–172, 198, 276
    in milk, 315
    nudging to lower, 16–17
    obesity caused by, 146–151
    and taxation, 242–244
    warning signs on, 198
Cameron administration, 328–329
Canada, smoker's regret in, 36
cancer
    ATF on fear and, 104
    behavioral modification to prevent, 101
    breast, 32, 116
    chemotherapy for, 119
    classification of, 69
    colorectal, 28, 103, 117, 119
    financial incentives to promote
        screening for, 223–224
    framing effects with screening
        messages, 322
    lung, 7, 109–110, 118
    and obesity, 273–274
    screening for, 116, 223–224
CAN framework, 17, 237–238, 245–260
cardiovascular diseases, 69, 109–110,
    274. *See also* heart disease
Center for Medicare and Medicaid
    Innovation, 225
Centers for Disease Control and
    Prevention (CDC), 242

fat
  claims on packaging, 6
  consumption of, by nutrition label
    readers, 276
  dietary vs. body, 313–314
  Facts Up Front labeling system on, 14
  in milk, 5, 187, 313–314
  and palatability, 314
  price and consumption of, 275
  saturated, 14, 242–243
  taxation of, 242–243, 274–275
  taxes on, 242–243
  "trans fats" banned, 274
fat shaming campaigns, 144
fear
  ATF on, 106t.
  with cancer diagnosis, 8, 103, 104
  and decision making, 102, 108,
    110–114, 116–118
  framing effects with, 113–114, 325
  graphic warning labels targeting, 14
  mixed with other emotions, 122
  in policy making, 120
  projection bias with, 48
  risk perception with, 8, 108, 110,
    113–114, 116, 120
fear appeals, 8, 325
feeling states
  blame, 106–107t., 109, 111, 118
  dread, 106–107t., 110, 116
  guilt, 33–34, 106t., 118, 124n.5
  pain, 10, 29, 48, 123, 179
  projection bias in, 48
  shame, 106t., 111, 118, 144
  trust, 106–107t., 111, 117, 328
financial incentives
  ACA endorsement of, 224–226,
    228–229
  for alcohol treatment, 37
  back- vs. front-loaded, 207
  for cancer screening, 223–224
  carrots vs. sticks, 229
  in Center for Medicare and Medicaid
    Innovation grants, 225
  for contraception, 220–221
  designing, for workplace wellness
    interventions, 18

  in discount rate calculations, 37
  discussion on, 203–231
  for eating healthy foods, 227–228
  escalating, 59, 209, 211
  ethics of, 226–229
  fMRI studies of brain activity with, 44
  framing effects with, 221–222, 322
  for habit formation, 79–81, 222, 227
  in hard commitments, 57–58
  incremental, 59, 206–207
  individual vs. group, 210–211, 216
  loss aversion with, 204, 207, 209, 213,
    219, 229
  lottery, 18–19, 208–209, 217–219
  vs. medical interventions, 230
  for medication adherence, 217–219
  "mental accounting" in, 209
  and motivation, 226–228
  for physical activity promotion, 41,
    221–223, 227
  process vs. outcome-based measures
    for, 228–229
  for public health promotion, 223–224
  public perception of, 230
  purpose of, 17
  salience of, 53
  size of, 205–206
  for smoking cessation, 18, 37, 58, 192,
    212–216, 230, 283
  and social norms, 227
  structure of, 206–209
  for substance abuse treatment, 37,
    217–218, 220
  for vaccination promotion, 223–224
  in weight-loss programs, 18–19, 192,
    204–212, 228, 230
Fish, Stanley, 333
Florida, Medicaid incentive programs in,
  225–226
flu vaccinations, 10, 21–22, 29, 54, 76
Food and Drug Administration (FDA), 14,
  119–120
food industry
  advertisements of, 4
  available, affordable, and attractive
    products from, 238
  dairy, 313–315

on exercise, 150–151
Facts Up Front labeling system, 14,
   172–173
information asymmetry with, 6
lobbying by, 14, 151
misinformation from, on obesity, 150–151
power of marketing by, 318
Food Marketing Institute, 172
4 P's Framework for Behavior Change,
   17, 177, 181–199
framing effects
   to alter perceptions, 321–322
   of competition, 332
   in decision making, 51, 320–321
   definition of cognitive frame, 320
   with dual-system theory, 302–303, 307
   with eating behavior, 322
   with emotions, 110, 113–114, 324–325
   episodic, 322–325
   with financial incentives, 221–222, 322
   gain vs. loss, 51, 110, 113, 116, 188,
      194, 320–321
   of healthcare, 333
   with intertemporal health choices, 51
   with labels, 322
   misleading, 5
   with multilevel theory, 307, 311–312,
      320–327, 331–333
   with obesity, 323
   as persuasive, 188–189
   with policy making, 322–325, 331–332
   with power, 311–312
   purpose of, 320–321
   with rationality, 332
   risk perception with, 110, 113–114
   with social determinants of health,
      322–323
   for socially beneficial options, 60
   thematic, 322–323
France, tax on soda in, 274
french fries, 11, 252, 256
"Friends Don't Let Friends Drive Drunk"
   campaign, 13, 163, 165
fronto-parietal system, 44
fruits
   availability of, for children, 183
   CAN framework on, 245–249

embedded triggers for, 165
financial incentives to promote eating,
   227–228
framing effects of messages on, 113
in grocery stores, 17
habit forming cues for, 79
in Half Plate guideline, 165–167
Healthy Start Vouchers for, 275
in lunchrooms, 183, 245–249, 253–256
marketing of, 327
in MyPyramid guideline, 165–167
obesity and eating of, 149
order effects for, 239, 240f.
policies requiring, 241
present bias in choosing, 47, 180
salience of, 253
in USDA Food Pyramid, 165
variety of, 254
vivid descriptors for, 187
functional magnetic resonance images
   (fMRIs), 44

General Electric smoking cessation study,
   212–214, 225
genetic testing, 116
gluten-free foods, 6, 197
goal-directed behavior
   action tendencies for, 108
   devices for (*see* commitment devices)
   and emotions, 102, 107t.
   enduring change through, 69–70
   in 4P's framework, 182, 188–192
   and habits, 71, 74–88, 93
   memory in, 77
   neural activities related to, 86–87
   positive vs. negative outcomes of, 74
   prompts for, 171
   and rewards, 79–80, 85–87, 207–208
   short- vs. long-term, 9
   strategies for, 39, 190–191
   and stress, 84–86
   tailoring of, 224, 229
good habits, 49, 74
Google case study, 193–198
grains, 165
gratitude, 102, 107t., 111,
   117–118, 124n.6

milk *(Cont.)*
    developing a habit for drinking, 76, 83
    dual-system theory and, 314–315
    fat in, 5, 187, 313–314
    location of, in coolers, 241
    in lunchrooms, 240–241, 242f., 250, 254–255
    and obesity, 314–315
    palatability of, 314
    plain vs. flavored in coolers, 250
    skim, 313–316
    vs. soft drinks, 243, 256
    USDA on, 165, 313, 315
Mill, John Stuart, 324
Mischel, Walter, 56, 88–89, 301
mistaken beliefs, 29, 47–51
moments of truth, 189–190, 198
moods, 124n.2
moral judgments, 119
moral licensing, 135
multilevel theory, 21, 303–335
My Healthy Plate initiative, 315, 332
myocardial infarction, 2
myopia model, 34
myopic loss aversion, 45
MyPlate guideline, 168–169, 173
MyPyramid guideline, 165–169, 173

naltrexone, 217
National School Lunch Program (NSLP), 240, 257–258
Nesta, 267
neuroeconomics, 44–45
New York City, "trans fats" banned, 274
New York State, outdoor smoking ban, 272
"No body shame" campaign, 143
No Child Left Behind, 333
noncommunicable diseases (NCDS), 69
Northern Ireland, physical activity study, 222
Nudge (Thaler & Sunstein), 267, 328
"Nudge Unit." *See* Behavioural Insights Team
nudging
    and autonomy, 329

    choice environment altered through, 16, 184
    context for, 271
    and dual-system theory, 302, 329–330
    enduring change through, 70
    ethics of, 329
    4 P's framework for, 17, 177, 181–199
    as libertarian paternalism, 54, 329
    vs. multilevel theory, 329–330
    through policy making, 54, 271, 329
    on portion sizes, 16–17
    as power to influence, 329
    through prompts, 171
    in lieu of regulations, 19–20
    skepticism and criticism of, 19–20, 329–330
Nurses' Health Study, 1
nutrition labels
    designing, 13
    effectiveness of, 276
    Facts Up Front system for, 14, 172–173
    numeric data in, 4–5, 13
    vs. price changes, 184
    purpose of, 275
    traffic light, 14, 172, 188, 197, 322
    understanding, 52
NUVAL shelf labeling system, 172

Obama, Michelle, food plate, 315, 332
Obama administration, libertarian paternalism of, 328–329
obesity
    and accessibility of food, 185
    anxiety and depression with, 274
    and beverages, 150
    and body types, 139–145
    calories as cause of, 146–151
    and cancer, 273–274
    Center for Medicare and Medicaid Innovation grants for programs addressing, 225
    communications on, 142–144, 152–153
    determinants of, 274
    and diabetes, 273
    diet as cause of, 6, 145–151
    and exercise, 144–151

risks borne by, 269
with self-control problems, 84
soft commitments by, 56–57
subsidizing healthcare costs of
  nonsmokers, 63n.4
valuation and choice by, 110
who want to quit, 36
smoking
  affect heuristic with, 7
  and affective states, 102
  attacking, 144–145
  bans on, 272
  Center for Medicare and Medicaid
    Innovation grants for programs
    addressing, 225
  cigarettes (see cigarettes)
  disgust leveraged in policies on, 114
  health insurance surcharge for, 225
  interpersonal attribution with, 111, 115
  legislation restricting indoor, 12
  lung cancer attributed to, 118
  as negative externality, 269
  obesity contrasted to, 144–145, 274
  passive, 269, 272
  peanuts effect with, 9
  peer norms and, 12, 111
  quitting (see smoking cessation)
  regulation of, 272–273
  sadness effects on, 114
  stigmatizing, 144–145
smoking cessation
  ACA on, 224
  and bans, 272
  Behavioural Insights Team on, 19,
    282–285
  decision on, 105
  delaying, as self-control problem, 29
  deposit contract for, 58, 214–216
  financial incentives for, 18, 37, 58, 192,
    212–216, 230, 283
  General Electric study of, 212–214, 225
  group counseling during, 214
  hard commitments in, 57
  implementation intention plans for, 82
  information on, placement of, 189
  medication adherence during, 217

policies supporting, 145
precommitment to, 9
relapse risk with, 89–90
social norms as basis for messages
  on, 283
Stoptober initiative for, 282–285
successful, 36
text-message reminders during, 15,
  53, 215
in type 2 diabetes prevention, 1
snacks
  accessibility of, 196
  cash for, 257
  container size impact on, 247t.
  habit of eating, 79, 83
  in lunchrooms, 254
  100-calorie, 248–249
  present bias in choosing, 180
  projection bias in choice of, 47–48
  serving sizes for, 197
Snow, John, 334–335
social cognitive theory, 325
social contracts, 285–286
social cost vs. benefit, 268
social facilitation, 137
social identity model of health, 139
social learning in habit formation, 77–78
social norms
  and alcohol/drug users, 133
  behavior influenced by, 12
  on body types, 141–145
  changing, 15
  definition of, 133
  in eating behavior, 12, 133–145,
    151–154, 180, 247t., 317
  emotional interpersonal attribution and,
    113–115
  and exercise, 133, 135
  and financial incentives, 227
  local/smaller vs. larger group, 152
  "magnetic middle" for, 135
  in obesity, role of, 133–145, 151–154
  in organ donation registration, 273t.
  in smoking-cessation campaign, 283
social proof, 134, 267
social referencing, 319, 326

socioeconomic inequalities. *See also*
low-income individuals and families;
the poor
behavioral economics and, 21
and cognitive biases, 30, 61–62
deaths attributable to, 331
and sin taxes, 61
and vaccination coverage gap, 22
soft commitments, 56–57
soft drinks and sodas
calories from, exercise to burn, 146
cash for, 257
as default option for beverage, 249, 256
free refills of, 185
marketing of, 311
vs. milk, 243, 256
payday effects on purchase of, 43
present bias for, 205
System 1 vs. 2 thinking on, 4
taxation on, 240, 241–244, 274
traffic light labeling of, 172
warning signs for, 198
South Korea, lay theories on obesity, 147
Spain, organ donation, 279
spillover effects, 289
stairs, 77–78, 91, 183, 189
Starbucks, 276
status quo bias, 10–11, 60, 117, 186,
209, 318
"stepped wedge" design, 292
stereotyping, 111, 113, 117
stimulus control, 89
strength model of self-control, 84
stress, 4, 84–86, 92, 144
"Strong4Life" campaign, 144
subjective norms, 12
substance abuse
addiction (*see* addiction)
alcohol (*see* alcohol users)
compliance with treatment for,
217–218
drug (*see* drug users)
financial incentives for treatment
of, 220
physiologic barriers to overcoming, 203
sugar, 314
sunscreen use, 8, 171, 321

Sunstein, Cass, 267, 328
Supplemental Nutrition Assistance
Program (SNAP), 42
surprise, 107t., 110
System 1 thinking. *See also* intuitive
processing
activation of, 300–303
on ADHD treatment, 330
advertisements appealing to, 4
availability bias with, 318
and bounded rationality, 4
with cognitive load, 178–180
communication addressing, 187
in daily life, 178–180, 302
as distinct process, 316
and dual-process theory, 335n.1
with emotions, 112, 325
4 P's framework for, 181–199
framing effects with, 302–303, 307
and habits, 317–319
heuristics in, 5–8, 112, 118
information processing in, 112, 118
and milk recommendations, 314–315
vs. multilevel theory, 303–309, 312,
316–321, 325–326
in power veiling, 312
and self-control problems, 45
self-control problems with, 162
vs. System 2 thinking, 3–4, 70, 162,
178, 299–303
temptation with, 178–179
System 2 thinking. *See also* deliberative
processing; systematic processing
activation of, 300–303
on ADHD treatment, 330
attention in, 162
availability bias with, 318
capacity constraints on, 162
with cognitive load, 178–180
communication addressing, 121, 187
in daily life, 178–180, 302
decision making with, 326
as distinct process, 316
and dual-process theory, 335n.1
with emotions, 325
4 P's framework for, 181–199
framing effects with, 302–303, 307

traffic light labeling system, 14, 172, 188, 197, 322
Transforming Your Life (TYL), 79
trust, 106–107t., 111, 117, 328
Tversky, Amos, 30
type 2 diabetes, 1, 273

"unit bias," 184
United Kingdom (UK)
　Behavioural Insights Team (*see* Behavioural Insights Team)
　Cameron administration, 328–329
　Debanhams' mannequins in, 142
　driving in, 90, 183
　economists in British Cabinet, 265
　Food Standards Agency in, 14
　Government Economic Service in, 265
　Healthy Start Vouchers in, 275
　medication adherence with psychosis study in, 218
　National Health Service in, 269
　Northern Ireland physical activity study, 222
　obesity in, 273
　organ donation in, 277–278
　Paxton's smoking cessation studies in, 214–215
　Pounds for Pounds program in, 210
　smoking in, 36, 73
　Snow in cholera epidemic in London, 334–335
　Stoptober initiative in, 282–285
　traffic light labeling system in, 14
United States (US). *See also individual states*
　ADHD medication sales in, 330
　dieting industry in, 151
　family food budget in, 238
　flu shot coverage rates in, 21–22
　GDP of, 151, 333
　Healthy People 2020 goals for, 21
　household debt in, 143
　lay theories on obesity in, 147–148
　Obama administration, 328–329
　organ donation in, 278
　overweight or obese adults in, 141, 204

　prevention and public health program funding in, 120
　regrets of smokers in, 36
United States Department of Agriculture (USDA)
　Dietary Guidelines for Americans, 165
　Food Pyramid, 162, 165
　on milk, 165, 313, 315
　MyPlate, 168–169, 173
　MyPyramid, 165–169, 173
　School Nutrition Dietary Assessment data, 257
　subsidizing school lunches, 252, 254
United States Preventive Services Task Force (USPSTF), 119–121
utility models
　discount (*see* discount factor)
　individual function for, 268–269
　in Laibson's β-δ model, 38
　with procrastination, 270–271
　simple lifetime, 31–33, 38, 270
　society function for, 268–269
　with uncertainty, 32–33

vaccination
　default effects on, 42
　financial incentives to promote, 223–224
　flu, 10, 21–22, 29, 54, 76
　payday effects on, 42
　as positive externality, 269
　socioeconomic gap in coverage, 22
valuation, 106–107t., 110–111, 113–115, 117, 120
vegetables
　availability of, for children, 183
　CAN framework on, 247t., 248t., 249
　as default side dish, 256
　embedded triggers for, 165
　financial incentives to promote eating, 227–228
　framing effects of messages on, 113
　in grocery stores, 17
　habit forming cues for, 79, 191
　in Half Plate guideline, 165–167
　Healthy Start Vouchers for, 275